*Nine women, Nine months,
Nine lives*

\
Nine women, Nine months, Nine lives

Dr Sandra L Wheatley

Potent

British Library Cataloguing-in-publication data
A catalogue record for this book is available from the British Library.

Copyright © 2001 by Dr Sandra L Wheatley

Published by Potent Limited, Leicestershire, United Kingdom.
E-mail: potent@hushmail.com
Website: http//www.potent.uk.com

All rights reserved. No part of this work may be reproduced or stored in an information retrieval system (other than short extracts for purposes of review) without the express permission of the Publishers given in writing.

Dr Sandra L Wheatley has asserted her right under the Copyright, design and patents Act 1988 to be identified as the author of this work.

Cover concept by Dr Sandra L Wheatley. Graphic design by Jacqui Morris.
Author photograph by Ian Moorcroft.
Printed and bound by Woolnough Bookbinding Ltd, Irthlingborough, Northants.

For my mum, from her first child

Nine women, Nine months, Nine lives

The Author

Sandra has been involved in research into the area of emotions in parenthood since 1993. She gained her first degree in Psychology from Royal Holloway, University of London in 1995. Her undergraduate research work "Partners in Parenthood – who needs them?" was received to critical acclaim in 1996.

This work found that those women who perceived that they were well supported by their partner throughout their pregnancy were at increased risk for developing postnatal depression. Not a comfortable thought and certainly not the established and generally accepted belief that being well supported by your partner protects you from emotional health problems at this time. The possibility that too much support could be just as damaging as too little when having a baby clearly required contemplation.

Whilst working as a Research Associate at the University of Leicester Sandra studied part-time and went on to gain her second degree (Psychiatry: Immediate award outright). She has specialised in researching women's experiences of having their first baby, and has carved a niche in the field with regard to emotional health promotion, in particular the prevention of postnatal depression.

Sandra is a member of the postnatal care and support sub-group, a team of professional and voluntary workers from Leicestershire who have instigated various much needed facilities in the area, and has also worked with Homestart regarding motherhood within the Asian community. Her research work has been published in various books and international journals to date.

If you have any comments about the book or would like to contact the author about your own experiences of having your first child, please email:

potent@hushmail.com

Contents

THE AUTHOR vii

INTRODUCTION: TO THE BOOK AND TO THE NINE WOMEN 1

FINDING OUT THEY WERE PREGNANT: ALL CHANGE! 7
The tryers... 7
And the not so trying 9
A moral dilemma 16

THEIR EXPERIENCE OF PREGNANCY AND BIRTH: WHAT HAVE YOU LET
YOURSELF IN FOR? 23
Pregnancy 23
Birth 27
Their experience of their partner's involvement during pregnancy and the birth . .37

THEIR EXPERIENCE OF EARLY MOTHERHOOD: NOW YOU KNOW WHY
YOUR MOTHER DIDN'T TELL YOU! 45
Imagination and reality 45
The highs and the lows 59
Their experience of their partner's involvement in early parenthood 61

THEIR EXPERIENCE OF MOTHERHOOD UP TO THEIR BABY'S FIRST
BIRTHDAY: TO TELL OR NOT TO TELL YOUR BROODY FRIENDS? 71
A life change 71
Changes within themselves 74
Their relationship with their partner's 85

THEIR IMMEDIATE FUTURE: WILL YOU HAVE TIME FOR ONE?! 97
  Hopes for the coming year 97
    Julia's hopes 98
    Emma's hopes 100
    Claire's hopes 101
  Building upon their new experiences 103
    To be developed... 104
    To be changed... 105

CONCLUDING THOUGHTS 107

ACKNOWLEDGEMENTS 113

INDEX 115

APPENDIX: OUR CONVERSATIONS 125
    EMMA 127
    TANYA 151
    HELEN 165
    CLAIRE 197
    SARAH 227
    AMEENA 243
    RACHEL 273
    SADIE 293

Introduction:
To the book and to the nine women

This book is written for all those having or recently having had their first child. Unlike most pregnancy and motherhood books, this one will not offer you a breakdown of the week by week or month by month physical changes that will be happening to both your body and your baby. This book deals with the changes that will be happening to how you are feeling. These are the actual and varied experiences of nine women having their first baby. From the moment they saw the blue line on the pregnancy test up until their child's first birthday their new lives and how they feel about them, as they tell them, will be presented.

The nine women who participated in this work are from nine very varied backgrounds. They were originally involved in my work with the 'Preparing for Parenthood' course run at Leicester General Hospital. This was part of my work with the perinatal research team based in the Academic Department of Psychiatry of the University of Leicester. Nine women were approached to contribute to this additional research, they all agreed to take part. The similarities and differences between the women are highlighted such that the common and uncommon themes and

Nine Women, Nine Months, Nine Lives

experiences are discussed. The book has a chronological structure, beginning at the beginning as it were, each of the chapters containing direct quotes from the women.

Chances are if you are currently pregnant with your first child and are reading this book you will have begun to wonder just exactly what you have let yourself in for! Expectations of the future can be double-edged swords. If we are overly optimistic we run the risk of being let down by reality. If we are overly pessimistic we can forget to treasure, or maybe even not notice, the small but important everyday pleasures of life. Trying to gain and maintain a balance between the two ends of life's spectrum is not the easiest of things to do, especially when you find yourself in a completely new situation.

Wondering if what you are feeling is normal is part and parcel of everybody's everyday life. Some wonder about it more often than others; most of us do it at some time in our lives. We are more likely to do it when we are in a new and unknown situation. You will have found yourself in a new and unknown situation when you found out that you were to become a mother for the first time. You may find yourself paying more attention to or noticing how you feel more often than you would usually do. You may also find that you compare yourself to others who are pregnant. Be it a woman at a bus stop, on the television, or on the cover of a magazine you may have found yourself wondering if she feels the same as you. This is a perfectly natural and very useful capability to have. This monitoring or comparing behaviour enables us to *adapt* to different situations *effectively*.

On the whole the women who took part in this book felt, with the benefit of hindsight, that too little information is given to women through the standard health care service about what to expect when you have your first child. They felt the information they were given by health professionals or that they had sought for themselves from friends, family and books was rose-tinted, inadequate or just simply inaccurate. Many of the hundreds of women I have spoken to over the years just want to know "is it normal to feel like I do?" This book will illustrate that there are many ways to be normal.

Introduction

The primary aim of this book is to reassure you about the range of emotions and experiences it is likely that you will feel and have when becoming a mother for the first time. Hopefully by reassuring you it will help you to be more resilient to, and adapt effectively to, your new day-to-day life. Research has shown that you are more likely to be relaxed and enjoy motherhood if your expectations are realistic because they are based upon the *actual* experiences of others.

If you are not currently pregnant but have "been there and done that" you will probably find yourself recalling your own experiences and comparing them with the women in this book. Whatever your individual perspective you are likely to find that you identify with one if not many of these women's experiences of becoming a mother for the first time. Should you find yourself particularly identifying with any one or more of the women, the conversations I had with them are provided in their entirety in the last part of the book – please note that the women's, their partner's (if they have one) and their child's names have been changed.

The extracts from the conversations which you will find throughout the following five chapters have been incorporated to illustrate the main text of the book and are abridged slightly, unlike the complete conversations at the back of the book. This was done to enhance the clarity of the point being made and to maximise the opportunity to present the variety of feelings of the women. The words spoken by me appear in italics.

The following nine paragraphs provide brief introductions to the women who contributed to the book. Let's meet them.

Emma was 31 years old when she found that she was pregnant. She had never really thought about having children. She has a long-term partner Neil whom she lives with and prior to becoming pregnant considered herself to be a career woman working as a Regional Company Auditor. Whilst being shocked and unsure about the pregnancy herself, her partner just incorporated it into their life together. Their daughter Lotte was very small and had breathing problems when she was born and spent the first month of her life in the Special Care Baby Unit at Leicester General hospital. Nevertheless, Emma and her family have survived to tell the tale and continue to grow stronger everyday.

Tanya was 19 years old when she found out she was pregnant. She had known the father of her child for a couple of years. She became single immediately after telling him she was pregnant. He has seen his daughter Katie once in a chance encounter in the street and had to be made to look at her. He does not contribute to either Tanya or their daughter's upkeep. Tanya would very much like to return to work (as a part-time sales assistant), but perhaps re-train to a job where she can be with Katie as much as possible.

Helen was 30 years old when she accidentally became pregnant. She and her husband Richard had been married for six months and have known each other since they were at school. She experienced a great deal of internal conflict about her decision to go ahead with the pregnancy, this continued well into the first few months of motherhood as she had never really seen herself having children. She returned to work as a long-haul Flight Attendant as soon as she could for her son Will's and her own benefit. This allowed her to retain her sense of self and give her best as a mother. As a consequence of her career she is away from home for half the week and therefore her husband is equally involved in their son's upbringing.

Claire was 25 years old when she and her husband Tom decided to start to try for a family. She had not even been married a month when she became pregnant! They had been planning to have lots of children but circumstances and ill health since the birth of Hannah have changed their initial feelings about parenthood. They have their own catering company and work together. Claire returned to work as soon as she could after having an emergency caesarean section.

Sarah was 29 years old when she found out that she was pregnant. She had been living with her partner Anthony for a few months and was not planning to have children just yet. However, they were both pleased and continued with their pregnancy. Sarah has returned to work part-time as a sales assistant, not to her original job as a Stable-hand, but wants to re-train so that she can spend more time with her son Jack and her partner. Having him has given her a new found strength and confidence

Introduction

within herself.

Ameena was 22 years old when she became pregnant after being married for two years. Her marriage was arranged through her family. She continued with her career in Social Services as a Contracts Assistant after marrying and indeed after having her daughter Ayesha. Although they had been trying for a child since marrying, she was glad it had taken two years to conceive as this enabled her and her husband Yusuf to get to know and grow to love each other. At the time of the interview she was experiencing a conflict within herself about the balance in her life between work and home.

Rachel was 27 years old when she found out she was pregnant for the first time. Her partner James was in the process of moving from London to Leicester to be with her and they decided that they would probably have started a family together in the future and so went ahead with their pregnancy. However, Rachel continued to feel unsure about having a baby right up until the day of the birth. She wanted to return to her job as a Nursery Teacher as soon as possible after having her son Charlie to continue building her career. When she had her son she left returning to work as late as she could and continues to feel a conflict between motherhood, which she unexpectedly found she loved, and her career.

Sadie and her boyfriend Paul were 17 years old when she became pregnant accidentally. He said he would support her so they went ahead with the pregnancy and moved in together. Two days before this interview took place, and eleven days before her first son Alex's first birthday, she had her second son. She was working part-time in a factory before conceiving for the first time but has not worked since that pregnancy. Her relationship with her partner was strained and on the verge of breaking down at the time of this interview.

Julia was 30 years old when she became pregnant after three years of trying to conceive and with her first attempt at fertility treatment. She and her husband Matt had been married for two years before she got pregnant. She found that motherhood was everything and more besides what she had expected it would be and so was very reluctant to return to work as a Care Worker for individuals with challenging behaviours and

Nine Women, Nine Months, Nine Lives

leave Daniel at home. However, her relationship with her husband has become very strained and at the time of the interview she was contemplating separation. Indeed, Julia requested that our full conversation was not included in the book for her own and her husband's personal reasons.

Now that you have been introduced, turn the pages and read about their individual journeys to their child's first Birthday.

Finding out they were pregnant: All change!

Like many pregnancies not all of those conceived by these women were intentional. A few of the women were trying to get pregnant. However, the majority were not. This chapter will recount each woman's reaction upon finding out she was pregnant and in most cases their partner's reaction to the news. In most cases the shock turned into pleasure, in some cases it did not. For at least one couple the decision to keep the baby was not a straightforward one and this is discussed in the final part of the chapter.

The tryers...

Out of the nine women only one of them was actively trying to get pregnant at the time and had been having fertility treatment. It worked for Julia on the first attempt after three years of marriage, anxiety and heartache. She went to the local chemists to do the pregnancy test and didn't tell anybody about the much longed for positive result until she had those she most wanted to tell all together.

Nine Women, Nine Months, Nine Lives

I've done that many tests, when you've been trying for three years, you know, and you... Because you worry and whittle and get yourself in a terrible state you delay your periods and what have you. Because I had always had completely regular periods up until trying to get pregnant. I used to like start on the same day, the same afternoon; I could be that exact. And then when I started trying they went all over the place. So no I didn't do a test at home I went to the chemist, and waited. And I was about, it was 48 hours after I was supposed to start, so it was very <u>very</u> feint. And yeah, I was over the moon. And I didn't tell anybody until the next day. Two days, no two days after. [Laughs]
Fair enough! [Laughs] So who was everybody then? Was that all your friends or...?
My mum and dad, and Matt.
Yeah, so the four of you together.
Yeah.
Oh right, I expect they were 'quite' pleased as well?
Oh yes!
Why did you wait for those couple of days, was it because you...?
Because it was extra <u>extra</u> special. And I really wanted the people who are most close to me to all find out together.
{Julia}

Two of the women were "sort of" trying. Claire was about to get married and had tried to take her pill in such a way that her period wouldn't fall during her wedding or her honeymoon. Consequently, she fell for Hannah. They had previously decided that they would start trying for a family straight after getting married and so were far from devastated at the prospect of a shotgun baby.

Were you trying to get pregnant at the time?
Sort of. Because we decided that when we got married we'd decide afterwards. So what happened was because my wedding and honeymoon were two weeks apart I messed about with my pill, so that I'd have my period in between and then I'd come off my pill afterwards and then get pregnant after the honeymoon. That was the idea! But because I'd messed about with it I actually got pregnant before I got married but I didn't realise until just after the wedding. So we were both, we were shocked, but we were both really happy, because we wanted a baby anyway so... yaay! [Laughs]
[Laughs] Yeah, you were happy?
Yeah we really wanted to have a baby anyway so it was just a month early.
Yeah, so it wasn't a problem at all?
No. Not at all.
{Claire}

Finding out they were pregnant

The other woman who was "sort of" trying had in fact been married for two years and had not been using any contraceptives throughout that time. As Ameena had not become pregnant she had begun to try to adjust to a future which might not include children. In fact, she couldn't bring herself to look at the result of the pregnancy test herself – her husband was the first to know! They were thrilled.

I, I somehow, felt pregnant. I don't know whether other women get that or not, but I just had that feeling. Not that I was expecting to get pregnant or feel pregnant but, after a while I thought I'd better do a test, but then I decided "No, let's leave it a week". I didn't tell my husband at first, I was acting a bit peculiar and he asked me if I was all right. It was funny because it must have been the first time I'd said "No, I'm not!" [Laughs] I reckon he thought I'd got backache or a headache from work! [Laughs] So I sat down and said "Look I think I might be pregnant"... Well! [Laughs] And then because he manages a pharmacy, he went back to work and got a test. Rushed back home, I wee-ed in the pot, and he looked and said it was positive and he was like "Oh wow!" Really happy! [Laughs] And then he had to 'phone everybody, he was thrilled!
That's nice.
Yeah, so, it did come as a little bit of a shock, but it was a nice shock.
So, why didn't you want to do the test? You said that you felt pregnant...
Yeah, I think it's, it's the unknown. I mean you hear about it don't you, "Gosh my life has changed."
...
So can you remember what actually went through your mind when Yusuf told you?
I was really happy, more than anything because I'd always thought I would never have children.
Why?!
Well because... [Whispered] We never used anything from when we were married and it just never happened, so... [Normal voice] I did want children but had gradually come to think that if this was the way it was going to be... If I'd pinned my hopes on it and then never been able to have any, that would have been devastating so...
{Ameena}

And the not so trying

Of the remaining six women, two of them had never envisaged having children. Helen had married her childhood sweetheart the year previously and did not look upon motherhood as a potentially positive experience. When she found out she was pregnant her immediate gut reaction was to have a termination. She knew that her husband wanted a family. They then went through a prolonged period of moral dilemma that resulted in them requesting a termination. However, following further contemplation, the turning point being a conversation between her best friend and her husband, she began to question the decision they had made. Following this period of extended contemplation, they went ahead with the pregnancy even though Helen continued to be less than certain about having a child until their son was a few months old. Their moral dilemma is discussed in detail in the next part of this chapter.

Conversely, although Emma had always considered herself to be a career woman, when she found out she was pregnant she felt confused. She was not unhappy but felt anxious about how her partner would react to the news. When he readily accepted it she was both relieved and pleased. With hindsight she thought that perhaps her and her partner had been scared to discuss with, or admit to, each other that they might want children, as they both happily and quickly adapted to the pregnancy and the prospect of parenthood.

Were you trying to get pregnant at the time?
No! [Laughs]
No, you weren't at all, were you?
No, no.
And you weren't planning on having children?
No.
Had you thought about it as a possibility? Were you dead against it?
Well, we weren't dead against it, just, we hadn't decided. Do you know what I mean? I don't think we'd even. We'd talked about it but we weren't… It wasn't like imminent that we were going to have children.
So would you say it was something you just hadn't thought about rather than something you'd decided you weren't going to do?
I think we'd both decided that we weren't going to do it, but I think we were both pleased we did! [Laughs] Do you know what I mean? [Laughs] When it came to finding out that I was actually pregnant we were both happy about it, yeah we were. [Laughs] We were both happy about it so… I think deep down we both really did want them but didn't really want to admit it I suppose, if that makes sense?
Yeah. Can you remember what went through your mind when you found out you were actually pregnant, when you saw those two lines on the test?

Finding out they were pregnant

"How am I going to tell him?" [Laughs]
...
So, that was your initial reaction, what did you then think afterwards? Was it the more immediate things like how am I going to tell him or was it more what am I going to do? Or rather what are we going to do?
It was "How am I going to tell him?" to start with, and I thought "Well, I'll get that over with"! [Laughs] I don't think we really doubted what we were going to do at all, it was "Oh fine" you know, and that was that.
{Emma}

Another two of the six who accidentally became pregnant had relationships that were currently undergoing a major change. Rachel and her partner had recently decided that they were going to live together and he had just got a job in Leicester and was in the process of moving out of London to be with her. She had only moved back to Leicester recently herself and was concerned about letting her new employers down. When she got pregnant she was shocked but her partner's positive view that they would have had a family together sooner or later swayed her decision in favour of having the baby. Nevertheless, she too continued to be less than certain about that decision until their son was born.

Were you trying to get pregnant at the time?
No. No, no!
Absolutely not?
Definitely not, he was a complete accident! [Laughs]
So can you remember what went through your mind when you found out you were pregnant? When you saw those two blue lines...
I couldn't believe how quickly the pregnancy test changed. I'd only moved here in the March [3 months earlier], and I'd only just started my job, so I thought "Oh my God what do I do?" And then we also had an OFSTED visit at the school, and I was like, a bit preoccupied with that, and I thought "Oh I'm going to let down the Head". Those kind of emotions really. And then James was at school as well for a parents evening, and I thought, "Oh God I can't tell him yet, not when there's all of these parents".
So James is a teacher as well?
Yes.
Right.
So, no he wasn't planned, it was a bit of a shock horror to begin with!
...
We went out for a meal that night to try and get things in perspective really.

Nine Women, Nine Months, Nine Lives

To try and sort things out?
We decided that we were in a good relationship, and the fact that we hadn't lived together yet didn't matter.
Yeah?
So once we'd recovered - that was that! [Laughs]
...
You were more keen for the baby than I was weren't you? [Talking to her partner James]
James: I'd got to thirty and thought well...
Now or never?!
James: Yes! [Laughs]
{Rachel}

In contrast, despite the fact that Sarah and her partner Anthony had barely begun living together she was pleased and excited about discovering she was pregnant. She was anxious about his reaction to the extent that she didn't tell him she was pregnant for ten days, wanting to be sure how she felt about it in herself first. As she expected he was shocked, but his shock soon turned to pleasure much to her relief.

So it was a completely unplanned pregnancy?
Yes.
Can you remember what went through your mind when you did the test? What was your initial reaction?
I was happy... Yeah, I was happy.
...
And what did you think about afterwards? Your initial reaction was happiness, did you then think "Oh my goodness!"?
I was shocked, mmm, a bit shocked. Well I was worried how my partner and my family would take it.
...
Initially, I was a bit worried, I mean, just on his reaction really. I mean I knew he wasn't going to desert me or anything like that, he's from a biggish family, so... Yeah, it was just his reaction really.
How he would take it. Did you think "My God how am I going to tell him?"
Yes! [Laughter] Yes. He was all right, he was shocked, took him about, he got used to it and he was really happy. I didn't tell, I told him first and then I didn't tell any of the rest of the family for a while, because I wanted to be sure, between ourselves, you know, before I told anybody else.
Were you living together at the time?

Finding out they were pregnant

Yes, yes we were, but we hadn't been living together very long.
Had you known each other long?
Yes, yeah we'd been together about 3 years but we'd only been living together about 4 months.
Oh right, so everything was new and different?
Yeah!
…
Right so you'd done a home test, then you went to the doctors and you still hadn't told anybody at that stage?
No.
How long did it take you between doing the test and then telling him?
From what when I knew positively?
Yeah.
I think it was about 10 days.
Ten days in total, so that's quite a while really. Do you think you were fretting a bit?
Yeah I think it, I was happy with it, I was happy with you know just being pregnant, but I was, I think I just wanted to get used to it.
In yourself?
Yeah.
To sort out how you felt? So perhaps you knew how you were feeling before you told him?
Yes, so I was feeling completely positive about it sort of thing.
Then it was just a matter of telling him?
[Laughter] Yeah!
{Sarah}

Of all the women, Tanya's partner reacted the most negatively. She had known him for a couple of years and was completely stunned by his immediate and sadly consistent reaction to "get rid of it". He threatened Tanya with violence if she named him as the father. He has never acknowledged their daughter, finishing their relationship when she told him she was pregnant. Despite this, Tanya was happy to find that she was pregnant.

Were you trying to get pregnant at the time?
No, no it was a complete and utter accident, yeah.
Can you remember what went through your mind when you found out you were pregnant?
"Oh my God, how am I going to tell my mum?"
Yeah?

13

Nine Women, Nine Months, Nine Lives

Yeah, that was it.
That was the first thing you thought?
Yeah, because I was on holiday at the time, and I thought "Oh my God I'm pregnant, how am I going to tell me mum?!" [Laughs]
So, did you think about it afterwards and did how you feel change?
When, when I was pregnant? I was happy.
…
And can you remember what your partners reaction was when you told him?
"Get rid of it. I don't want nothing to do with it."
…
And how did you feel about your partner's reaction?
I was really upset.
Had you known each other for a long while?
A couple of years, yeah.
Yeah? What did you think his reaction was going to be? You said your first reaction was your mum…
Yeah, and then I thought about him after, but, I don't know, I don't know what his reaction, I don't know what I was expecting from him. I didn't expect him to say what he said, but at the end of the day it's his choice isn't it? I thought he was more mature than what he was, so…
…
So, has he ever seen Katie or…?
He's seen her once but he didn't, I mean, I had to turn the push chair round so he could see her because he weren't going to, so… I thought "Yeah - you look at how beautiful she is!" [Laughs] "See what you are missing out on!" But he just didn't want to see her.
Did he speak to you?
Yeah, he spoke to me, he's fine with me, it's just Katie.
So he wanted you to have a termination?
Yeah.
And did you consider it?
No.
Not at all, not for a moment?
No, I don't think I'd have been able to. I mean don't get me wrong, if people, if that's what people want to do then that's up to them, but I couldn't do it myself. I just don't think I'd be able to live with myself. So, it was just, I didn't even think about it, that's the way I've been brought up, so…
And what did your mum say?
She cried a lot! [Laughs] And then she cried even more, so I cried, and then, what did she say? She said, "Who is the father?" And I said, "I don't want to tell you".
Was she upset about that?
I think so at the time but, my ex-boyfriend he'd, he'd, oh what's the word…? He told me

Finding out they were pregnant

that if I told anybody that it was his baby he would beat me up. So I don't know where I'd have stood, if I'd have told my mum then, because he got on quite well with my mum and dad.
Oh, did they not realise...?
I think they realise now, but they still don't know till this day, but I couldn't...
No, not for sure.
But they think it's him. I don't know (whether they know for sure).
So, you don't get any support from him at all, maintenance or anything?
No, no nothing.
That must be very hard.
Oh it is. Definitely. On the benefits I get it's crap. I get the money on a Monday and nearly all of it goes on bills. It's hard. I get nappies and food for her, and then I've got like five pound left for myself. So, I mean, well my mum and dad have been helping me out as much as they can, which is really good of them, but you just have to get on with it don't you? I suppose.
Yeah, and do you think you made the right decision?
Yes, I do.
You seem very sure.
Yes, oh yes, I just don't know what my life would be without her.
{Tanya}

As the youngest woman of the nine, Sadie at just seventeen was scared and upset when she found out she was pregnant. She decided to go ahead with the pregnancy after considering all her options and her partner said that he would support her in this decision. She and her boyfriend were not living together at the time but now do. In the year since Alex was born they have had another child, Nathan.

So it was unplanned?
Yeah.
OK. Can you remember what went through your mind when you saw the blue line on the test?
I was scared, worried.
Was anybody with you?
Yeah, my boyfriend, and my friend, I was just upset really.
Yeah, so did you, had you thought before hand that you were pregnant or did you...?
Yeah I did have an idea.
...
And your immediate reaction was to be scared and upset. And what did you think

Nine Women, Nine Months, Nine Lives

afterwards, when you'd got over the shock as it were?
I didn't know whether to keep it or have an abortion. But I decided to keep it in the end.
So you were thinking about whether it was actually possible?
Yeah... It seems so long ago now!
Yeah, so it's not really fresh in your mind? [Has just had – in the last 48 hours- her second baby]
Not really!
So your partner and your friend were with you when you did the test. And can you remember your partner's reaction when you found out?
He was shocked but he said he'd stick by me, he were, he didn't really say much.
Is that unusual for him or...?
Probably for a lad, yeah! [Laughs]
So you told him that you were possibly...?
I didn't actually tell him. Well I did tell him a week before I done the test, so he knew what to expect.
Right.
So he knew I might be pregnant.
So he'd had a while to think about it?
Yeah, but he was agreeing with whatever I wanted to do.
{Sadie}

A moral dilemma

Helen's personal experience of suspecting she was pregnant, finding out that she was pregnant, and the decision process that she and her husband went through regarding whether to continue with the pregnancy or not are presented below in full as she described it herself. She thought that it was probably the most she had ever questioned her morals in all her life. It was not a comfortable or an easily forgettable experience.

If you could think back to when you found out you were pregnant. OK, were you trying to get pregnant at the time?
No!
Can you remember what went through your mind when you found out? When you did the test, when you saw those two blue lines on the...?
<u>Anger,</u> absolute anger, fear and frustration at having got myself into that situation.
Because wasn't it something like you were on the pill?
Yes, yeah I stopped that whilst I was on a course in Germany, and I thought "Well I'll

Finding out they were pregnant

start having a break then." So I stopped taking it not thinking that Richard might come out and visit. He came out to visit and because I had been on the pill so long I thought... And I'd really taken it very haphazardly.
Yeah I suppose it must be difficult flying and that, [works as a Flight Attendant] working out the time zones and that...?
Oh yeah, well I'm a bit dizzy anyway, I mean I'd take none for two days and then take two the next day and stuff. So I thought, I really thought "Oh I'm immune to it". And then flying as well messes about with you so I thought "Well it must be OK, there's been no reason to think that it could happen". Which was so so stupid and I was just <u>so</u> livid when it happened. So... That was the situation. Didn't expect it. Made a silly mistake and...
Because you weren't planning on having any kids at all were you?
Well, it didn't figure in my life, I knew that at some point it would probably figure in Richard's. I'm sure it did. To be honest, I'm sure it did. And I really wanted to hold out as long as I could. It really wasn't on the agenda, it's not something that we thought "Right we'll do that in so many years". I really thought I could last out until I was almost forty, but whether that was my dream...
Well maybe, maybe not. I mean you know it's not impossible, it could have been like that. There's no reason really to say that it wouldn't have been.
Yeah it's probably just something I'd put to the back of my mind and thought "Well maybe at some stage in my life I'll want to do this but I really don't want to start talking about it or doing anything..."
So was anybody with you when you did the test?
No, no I was on my own.
Was that what you wanted to do?
Well it was during the day and Richard was at work and I just knew I had to get this test over and done with, because I knew otherwise...
Were you late?
Yeah, and... I felt, I'd just been to my cousins wedding and I'd felt really ill for about a week after that.
Really?
Yeah, I was sick and oh! I was thinking "This is some hangover, one or two days is fine but [Laughs] not a week!"
Oh my God!
Yeah, and one of my friends said to me "You know you've been sick and well, you should really find out for definite". I must admit the thought had entered my head but I thought "No it <u>can't</u> be true, it really can't be true" and then when I did the test... It was a real effort to get out of bed in the morning to go and get the test, I mean I haven't done a pregnancy test for years, I still thought that you had to do it first thing in the morning.
Oh right!
So that shows you how long! So I ran down to the chemist, ran back, did the test, and

17

Nine Women, Nine Months, Nine Lives

that explained why I was late.
So how late were you? Were you like a week or two weeks?
I'm not quite sure but I'd say it was probably about two weeks. Yeah, which is kind of major, but then I didn't really pay much attention to it because I'd just stopped taking the pill and I just thought well, my system and everything will be completely messed up.
And you'd expect there to be some kind of adjustment anyway?
Yeah exactly and plus two years prior to that what with the wedding and the travelling and... I'd worked as much as I could work right up until Christmas, I'd got all my hours in before Christmas. So that the day after I'd finished work we went off to Australia, and I didn't have a period that month, so it wasn't until the following month, so it, that was strange. So I just thought "Oh it's all messed up, I've been working a lot" which does sometimes happen.
Yeah exactly.
So it really didn't worry me until I was still feeling ill after this wedding.
Your 'mysterious' hangover!
Yeah, yeah, so then I knew what it was likely to be, yeah.
And what was Richard's reaction? When did you tell him? Did you tell him straightaway?
No... No, I told him that day but he was very late coming home from work. And... It all just cascaded out, it'd been going round and round in my head that day, and oh! [Laughs] It's just that, when you know that you're all emotionally... So it came across from me as being the <u>worst</u> thing possible and, and I just blurted it out. I was just <u>the</u> most miserable sobbing wreck. So his reaction was pretty negative as well, but that was tinged with shock. Yeah and I, beforehand, if I'd ever imagined telling him something like that I'd thought well yeah... But as it was he wasn't as overjoyed as I thought he would be, so that was good for me, personally. But he took it really <u>really</u> strangely, and that wasn't...
Well yeah, I suppose, I mean, did you get the impression that he was reacting to you more than reacting to the fact that you were pregnant?
I don't know, a bit of both really. I mean we'd only been married six months, and although we'd been together for so long it...
Oh yeah, because you've been together since you were at school?
Yeah, and I think all the things that we could do together, you know, get off and do some more travelling together instead of doing it separately, which we had done, and... That was all in the forefront of my mind. It just seemed to be at the wrong time, and also knowing how I'd always felt about having children he knew that that was a bad thing. And initially he just said to me "Just do what you think, what you want to do" and that was a hard thing for him to say, it was a <u>hard</u> decision to have to make.
So do you think he handed over the responsibility?
Initially, initially, as I say it was, well it was really just that day. By the next day it was like "No, <u>we've</u> got to decide what <u>we</u> want to do". Then that changed over the next fortnight, I knew what I felt, that I wouldn't want to, but... And I think Richard knew that and he kept saying "It'll be OK" and then it'd be "No we can't do this, we can't have

Finding out they were pregnant

a baby, it will change everything." To the point that at the end of that fortnight... We came to a decision at the end of that, because we had to put a time limit on it, and then we talked and he said that we would do whatever I wanted to do. And he knew what I wanted to do, I wanted to have an abortion and that he was saying it was OK with him... And so that was what we decided to do, made another appointment to go and see the doctor... To get it arranged basically.
To go and get the blue slip and...
Yeah, that's right... Then my best friend called that night and she asked me if we had come to a decision.
So you'd talked to her about it?
Yeah I'd talked to her as she was my best friend. And I said "Yeah" and told her what we'd decided to do and she said "How does Richard feel about that?" And she's known Richard for probably about the same length of time as I've known him. All our adult lives anyway, and I said "I'll pass the 'phone over to you he's, he needs to speak to somebody else, he's only spoken to me, nobody else has discussed it with him, nobody else knows the situation" and I was sat on the stairs listening. Which was a strange thing, it was quite open, and I was sat there waiting for him to come off the 'phone so I could speak to her again. And... I understood that what he was saying wasn't in line with what he had told me. So really it came across that you know he, that we would go ahead with the abortion to please me. I, I didn't discuss it any further at that point, I just thought maybe I need to rethink this. Because I'd spent all my time thinking "I can't do it, there's no way I can do it" and I had never swayed in thinking that until this 'phone call.
How long after you found out did you decide that you were going to have an abortion?
Straightaway.
And then how long after that was this conversation, was it a week or two weeks?
This conversation, the conversation with my friend was two weeks later and in that time we had both gone to see our doctor. Richard's now registered with my doctor so we've all got the same doctor. And his reaction was initially "Well you'll have to pay for it yourself." Which, at the time was a bit of a strange thing to say.
Particularly for a GP.
It's not as if we had done this willy nilly...
It's hardly as if you used it as a form of contraception!
Yeah, <u>quite.</u> Well, we said that was fine and he said "And then of course there's your age". Which kind of shook me.
How old were you?
I was 30 just under 31, yeah I was 30. And that really shook me. Because sometimes... Because we'd always been together you just think of yourself as being 20 or whatever and then all of a sudden it was like "Oh I'm 30!" One minute I was at school and the next minute I'm too old to have children! And it really effected me that way and... I knew that was rubbish I just thought "Thirty's not old! I know what you're saying, I know the biological clock may be ticking but I still feel too young to do it. I don't want to do it, I

don't feel responsible enough to do it."
Yeah, but if you feel too young then, well perhaps you are...?
Yeah, and then it did make me have a rethink. I'm trying to remember exactly how he worded it but he, he was implying that it wasn't always the best physical move to make for your body if you want to have children after that. And... Once again I kind of decided that that was something that would be...
So if you perhaps decided that you were going to in the future then...?
Which I always think of as a scare-mongering tactic. That if you have an abortion then...
Yeah, I would say that I agree with that, you can have a balanced opinion. GP's don't need to have an in-your-face extreme...
Yeah, he came on quite strong, trying to dissuade me. But it did initially, the day after the doctors. Yeah, so that, that was very strange, I did the test on the Friday and we went to the doctors on the Monday, it was either the Monday or the Tuesday. Yeah because I'd already booked an appointment at the doctors, but then at the end of the conversation at the doctors he said "I think you'd better go away and make up your minds, come back in a week". So I had this time limit. "If you can't get back here in a week, get back here as soon as you can, because you need to decide either way". I'm glad we did that, and I think it was better to have the time. And then before going back was this turning point, the 'phone call from my best friend. And I didn't say anything to Richard at the time, I thought about it over-night and I was going back to work the following day. And I said "I think I've changed my mind, I thought maybe this is the only way, this is for the best, but it will happen again" - which is more to the point. What would I do if it happened again? I can't be picking and choosing having one abortion or more.
Yeah, it's kind of like the consistency of your decision isn't it?
Because I'm so haphazard, I always have been haphazard with the pill which is why it never scared me that I would ever be pregnant I think.
Yeah because you kind of feel safer once you've been haphazard for so long. You kind of think, well I'll be fine. I mean I'm on the pill, the times that say I've got up late, say half past ten and I think "Oh it's only three hours, I'll be all right..."
Which never phased me at all!
No, exactly.
If it was only half a day late, that was normal. Or I'd take it at four o'clock in the morning and then again at 8 o'clock at night, when I was away on trips you know. So yeah it never really bothered me. So I thought I was safe, and as much as this has frightened me, it's going to happen again, I'm sure it is, because I will just think "Oh I'm OK". Which is why I've not gone back on to the pill again, because it's just too stupid.
There's always going to be the possibility of it happening again.
Yeah, exactly and I can't let that happen again. Because there's no way I ever want to have to make that decision again, no way. I know that I thought that this might happen again this time, so in the end I thought right just get on and do it... So will that do (as an answer to the question) ?! [Laughs]

Finding out they were pregnant

Yeah, yeah! [Laughs]
And when I called Richard, on his mobile it was, to talk about me having changed my mind... I'd actually left a note on the pillow, and he hadn't been home yet, and I told him and he said he just couldn't take it in, his reaction was just so positive "It'll be OK, I'll look after your baby, I'll do everything!" So it was <u>so</u> positive.
Really, <u>really</u> positive.
I knew then that what he had said to me was <u>very</u> different from what he was feeling. It was amazing, unreal, to think that he cared about me that much! [Laughs]
Yeah, well that's it, you know no-one's ever really certain all the time...
No, but, I wanted to talk to him about, not practically, day-to-day but, what would happen, <u>how</u> would we look after a baby? When would I go back to work? Richard's work? We talked about the realities of it all, and he just kept saying "It'll be OK". And he has been great, I mean the times that I was in a real state, that I'd been on a flight with loads of screaming children, I would come home and close the door, I just felt like I couldn't deal with it. And then he would say something like "It'll be OK, yours won't be like that" [Laughter] And I was like "Oh yeah, and how do <u>you</u> know?!"
Oh really?! Yeah mmm.
I was like, because he is so laid back and so am I, but he was convinced "No they won't be, they won't be highly strung or anything like that" but I wasn't so sure!
Yeah, well everybody has their good days and their bad days. And so do kids, every child is different, so you know, it's true what he said, yours might not be like that! But then again... [Laughs]
So... Even, I think even up to the end I wasn't sure if I was doing the right thing. But... you can only do the best that you can, and I was trying to cope with it, thinking "I am going to have this baby - it's too late now".
Mmm, kind of dealing with it then, knowing that you were going to have to deal with it at some stage...
At some stage, yeah. It was a case of really, but I've <u>never</u> questioned my morals like that before <u>ever.</u> I always knew exactly what I would have done. Say if I'd got pregnant at twenty, it would have been a different situation but I would always know that if the situation arose... The main thing that made me step back from it was the fact that I was married, I couldn't justify it as much as if I had been single.
Really?
Yeah, which is ridiculous but yeah, and I don't think that marriage is this big thing, I don't think you've got to be married to have children, but the fact that I was married in that situation...
Do you think marriage perhaps reflected security almost?
Mmm, yeah. Yeah maybe but I just felt that I couldn't, because I could have done it when I was single. Because Richard said at one point "If we hadn't have been married, even if we had been living together, and you'd got pregnant, you wouldn't have told me would you?" And I wouldn't.

Nine Women, Nine Months, Nine Lives

No, it would have been a different situation.
I mean he knew me well enough, and knew what I would have wanted to do, but... Yeah that's the way I would have done it.
Yeah, if that's the way you feel then...
But I think it did make a lot of difference the fact that I was married, I <u>couldn't</u> justify what I wanted to do, other than for selfish reasons and feelings on my part.
Yeah, it is quite a big-ee
Yeah, definitely.
{Helen}

Curiously enough even though only three of the nine women were not making strident efforts to prevent themselves becoming pregnant, of the six who were actively avoiding pregnancy, in the event only one of them seriously considered having a termination and viewed the prospect of motherhood with disdain and despair. In the next chapter I will relate the women's actual experiences of pregnancy and birth and their partner's influential role throughout that time.

Their experience of pregnancy and birth:

What have you let yourself in for?

This chapter will move along through time to look at the women's expectations of pregnancy and birth and compare those imaginings with the physical and emotional experiences that they actually encountered. We will also explore their hopes for their partner's involvement and whether his actual support (both practically and emotionally) lived up to his anticipated behaviour.

Pregnancy

Very few of the women had ever contemplated what pregnancy would feel like *before* they got pregnant. Unsurprisingly as they weren't planning to have children, neither Helen nor Emma had previously thought about it. Equally unsurprisingly, as she had been trying to get pregnant for several years, Julia had imagined how pregnancy would feel. She thought it would be wonderful.

Nine Women, Nine Months, Nine Lives

Oh all floaty and lovely and you know! [Laughs] I really, I mean I thought the worst bit would be morning sickness and then I thought obviously the labour. I just didn't imagine there would be so many other things. Not majorly awful things but just things like, that I just hadn't imagined.
{Julia}

    Claire was another woman who looked forward to being pregnant and anticipated that it would be a "wonderful experience". Interestingly she too was planning to start a family in the near future, soon after she was married. Ameena was the other woman who was "sort of" trying to get pregnant at the time she conceived. However, she said that she had "never really stopped to think about it" beforehand and continued to not wonder about how the pregnancy would make her feel throughout the remainder of the nine months.

    Although Sadie was not planning to get pregnant so young she had spent some time imagining what pregnancy would be like. She thought it would be a good experience and had focused on the physical aspects of pregnancy, looking forward to being "big and fat!" Similarly, Tanya had thought about the physical aspects but admitted that despite always feeling as if she wanted children, she didn't really know what would be involved in pregnancy. Again her thoughts had concentrated on the physical aspects of her body's changing shape and size.

Well I've always wanted baby's since I was young. I've always loved kids but I didn't know what it would, I mean, I knew obviously that your belly got bigger and your bum got bigger and you know you just got bigger, but, I didn't really know what it entailed until I actually got pregnant.
{Tanya}

    Rachel expected that she would be like her mum, knowing that her mum had been sick throughout her first pregnancy, and so didn't have a particularly positive viewpoint. Sarah did not "know what was going to happen or what it was going to be like", but once she found out she was pregnant she began to wonder a little about what was going to be involved. This was unusual in this group of women as many of them, even

Their experience of pregnancy and birth

when they had had their pregnancy confirmed, didn't stop to wonder if how they would feel in the later stages of pregnancy would be different from how they felt in those early days.

So, was how they had expected to feel anything like what they actually felt? The answer to this question was a resounding "No!" For those who had thought about it prior to getting pregnant, thus excluding Emma, Helen, Sarah and Ameena, their actual experiences were very different both physically and emotionally. Several of the women, whether they had planned the pregnancy or not, did not enjoy it at all. Helen who had not planned it and was not looking forward to it did not enjoy her pregnancy. Claire who had "sort of" been trying to get pregnant and was looking forward to being pregnant found that "everything seemed to just drag on". The one woman who had really been trying to get pregnant and had sought fertility treatment, Julia, even went as far as keeping a diary in the long sleepless nights she encountered in the months before the birth to make sure she never forgot how dreadful she felt. She joked that she thought this might come in handy "To put me off ever having children again!"

Not one of the women told me that she had totally enjoyed her pregnancy. Many of them felt bad about this and wished it had been different. If they had had realistic expectations of what pregnancy actually involves they may have enjoyed it more or perhaps not disliked it so much. Unfortunately, knowing about the possible experiences you may have will not prevent or remove those feelings. However, it will help you to incorporate those feelings into your life as part of your very personal idea of what it is natural to feel and encounter when you are pregnant.

The list below describes the experiences that one or more of this group of nine women had at some point in their pregnancies, whether they had expected to have them, or feel that way about them, or not. Who experienced what is shown in brackets so that you can see which were experienced most commonly amongst this group of women. If you are currently pregnant, try not to worry too much about the length of the list, remember these are nine women's collective experiences, it is highly

Nine Women, Nine Months, Nine Lives

unlikely that you will encounter all of them. Nevertheless, you will probably feel some of them. Note how many of the experiences listed are of a negative nature. Mostly these seemed to be the unexpected ones.

- Sickness – when hungry and/or tired, day and/or night, in some cases up until about the sixth month of pregnancy {Tanya, Claire, Rachel, Emma, Helen}
- Going 'off' some foods {Tanya}
- Tiredness and exhaustion {Helen, Rachel, Julia}
- Physically limiting – for example not being able to walk as fast or bend in the middle {Helen, Sarah, Rachel}
- Clothes no longer fitting – including underwear {Helen, Rachel}
- Itchy skin {Helen}
- Feeling physically unwell and not being able to take any medicines to alleviate it {Helen}
- Lack of control over their own body – changing size and shape very rapidly {Helen, Claire, Ameena}
- Becoming public property – no respect for your personal space as complete strangers happily touch your belly {Helen}
- People volunteering their embarrassing and unwanted "horror stories" – men and women {Helen, Emma}
- Breathlessness {Helen}
- Water retention – everything was swollen {Claire}
- Over-sensitive and tearful {Sarah, Rachel, Sadie}
- Not being able to sleep even when thoroughly tired {Ameena, Julia}
- Leg cramps {Ameena}
- Obstetric problems and imminent hospitalisation – bleeding {Rachel, Julia, Emma}
- Stomach pains {Rachel, Julia}
- Backache {Rachel, Julia}
- Worry – is the baby OK? {Rachel}
- Putting on too much weight {Rachel}
- Irritable {Sadie}

Their experience of pregnancy and birth

- Depression {Sadie, Claire}
- Pleasure as baby begins to move around {Sadie}
- Uncomfortable as baby's head engaged in the pelvis early {Julia}
- Painful due to ligaments in joints softening {Julia}
- And finally; Panic attacks/anxiety - about the birth {Julia, Ameena, Tanya, Emma}

As all of these women's experiences of pregnancy differed from their expectations, the value of imagining what pregnancy would be like beforehand could be questioned. To increase the value of anticipating how we will feel, i.e. to increase the likelihood of our actual experiences matching up to our hopes, we need honest and matter-of-fact sources of information to base our hopes upon. This book aims to fulfill these criteria and so by reading this you are helping yourself to not feel disappointed in the way that they did.

The majority of these women avoided finding out about unpleasant possibilities, shunning personal "horror stories". Whilst it is only natural to protect ourselves from hearing about potentially panic inducing scenarios, particularly as they may not actually happen to us (making them a source of needless anxiety), sometimes we need to hear the negative aspects as well as to hear the positive aspects. If this is done, and it must be done sensitively, we will have a balanced view of the situation and therefore be able to cope with most of the eventualities of life more comfortably than if we had expected to experience *only* the positive or the negative. Obviously this applies to every area of our lives, and is of particular relevance to the next part of this chapter, the birth.

Birth

One woman out of the nine said that the birth was as she had been expecting it to be. Sadie was scared because she expected it to be painful. It was. The other eight women had a great variety of experiences. No-one looked forward to it, some accepted it as an inevitability, some dreaded

Nine Women, Nine Months, Nine Lives

it, *all* survived it.

Anxiety about the birth was focused on the pain they would feel, the side effects of the pain relief they were likely to be offered, what would happen if they went over their due-date and had to be induced, and the likely method of delivery of their baby. Most had sought some information about what would happen during the birth and consequently knew what they did and did not want. Julia had found out in great detail about every eventuality and reflected that she thought she had succeeded in scaring herself unnecessarily. On the other hand, Helen had gone out of her way to avoid knowing anything about it until she had a show! Each woman coped with the prospect of birth very differently, and indeed, each birth was unique.

Nearly all of the women mentioned the fact that they were scared of the pain that would be involved in giving birth. Ameena was particularly worried as she felt that she did not handle pain very well at the best of times. Somebody had told her that "labour pain is ten times worse than period pain" and she had always had bad period pains. However, as it came closer to the birth and she passed her due-date she became less and less terrified of the birth and just wanted to "get it over and done with!" She did in fact surprise herself and her family. She had to be induced because she went two weeks over her due-date and found that having her waters broken was actually more painful than having the contractions! Once labour was established she decided to try and do without the pain relief her husband was encouraging her to have. And she did. She found that she could cope without it and that the pain was not as bad as she had imagined it would be. As an aside, she also feels that her period pains are now not as bad as they used to be.

I mean the minute we got into the delivery suite, Yusuf was like "Quick, quick, where's the nurse? Who do we talk to for an epidural?" And I was like "Yusuf, hang on a minute!" [Indignant] And he just looked surprised. I think he felt sorry for me more than anything! I think he thought "Oh she has to go through all that pain!" he just wanted me to have the epidural. I didn't, I wanted to do it, I wanted to prove it to him! [Laughs]

…

But, the labour pains, a <u>powerful</u> pain, but it was, it was an enjoyable pain. I don't know

Their experience of pregnancy and birth

whether it's psychological, that you can see that at the end of all this that... I mean it's going to be over soon, and at the end of it you get a lovely baby.
So you felt like you were working towards something? Something that was worthwhile?
Yeah, yes, yes, exactly! You're working towards something. I quite enjoyed the pain [Sounds surprised] it sounds a bit daft but...
Would you say that you actually enjoyed the pain itself, or what the pain was leading you towards?
I actually enjoyed the pain. It sounds really stupid but, I, I saw it as a challenge. People always say it's bad. Mum used to say "Don't worry about it, but yeah, it's really bad". Until I had actually experienced the pain I was terrified, but I did, I liked it! You must think I'm mad! [Laughs] Yeah, yeah I enjoyed it!
{Ameena}

Another woman who was dreading it from the point of view of "How on earth do you survive? Why does that not kill you?" was Julia. She did not want to have an epidural or an episiotomy and did in fact have an episiotomy and stitches but no pain relief at all - "I didn't even have gas and air!" She also found that she actually enjoyed her labour.

No it was nowhere near as bad as I thought it would be. Yeah... In fact I enjoyed my labour. I know that sounds silly, but I actually enjoyed my labour! Just the fact that, you know, that with every push you know you are nearer to getting your baby. And you think as well, if you've not had a baby, you think that the whole part of the labour is, is absolute agony and it's not! It's only when you are actually pushing, and that's not agony... The pushing's not very pleasant but.... The contractions, they're really nothing at all, and once they get too bad, you tend to go on to the pushing stage anyway. And the only time it is painful is when you are actually having that contraction. I mean in between times we were, we were laughing and joking.
{Julia}

She tried to stay at home for as long as possible because she was worried she might get to the hospital only to be told to go home and come back when she was 'properly' in labour. She thought on reflection that it might not have seemed so bad in reality because she had been *so* scared of it beforehand. She was so scared that she could not even watch any of the videos that they had borrowed from the antenatal classes about birth, telling her husband Matt that he could watch them as many times as he wanted "but don't watch it when I'm there!"

Nine Women, Nine Months, Nine Lives

Claire had just begun to enjoy pushing with the contractions when her baby turned on to its side, blocking it's own exit as it were. The midwives and doctors tried to turn the baby but couldn't. As she had been induced and the contractions had become very frequent very quickly she had had an epidural. Prior to the labour she had not wanted one as she had been led to believe that "They're horrible, they hurt and they're dangerous". However, what she described as her "strange but horrible" contractions had been so bad that she didn't even feel the needle going in to her spine. In fact she had no ill effects from the epidural.

As the baby had turned on to it's side and could not be moved back into position using a ventouse suction cap, she was offered an emergency caesarean section. She had been in labour for several hours and was very tired. Although she consented to the caesarean she began to panic and shake as she knew she would have to be awake for it (due to having had the epidural). She had originally decided to be induced with an open mind about the labour and the type of delivery she would have, but was still shocked to have to have a caesarean and concerned about what that would mean for those first few days after the birth.

So do you think it lived up to your expectations? Do you think it worked out for the best in the end or not?
No, no. I wanted to have her naturally. I didn't want to have a section at all.
Why did you want to have her naturally?
Because, because… It took me ten days to get over the section, whereas if I had had her normally, OK I might have had stitches, but if I had had her normally, I might have been up and… You know when you are lying there you can see the other mothers that have had their babies, they were up and about, and I couldn't do that. For two days I couldn't get out of bed, I just, I just, I wanted to get on with it and I couldn't, it was like being held down.
{Claire}

Tanya also had an emergency caesarean section because her baby was not in the right position. She had been in labour for 48 hours, and the baby was beginning to show signs of distress – as was Tanya after two days of regular contractions! Tanya had read about the various methods of vaginal deliveries and was "*so* petrified" of them. She actually wanted

Their experience of pregnancy and birth

a caesarean and would have requested one had she known that that was possible. Although she was relieved that she was to have a caesarean she was also a little scared of the actual physical process of this method of delivery. After all, it is a major abdominal operation even if it is carried out with the aid of an epidural so that the woman can be awake throughout.

> I was like "Well, what does it involve?" So they told me, but it was like in one ear and out the other! Because I was [Laughs] in the sky but I was like "Yeah, go for it then". But I wanted just what was best for her at the end of the day, I didn't want her to be hurt or anything. I just wanted to make sure she was all right, and worry about me later! [Laughs]
> {Tanya}

The anaesthetic made her feel queasy and she was in fact sick on the anaesthetist's hand and not into the kidney dish he was holding for her – it's not easy to be that accurate when you are numb from the chest down! Unlike Claire she was up and about the day after her caesarean and didn't find that the operation had limited her too much in those early days.

As mentioned before Helen had read nothing about the birth and did not even know what pain relief was available "until the contractions were happening". She did know that she did not want a vaginal delivery and like Tanya would have requested a caesarean had she known that that was possible. Despite the fact that she was still feeling uncertain about her ability to be a mother, she found that the birth was better than she had been expecting it to be. The pain wasn't too bad and what she considered to be her labour "from when I had real pain, which was literally right after the drugs I was still having pain, so that to me is *real* pain", lasted only about an hour and forty five minutes. However, it was more exhausting than she thought it would be, so exhausting that she did not even have the strength to hold her new baby shortly after the birth.

> But there was just the midwife, yeah... The midwife, Richard and myself. Apart from when they brought in the anaethetist, it was just the three of us, which was so strange. I'd never really expected that so I'm glad I had no expectations... Well the only expectations that I had were negative. Because it was far better, from that point of view,

with just the three of us. So it was quite a private, nice thing. Well, it wasn't nice, but you know.
It was nicer?
Yeah, you've still got to do what you've got to do at the end of the day but it was loads better the way it was done. And… Everybody says that at the end you want it out and you will do anything to do that, but that's for a short time when you feel like you just want it over. I don't think I realised how exhausted I was going to be… Because I had felt exhausted, well not exhausted but… Doing a job on a daily or a weekly basis but you knew that if you pushed yourself too hard at each end (of the flights) then it would catch up with you. So I'd kind of thought that it's probably going to be like that. But it was much more, I was ab-so-lutely exhausted, because you are. I was in the room and the nurse came into the room with a bottle and I thought "Oh no, I can't!"
You'd no strength to hold him and feed him?
Yeah exactly, I thought "What am I going to do? And I just, I can't do it!" Thank goodness they had no intentions of giving him to me. They went straight to Richard, which was lovely! [Laughs] I was just so relieved! [Laughs]
Yeah, there's all these things that you can't know until you've been there and...
Mostly I just felt relief, relief it was a boy, and relief that I don't have to do it again! [Laughs]
{Helen}

Like Ameena, Rachel had gone over her due-date and had been told that she may have to be induced. In the small hours of the morning that she was booked to go in to hospital to be induced she went into labour, this was quite a relief as she "really did not want to be induced". She had been to the standard midwife led antenatal classes and had also attended the local NCT (National Childbirth Trust) course, consequently she had a pretty good idea of what she did and did not want to happen during the birth. Like Julia she did not want to get to hospital and be sent home having been told that she wasn't 'properly' in labour and so had hired a TENS machine to help her through the first stage prior to getting to the hospital.

I had a TENS machine which I think kept me at home for quite a long time really. I'd been in labour about nine hours by the time I'd gone in, I think that just kept me at home longer than if I'd, not that it actually stops the pain it's just I think that, psychologically, you feel as if you are almost doing something with your body.
So that was good then, being at home?

Their experience of pregnancy and birth

Yeah, James was quite agitated to get going, but I didn't want to get sent back home (after being) told "You're not in labour!"
{Rachel}

She remembered that when she realised she was actually going into labour she felt a mixture of emotions. She felt anxious about her ability to cope with it and yet excited at the prospect that it was finally starting. Unfortunately, the pain relief she wanted did not agree with her – the gas and air made her feel really drunk and out of control and her mouth went numb which made making decisions and asking for things difficult. She decided to try an epidural instead and, despite her reservations about the possible side effects, experienced none herself. However, when she was fully dilated and wanting to push she found that she couldn't manage it. They broke her waters to help her along and noticed by the colour of the waters that the baby may have been in distress (the baby had opened his bowels). She was offered a ventouse and accepted it with relief. Although her birth was different to what she had expected, it was still quite a positive experience for her.

Sarah also had an assisted delivery and didn't react well to the gas and air she had decided to try as pain relief. She felt like she was out of control - "I wasn't in charge of what was happening". She said that after the birth she felt inadequate because she had not had her son 'naturally'. However, she was extremely relieved that he was "in one piece".

But I felt, because he was an assisted delivery, I felt like I hadn't done it.
Oh right... So what, was he a forceps delivery?
Yes. I kept saying "but I didn't do it" or something like that, I felt that, yeah... I can't think of the words to put it in to, but I felt like I wasn't, that I hadn't done it all myself sort of thing. Inadequate, I felt a bit inadequate, in the delivery sense because I'd had the forceps.
{Sarah}

The woman who probably had the most traumatic birth experience out of these nine women was Emma. She had the usual concerns about how she would cope with the pain, she did not want to have a caesarean, and had the extra obstacle of being needle phobic. Emma's labour was similar in many ways to those already described here. She was induced to try and speed up the labour when 27 hours had elapsed since her first contraction and she had an epidural to help with the pain. Like Rachel her baby began to be distressed which could be seen from the colour of her waters when they broke. This is known as 'meconium stained liquor' and the green/black evil smelling meconium, the baby's first bowel movement, is particularly toxic if inhaled by the baby in the process of being born. This is precisely what happened. In addition to having inhaled this life-threatening noxious fluid, Emma's daughter was very small when she was born, weighing in at 4 and a half pounds. She rapidly developed breathing problems after the birth and was rushed to the neonatal intensive care unit.

Emma can't really remember holding her baby for the first time straight after the birth – she only knows that she did because her partner Neil told her she had. She feels that she missed out on having that special time together and also that she didn't have the opportunity to show her off whilst they were in hospital. It was more than a week later when she finally got to hold her child for the first time, that she could remember.

I don't remember much at all to be honest! I know I held her and that's all I know and that's because Neil told me. And then she started to have breathing problems again so they took her. She was 6 days old before I held her. She had wires and things coming out of her and I think I was more worried about pulling them out or making something go off than holding her close. I didn't hold her for long. Yeah it was 5 or 6 days I think it was.
And you felt pretty scared about the fact there were all these wires and things coming out of her...?
Yeah, and she was so long and so thin that I thought if I hug her tight I might break her. Does that...? [Laughs]
Yeah, yeah, of course! [Laughs]
She was really really really really thin, I thought I'd better not hug too tight. But I wanted to.
Yeah, to hold her and squeeze her.
To let her know "you're all right".
Yeah, as reassurance.
Yeah that was what I was worried about. But... They were very good all around me. [The staff at Leicester General hospital] So, yeah, they were very good.

Their experience of pregnancy and birth

So when was the first time, would you say that you really got to hold Lotte?
Probably after she, when she was about 8 or 9 days old really. Yeah, she still had the nasal thing in but she wasn't, there weren't heart monitors, well there were but you know it was a lot easier because they would all tuck up, so yeah, she was about 8 days old.
And how did that feel?
Lovely! [Laughs]
Yeah, I'll bet.
{Emma}

You may find it surprising that most of the women couldn't really remember the first time they held their baby. Of those for whom it was a little vague Julia remembered it being "just all magical"; Sadie remembered being "a bit shocked really to actually have him. The real thing! I was scared, but I loved it!"; and Sarah "was just really happy seeing him". Unfortunately, Helen continued to feel like a fly on the wall for the time immediately after the birth and for the next few weeks and months, as if the whole experience was happening to someone else - "How can I be in this situation?"

Rachel clearly remembered the way she was introduced to her son, and the way she felt when she had actually held him properly for a while.

He was thrown on my stomach when I wasn't quite expecting it and then whisked away straightaway. I thought that was a really horrible way to be introduced to your baby. He was just slapped on and then gone straightaway, you know.
...
How did you feel when you first held him? You said that he was kind of slapped on to your tummy and then whisked off, that's not really holding him, so...
No, I think it was almost like "This is your child" sort of thing. And then... He had some oxygen and then he was wrapped up and then, they bathed him first and then they got him dressed and then I held him. And he was squealing, you know crying, for about an hour, but it didn't seem to matter! And then I breastfed him, and he just went to the breast and...
And was that all right?
Yeah, that was fine. It was quite painful at first but after a bit it was, yeah it was fine. Yeah it was quite nice really, because I'd had him at like half four in the afternoon so I was in time for the auxiliary nurse coming with the tea round! [Laughs]
[Laughs] How convenient!
Yeah it was very convenient! But it was really nice that I could actually show him off

35

straight away, I was tired but... [Laughs]
So, when you were showing him off, how did you feel at that time?
Proud. [Shows in her face too]
{Rachel}

Due to having a caesarean Tanya didn't hold Katie until they had sewn her back up and she was taken into the recovery room of the operating theatre, some 45 minutes to an hour after she was born.

That was the first time I really held her and that was, and that was, oh, that was just lovely!
It was really good?
Yeah, yeah it was, I was just crying my eyes out. [Laughs]
So you remember it very clearly when you first held her?
Yeah, I was just lying there, and she was lying next to me and I was saying "Hello darling, I'm your mummy". And I was just you know, gabble, gabble, gabbling away. I'll never forget that moment.
{Tanya}

The other woman who had had a caesarean was Claire and she remembered that she was "absolutely shattered" by the time they brought her baby to her to feed, "but it was wonderful". She was extremely pleased to have a daughter having secretly hoped for one throughout her pregnancy. "It made it all worth it, you know the pregnancy and everything, it just made it worth it having a girl".

Ameena had also secretly wanted a daughter and held her about five minutes after she was born. She was also surprised at how tired she was and found that she just could not carry her. Despite her reservations about sharing her desire to have a daughter with her husband due to her experience of general Asian cultural perceptions of gender, he was also thrilled with Ayesha.

Wonderful! It was such a relief to have her out, but other than that I just felt so tired. And I always wanted, secretly I always wanted a girl. And I know in the Asian community it's always "Boys, boys, boys, boys, boys and I hate girls", you know, but gosh! I was so thrilled. I can't, I can't express myself I was so happy, so relieved! [Laughs]
So it was an intense high then really?

Their experience of pregnancy and birth

Yeah, yeah it was, definitely. But yeah, he held her first, and he was just, because she looked so much like him he was just... [Puffs herself up with pride in imitation of him and laughs] <u>Very</u> chuffed, very chuffed "My girl!"
{Ameena}

So, two women had caesareans – both of them emergency caesareans, one woman had a forceps delivery, one had a ventouse delivery, two women were induced and the rest were straightforward vaginal deliveries. Those women who seemed most satisfied with their birth experiences appeared to be the women who had the type of birth they most wanted to have, whether it was a caesarean or a vaginal delivery.

So if you are currently pregnant and you think you know what you might prefer when it comes to giving birth, make sure that you talk to your midwife about it and record it on your birth plan for the day (or night as the case may be!). You could also talk it over with the person you want to be with you when you are giving birth. The assumption that most people make is that this is likely to be your partner. However, he may or may not be the best person to support you at that time.

The next part of the chapter describes these nine women's experiences of the support they hoped their partner would provide throughout pregnancy and birth, and the support they actually received. They did not always match up. Those who were realistic about their partner's capabilities seemed the most satisfied with his support – some good evidence for the benefit of realism for our future happiness. Feeling pleased with the support their partner had given them made all the difference in the world to how they felt about one of the biggest milestones of their lives.

Their experience of their partner's involvement during pregnancy and the birth

The majority of the womens partners' were involved in their pregnancies. Only three took little or no interest at all. Sadie's partner was not very supportive during her pregnancy to the extent that he did not understand her mood swings. When she tried to explain to him that they were mostly due to her being pregnant he did not want to listen - "talking to him is like talking to a brick wall". She thought this was most probably due to him being so young. However, they were *both* seventeen at the time.

Julia and her husband had been planning to have children and were trying to get pregnant when she finally found that she was expecting. Perhaps it is a little surprising then to find that Julia describes Matt as not being supportive or caring enough (for her) in the practical or the emotional sense during her pregnancy. He did go to some of the classes with her but seemed to fail to relate to the changes that Julia was going through, particularly physically.

Probably could have done more. Definitely, yeah.
And can you think now, in the future, what those things would have been?
Just generally accepting that I was pregnant, and what pregnancy actually involves. Because I think Matt just took it as me being pregnant and not any of the pregnancy aspects, do you know what I mean?
Sort of...
Not that I was actually pregnant, that I was having a baby but that I wasn't experiencing any of the things that you experience in pregnancy.
That it would just happen? You'd just have the baby and you wouldn't be any...?
Yeah, I mean like he was useless when I'd say "Oh my back aches" you know silly things like that. Which he now feels bad about when I remind him.
{Julia}

Much to Tanya's disappointment her partner was not at all supportive of her during her pregnancy. He also walked out of her life. She had hoped that they would be able to talk about the pregnancy and that he would be involved in some way. He did not want her to have the baby; she told him that she was going to have the baby. She had not expected that they would bring Katie up as a family, but she had hoped for a little more support than she got.

Despite Emma's initial fears about how her partner Neil would react to the news that she was pregnant, he was very supportive both practically and emotionally. Throughout the pregnancy he was curious

Their experience of pregnancy and birth

about her feelings and her changing body; he accompanied her to the ultrasound scans and the hospital tour but couldn't get time away from work to go to the antenatal classes with her. This was far more than she had dared hope for.

Helen was concerned about how her partner would react to her being pregnant for different reasons to Emma. She thought that he would be positive but knew that she did not want to have the baby. As described earlier they decided to go ahead with the pregnancy, with Helen continuing to feel unsure about the wisdom of that decision for many months. Throughout her pregnancy she needed additional emotional support from Richard and she felt that she did get it when she needed it. She acknowledges that it must have been hard for him to hear what she had to say at times, regardless of this "he was totally supportive all the time".

Rachel also experienced a great deal of uncertainty about whether her and her partner James had made the right decision. It was not easy to talk to him about her feelings of guilt that continued throughout her entire pregnancy due to him being "more keen" than her to have the baby. She felt he was very supportive emotionally. Practically, he attended the NCT classes (offering some original if embarrassing contributions to the couple discussions) and the ultrasound scans, he also accompanied her to the hospital when she had a bleed seven weeks before she was due to have their baby.

And I would talk to him about things, and he was involved in the NCT classes, he came when the other couples were there and took part in the cross-couples exercises and that was, that was quite good too. And also it allowed us to have an opportunity to say how we felt in a supportive context, without it being confrontational. I remember James at one point wanted to bring the placenta home, he wanted to bury it in the garden! [Laughs and rolls her eyes] I was like "Don't be stupid!" [Laughs] I was like really shocked because it wasn't something that we had talked about at home! So… [Laughs] But yeah he was really supportive, he was involved quite a lot.
{Rachel}

During her pregnancy Sarah considered that her partner Anthony's support was good both practically and emotionally. He found it harder to understand the emotional things she was going through; he didn't ask questions but he did listen when she wanted to talk about the various things she was feeling. Nevertheless on reflection she thinks that maybe he could have done more. In his defence, she did explain that she thought he was reacting to her desire to carry on with their life in as much the same way as it had been before she was pregnant. Consequently, next time she has a baby she would "like it to feel a bit more special".

Until Ameena's bump began to show she did not really notice any change in her husband Yusuf's supportive behaviour. In fact prior to being pregnant Ameena had rarely ever asked him for any support or help of either the practical or emotional kind. However, with her becoming pregnant "he had to change". She felt that his support during her pregnancy on the whole was "a tiny bit more" then she had hoped for – like Sarah's partner Anthony he was better practically than emotionally.

Uniquely in this group of women Claire felt that "there's not much a man can do is there?" Her husband Tom came to the ultrasound scans with her and tried to be supportive when the pregnancy began to drag and she became more and more uncomfortable. Her expectations of him were fairly low and she got the amount of support from him that she expected. She was also amused by his reaction to her changing body.

He was scared! You know like if he knocked me or anything he'd go "Is the baby all right, is the baby all right?" [Laughs] Just things like that you know. I think he was very scared of my bump, very delicate around it.
{Claire}

Moving on to look at their partner's support around the time of the birth, if the women were afraid of the pain, the majority of the men were quite simply afraid of the birth! When Claire had originally asked her husband Tom if he would be with her during the birth he said yes, but she got the distinct impression that he was less than keen. Throughout the pregnancy she gave him the opportunity to change his mind or at least talk about it with her, "I kept asking him because I got the impression that he was very scared". He never admitted it and was in fact present at the birth and was very supportive too. This was more than she had hoped for.

Their experience of pregnancy and birth

The main reason that Emma wanted her partner Neil there was because she was scared. They had not made a definite decision about whether he would be there or not right up until their daughter was born. Like Claire's partner he was not eager to be there, and Emma did not expect him to be there. In the event she was glad that he was for his emotional support, particularly as their daughter Lotte's first few hours of life were so precarious. She thinks that the reason he came to the hospital to be with her had a lot to do with her admitting to him how she was feeling.

Were you glad he was there?
Yes and no actually. He wasn't much of a help! [Laughs] But then I wasn't expecting that anyway, I think it was just because I was a bit scared towards the end and I had been in labour for so long that I just wanted somebody there that I knew really.
...
You were expecting him to stay out of the way?
Yeah, (but) he came back and stayed, only left the room once.
Do you think he came to support you? Do you think he came because he thought this is only going to happen once, the first child?
I think he came for me, yeah.
Because he thought you'd been in labour for such a while?
Well I didn't go straight onto the labour ward, because it was full. I went onto the ward and pottered around, had a few baths. And... I said (to him) "I am absolutely terrified" and I think it was because I actually admitted that to him, that he thought "I'm going to come back".
And has he said anything since the birth?
No because he knows I get upset about it.
Did you get the feeling that he was glad he had been there?
I think so yeah. Just the once he had to go out when it started to get a bit scary, they were taking some blood off Lotte's head with a needle or something because she was in distress and he said he couldn't handle that so...
It was understandable?
Yeah, so he went out which was obviously before she was born, but he was there when she was born.
{Emma}

Sarah's partner was not sure if he could cope with being there for the birth. She wanted Anthony to be there "and it did help knowing he was there, just a nice hand to hang on to!" He was pleased he was there throughout and said to her afterwards that "he couldn't have left anyway, he said he couldn't have just walked out on me".

Although she did not want her mum there, Ameena's husband Yusuf had taken the precaution of asking her to be at the hospital when she was induced in case he could not cope. Ameena wanted him to support her and he was willing to try. However, he did have a tendency to panic. Therefore, asking her mum to be there turned out to be a very wise move as Yusuf was not much practical help during the birth, although she described him as "quite comforting". She thought that his practical support was less than she had hoped for.

He was worried that he would faint and he thought "God I can't cope!" He was more worried about himself, not being supportive towards me so, my mum was there. She was the main one, if she hadn't been there I wouldn't have been able to do it. He was very comforting, very supportive, he was doing the things she was doing as well, and if I didn't decide to have him there next time I would definitely take my mum! [Laughs] And I'd say to Yusuf "Don't worry about it, you don't have to be there, don't worry about it, go to work and I'll let you know when it arrives!"
Yeah?! [Laughs]
But my mum, she was brilliant. You know it's funny, I thought it would be the other way around. I thought he would be rubbing my back and saying "Don't worry darling everything is going to be OK", he was just, well he was just not up for that!
{Ameena}

In the absence of her partner, Tanya's mum was with her throughout her labour and was the first person to hold her daughter Katie. Sadie may have felt that she would have been better off with her mum instead of her reluctant partner. He was scared to come in with her, but did and he was more supportive during the labour than during the pregnancy - "He'd wised up by then". Nevertheless his support was much less than she had hoped for.

Only three women's partners did not appear, to them, to be scared about the birth. Helen did not want her husband Richard to be there for the birth "I just wanted to go away, get it done, and come back with a baby!" However she was glad that he was there - "he was brilliant". She felt that she was so caught up in herself at the time that that was why she

Their experience of pregnancy and birth

hadn't been expecting him to be as good as he was.

Despite feeling that her husband Matt was less than supportive during the pregnancy, Julia felt that he was very supportive both practically and emotionally during the birth. They even managed to laugh!

I mean if you'd seen Matt! Because I spent most of the labour at home in the bath, because I didn't want to go to the hospital and be told to come home. So, I wanted to leave it to the very last minute. And… We did! Within three quarters of an hour of getting to the hospital, I was pushing so… But, I sat in the bath, and the only thing I'd asked Matt to do all the way through the pregnancy was help me with my breathing. All the way through my parentcraft classes I couldn't get the breathing right, and that was the only thing I asked him to help me with. Well, when it came to it Matt sat there timing the contractions, and a notebook trying to tell me how to breathe. Well! If you try and write breathing down on a piece of paper it just doesn't work! And there he was, trying to time these contractions and he didn't know when I was starting and when I was finishing! [Laughs]
{Julia}

Rachel's partner James was as informed about the birth as she was but he deferred to her in the decisions that were made during the labour. She felt that his support was "what I'd hoped for, I think I'd expected him to be as supportive as he was". She thought he had had a surprise though.

When I had the ventouse you had to push down with the contractions and he got a bit of shock then when I was gripping him! [Laughs]
{Rachel}

Overall, the nine women were pleased by their partners' support. In some cases they were quite surprised and in others they were quite simply disappointed. More often than not their hopes were not dashed and their fears were allayed. However, what would their partner's support be like in the future? The birth may have been the first time that they had met their baby's, but the next few months would be the time that they would get to know them. The first few months are a time of enormous change and a great deal of flexibility is needed all round. The following chapter describes this exhausting but exciting period in their lives.

Their experience of early motherhood:
Now you know why your mother didn't tell you!

The first few months are often a time of mixed emotions. The joy of having the baby you have been carrying for nine months in your arms at last, is often combined with the everyday frustrations of meeting the needs of this little, but very loud stranger, who hasn't had the courtesy to arrive with a set of instructions. This chapter explores the nine women's expectations of the first few weeks and months of motherhood. Their imaginings are compared with their newfound reality - the highs *and* the lows are described here. Their partner's involvement in their child's early life, whether this matched up with the anticipated commitment of their partner's and the actual day-to-day division of parental responsibility are also presented.

Imagination and reality

In their imaginings of how early motherhood would be for them few of the women had contemplated that some of the physical and emotional aspects of pregnancy may linger on into early motherhood. The most

commonly experienced aspects of pregnancy that did continue over into the early days are shown below, and the women who reported having them are shown in brackets.
- Water retention {Emma, Tanya, Claire, Ameena}
- Tiredness/exhaustion {Helen, Ameena, Rachel, Sadie, Julia}
- Depression/feeling down {Claire, Helen, Sadie}
- Back ache {Ameena}

The same was true for the birth. When considering which method of delivery they preferred very few of the women contemplated the effects of the birth upon the early part of motherhood. Their main concern during their pregnancies had been how the pain and the possible anaesthetic/pain relief were going to affect them, and their babies, when the time came. Even those women who really wanted a caesarean birth (Helen and Tanya) hadn't thought about the physical limitations that method of delivery places on the individual for the first six weeks after the birth. Claire, who did not want, but did in fact have, an emergency caesarean, had thought about it previously. It was precisely those physical restrictions, the feeling of being held down described in the preceding chapter, that she wanted to avoid. She found that they placed a considerable additional strain on herself and her husband in those early weeks.

The most commonly experienced problematic side effects of their births that arose in the early weeks of motherhood are shown below and the women who reported having them are shown in brackets. As a brief reminder, a summary of the nine women's births follows. Both Tanya and Claire had emergency caesarean deliveries; there were two assisted deliveries - Ruth had forceps, Rachel had a ventouse; two women were induced, Rachel and Ameena; and Emma, Helen, Sadie and Julia had straightforward vaginal deliveries, although Emma's daughter inhaled meconium during the birth, and Sarah and Julia had to have episiotomies. The side effects of the birth they, as a group of women, experienced were:
- Depression/feeling down {Emma, Claire, Sarah}
- Physical restriction due to being told not to carry/lift anything heavier than the baby for six weeks {Tanya, Claire}

Their experience of early motherhood

- Feeling they were dependent on others, predominantly partner/mother, for practical help {Tanya, Claire}
- Risking their health - by lifting/carrying heavier things than the baby when no-one else was around to help {Claire}
- Exhaustion {Helen, Claire, Rachel}
- Uncomfortable and sore – been "pulled about" {Helen, Rachel}
- Stitches – painful to sit and/or walk {Sarah, Julia, Ameena}
- Constipation – fearful of tearing stitches {Ameena}
- Bleeding – longer and heavier than expected {Rachel}

As mentioned in the previous chapter regarding the list of experiences the women had during pregnancy, it is unlikely that you will experience all of these side effects of the birth. If you are currently pregnant, try not to worry too much about the length of the list, remember that these are nine women's collective experiences, it is highly unlikely that you will experience all of them. Nevertheless, you will experience some of them. Which of them you experience will almost certainly be determined by the type of delivery you actually have.

So, if the women had not imagined that their pregnancy and/or birth might have an effect on their experiences of early motherhood, how had they imagined early motherhood to be and what had they based those ideas upon? Many pregnant women I have spoken to over the years say that their confidence in their own predictive abilities regarding their feelings, were severely shaken during their pregnancy. This was as a direct consequence of their actual experiences of pregnancy turning out to be so different from what they had imagined their pregnancy would be like. They felt that if they had been wrong in the past about their feelings during pregnancy, they could definitely be wrong about future ones regarding motherhood. And it was too late to do anything about it. They were going to have a baby and they were no longer sure of what the future held for them.

Try not to worry if this thought has flitted through your mind; you are actually helping yourself to adjust to the possibility that the future may be different to what you had imagined by reading this book. Most importantly, you will be able to base your imaginings of your own future upon the *reality* of these nine women's experiences.

Emma sought information and tried to be realistic about the future by partly basing her own expectations of early motherhood upon contact with her sister and her daughter Abigail who was a relatively relaxed and quiet baby and (curiously enough) exactly a year older than Lotte. Similarly, Sadie had imagined what her baby and motherhood would be like and had tried to be realistic about it by basing her own expectations on the first hand experience she had had with her younger siblings and of her friends lives with their young babies. As a single parent Tanya "knew it was going to be hard" and tried to remain realistic throughout. Helen on the other hand had not wanted to think about it and did not imagine it at all. If anything she avoided thinking about it and had only negative expectations of what life would be like with a newborn baby – she was scared.

As with pregnancy Julia thought that early motherhood would be "all floaty and lovely", "the worst thing I could imagine was feeling desperately tired". Claire hadn't spent much time thinking about it and said that she "just thought you'd have this baby and feed it and change it and play with it and it'd be good!" Sarah hoped her baby would be all "smiley and gurgley" and she was looking forward to "going round and showing off my new baby".

Ameena wasn't sure if she had ever imagined being a mum whilst she was pregnant, "I probably did but I can't remember whether I had thought how I would feel". Rachel had imagined it would not be for her. She thought she would want to get back to work as soon as possible because she would be isolated at home with a young baby, and that any socialising she would have the opportunity to do would be at cliquey mother and baby groups, "I don't particularly bond with those kinds of people… I'm not like that at all".

As a group they were positive about the experiences that lay ahead of them, only Helen and Rachel were openly pessimistic. A few of them had tried to be realistic, however, some were quite clearly overly optimistic. Every single one of them found it harder than they had imagined, but like the birth they all survived. Some positively enjoyed it and some just got

Their experience of early motherhood

through it. Would you like to predict who falls into which category before you read on? Let's see if your own expectations of them based on what you know about them so far matches up with their real-life experiences.

Rachel found life with a newborn baby more tiring than she expected but also more rewarding, she had been really quite pessimistic about the prospect of motherhood. The main conflicts she experienced were to do with breastfeeding and visitors. The pleasures for her were the reward of seeing him develop and react to her. She could not believe the depth of pride and love for him that she had.

I'd have a shower and, I always used to think I could hear him cry, even though James had him I thought I could hear him cry, I used to think "Is that him or not?" And I spoke to another one of my friends, and she felt the same, she thought she could hear her baby crying in the other room, so it was really strange, a strange instinct really. And I couldn't believe how much I bled afterwards. I expected to bleed but not for as long or as heavy. And one thing I really didn't like about breastfeeding was that once you'd have a shower and you were clean, then you'd start leaking and you'd feel really dirty again. I had a feeling of being dirty for quite a long time, and of feeling quite sore and bleeding and then he would want to comfort feed from about eight until one which was hopeless because I was feeling so sore as well. I think, I think you feel really proud and excited but it's like all the people who come to visit you, you either feel like you're being the hostess and you're not seeing to the baby or you just like… No time for it really. I mean you're trying to keep everybody you… Like because James's parents live away from here, so trying to give them an opportunity to come and see him. Whereas with your own family it's different. They had spent longer travelling and wanted to stay for longer, do you know what I mean? You would try to be fair but you'd think "Oh God!" And I think, my mum and James's mum, they'd both bottle fed us, so they didn't accept, my mum especially because she'd seen me sore with feeding. They'd kind of ask me "When is he going to have a bottle?" and "Are you sure he's hungry again?" and not realising, you know, that breastfed babies do it like that. Do you know what I mean? They were always trying to put pressure on to not breastfeed. You always have to justify why you are breastfeeding. And it wasn't always said in a negative way but, you know, you get the… That was, not a pressure but something that was a bit tiring at times.
…
I think it's more tiring than you ever imagine. And you wonder how you'll get things done. But I think it's more rewarding than you think. I was really kind of not keen on the idea of the actual baby stage when you'd be doing things for him, but the actual bond and love that you have for them is far more than I could have ever imagined really. [Laughs] {Rachel}

Nine Women, Nine Months, Nine Lives

Helen thought that although the only way she had prepared herself for those early days was by thinking "that it was going to be bad, it was still a shock…not nice". Like Rachel, she also experienced conflict regarding visitors. She did not enjoy the early months of motherhood, but managed to get through it by trying to use common sense in the absence of any information about caring for a young baby, which she had resolutely avoided for the vast majority of her pregnancy. If she was cold, it was likely that Will was cold; if she was bored, it was probable that Will was bored; and so on.

The constant lack of sleep, and the fact that there was no let up. And because people were continually around, there was no let up when there should have been. And, and, while it frustrated me and I was trying to sort myself out and deal with it and like say "Don't come round" I also didn't want to upset anybody because I was so emotionally unbalanced at the time, I couldn't. I think that it just frustrated me so much, and the lack of sleep. Because normally as I say, when you can catch up on your sleep, fine. It's a different day, deal with it, but it was constant, constant, constant.
…
Richard's mum was fantastic she'd turn up and say "I've brought you something to eat, just plonk it in the microwave; I've put the washing in, I've taken it out, there it is clean". My mum would come round, play with him, and then go home about half an hour later!
Yeah? Just what you need!
Yeah! [Laughs] That happened time and time again, ridiculous, awful! My dad thought it would be a good idea for my mum to come and help me in the first week but that just wore me down. And the emotional situation as well, the fact that it was just such an alien thing to have this little thing in your home, it wears you down.
And there's nothing that you can contemplate it like being.
So you've got the emotional tiredness, the physical tiredness, purely because of the things that need to be done.
The things that have <u>got</u> to be done.
Yeah, yeah. I'm sure whether you are breastfeeding or bottle feeding you would have the same exhaustion. You've just got to do it and there's no escaping it, and when there is someone who will do things for you there are still twenty things down the line that you've got to do. To eat yourself, to get some sleep, you know, but that's way down the line, because firstly you've got to look after this little baby so... Yeah so exhaustion I think was the thing, because I, I tend to… Prior to this, in my life I just pushed myself, I just pushed myself, I'd get by, I'd be OK, I would tend to think "Oh I'll sleep later on".
Yeah or catch up in the week?

Their experience of early motherhood

Yeah, whereas with this there is no catching up. There's always a feed or something.
...
I think I blocked it out of my mind because I just couldn't imagine what I would be doing. So everything was, each day was, was, I just ended up applying common sense to, that was how I got by.
Yeah, I remember you saying when I saw you before.
I remember Richard saying early on he was like, "well if you're hot then he must be hot".
Oh yeah!
And that, yeah, I just kept thinking that all the way along. It was just such a simple thing. You know, I need to eat every three hours because I've, I've got low blood sugar but I have, and I need to eat on a regular basis, and I thought "Well yeah, If I need that then he needs it!"
I mean he's not an alien, you know he's a human...
Exactly, exactly! So that was how, you know that kind of got us by. Prior to that I just hadn't given it a thought.
...
A shock but then, then you surprise yourself and think as the weeks go by "I think I can deal with this, you know, it's OK. I did that last week so I can do it this week. And this week is better than last week, or this day is better than last week", and then all of a sudden you get a day that is just crap. And I'd think "I hate it I don't want to be in this situation, how did I, why did I decide to do this? How can I get out of it now? Right now!" [Laughs] "Can I just go?!"
{Helen}

There were four women who were unrealistic and perhaps overly optimistic about life with a new baby. These were Claire, Sarah, Ameena, and Julia. Claire was shocked by how hard day-to-day life was, particularly by how "naughty" and demanding her baby was, "I wanted such a brilliant baby and she was such hard work, she wasn't like they tell you". It was much more frustrating and she found it hard to cope with these feelings of resentment towards the baby.

That's it, it's like when we were doing the classes, everyone was saying "No-one expects you to have a perfect house, you won't have a perfect baby" and you sort of accept that. But you don't accept it! Because... I'd kept my house so clean when I was pregnant that when she came it was such a mess, and I couldn't handle the fact that the house was a mess. I had to clean it yet I had no energy or time to clean it. And she was so naughty and I used to think "Well what have I done wrong to have such a naughty baby?" [Laughs] "What am I doing wrong?" You know, that's how it makes you feel because you try and do so much. It's not because anyone expects you to, it's because you in yourself

expects you to even though you know... And it's like they were saying as well that... If you are feeling down you should call someone. When you are feeling down, you don't want to call anyone. When you come out of it you think "I should have called someone" and you know you should of, but you just don't when you are actually in that situation.
Did you ever have a time when you were feeling down and somebody dropped in to see you or, phoned you or something like that?
I was relieved.
Yeah?
Oh yeah definitely but I wouldn't have, I wouldn't have...When I was really really down I wouldn't have called anyone to say come round or anything. Because I was always like ashamed of feeling down, and I never got, well sometimes I used to sort of shout at her but I'd never, I'd never get angry angry with her. She never got me to that stage, I'd cry if anything. I'd cry with anger rather than...
You were frustrated?
Yeah, you know.
Were you angry with yourself or were you angry with her?
I think myself really because I kept thinking "I must be doing something wrong" for her to be like this. But like I say, by the time she had reached eight weeks she'd really started to calm down, she wasn't as bad. As the weeks went by she just calmed down even more until she was like she is. I think her problem was, she was too active, she wanted to be moving, once she'd started rolling around and crawling she was better, and now she can crawl and she's trying to walk she is better again. I think that was her problem, she didn't like lying still, she wanted to be, she's always wanted to be standing on her feet and I think that was half the problem, she just didn't like lying down. She was just too demanding! [Laughs]
{Claire}

Sarah found that it was much more chaotic than she had imagined, and like Claire that it was so much more demanding than she had expected. Her son Jack had colic for the first few months, which made life harder, and she felt that the fact he was so agitated because of the colic put visitors off leaving her feeling isolated and down.

It was more chaotic than I thought it was going to be! [Laughs] I wasn't quite prepared for how regularly he would want feeding and just the amount of attention that he needed really, I wasn't really prepared for all of that.
The 24-hour care?
Yeah, and if you wanted to go anywhere. Well, I particularly felt a bit stuck here with him for a start. I felt a little bit isolated with only a pushchair... I didn't, we didn't have a car for a start so that was, well an obstacle to doing things. I felt shut in.

Their experience of early motherhood

Right, so did any of your friends live locally or...?
No, none of them.
What about your family, sisters?
Well, two are in Melton, mum is twenty minutes away. She'd well, she'd come over and see us now and again, she didn't like pressure us, she didn't like just pop over.
She didn't just drop in?
No, no! She'd come over a couple of times a week, which was nice. It was nice when people did come, I was pleased! [Laughter]... Sorry I keep forgetting what the question was!
No, no you just tell me what you think and we'll carry on from there, don't worry at all! OK so how you'd imagined early motherhood, do you think it turned out to be the way you had expected?
Not, some things yes.
And some things not?
Yes, it wasn't, it would have been better if I'd been prepared for the colic. I had a job keeping him quiet and happy, so that sort of, I think that upset me a lot, I thought things would be a bit happier and a bit smoother. And... I was looking forward to going round and showing off my new baby and things like that, and I felt like I couldn't because he was so colicky and crying, you know you couldn't.
Not very settled?
Yeah, even when people came here he would scream the place down, and I used to look at him and think why couldn't he be a bit more smiley and gurgley and then people might come more often! [Laughter]
Yes! But, how long did it take to get the colic sorted out?
Well he got a bit better after a few months, the GP couldn't really prescribe anything for him. It didn't go until he was nearly four months old.
{Sarah}

Ameena found that having a newborn baby was totally different from what little she had imagined, "you picture a scene where the grass is green, and then you have them and she has eczema and asthma and then it is a totally different story." She felt as if she didn't have the time to live life the way she wanted it to be, and when she did have the time to do anything she was so exhausted that she just couldn't do it. She experienced a great deal of guilt from thinking that maybe she could have stopped Ayesha from having baby eczema.

Ayesha used to give us lots of sleepless nights, she used to cry and cry and cry a lot. And then she got into a pattern whereby she would sleep for two and a half hours at a time

and during those two and a half hours I used to be trying to do everything, and oh!
Oh yes, I remember now, when I saw you before...
I remember being so exhausted.
...
So would you say the first three months have been different from what you'd expected?
Yeah, I was really tired. I mean I remember being, I mean I'm always tired now, always needing to sleep, can't sleep but want to sleep. The house was always a tip...
Oh good Lord!
Yeah but the things like that ... But (a) I don't have the energy, (b) I don't have the time and, I didn't, she's ever so ever so demanding during the day, and at night. That's one of the reasons why I've decided to go back to work full-time, so that I can get even more of a break from her! [Laughs] Because I'm like, she's not up, physically up most of the night, but she is awake, you can hear her being awake and well her back is quite sore so she's not comfortable. I went to see the doctor and he suggested I took her to see a specialist and she was to have some medication. It helped, but I can't afford to keep going back and forward to it. And then some nights you think "Ooohhhh!" and you just get so fed up. And Yusuf can't feed her so I'm there doing it. It just gets so much that you just want to dump her in the cot. And when she falls off to, when she does finally fall to sleep, you put her in the cot, and then in the next minute or minute or two, you think "Oh maybe she'll be all right". But then she's up again because she doesn't want to be in the cot.
...
Yeah and another was the eczema. I mean you hear about dry skin, these days a lot of babies are suffering with that condition, but when Ayesha actually had that, I thought "But how? But why? Is it because I, is it something that I've done wrong or..." I don't know you just... I sort of went through a guilt trip. Because I know initially that her skin was dry when she was born, but that was because she was late, she was overdue, and it was improving and it became very nice and soft. And after three months following the medication, I did, I did see her skin getting quite dry but, I carried on giving her a bath everyday, using baby powder, I used baby powder. I keep thinking in my mind that it was the baby powder that made her worse because of the talcum powder. I thought "Well maybe that if I'd just stopped using that...?"
{Ameena}

The last of the four women who were unrealistic about new motherhood was Julia. She found that it was harder than she had imagined mostly because she didn't know what she was doing, and instead of asking for help or admitting to these feelings of panic she just kept going. There was a family row during the early weeks. In addition, her husband Matt had an operation when Daniel was seven weeks old so

Their experience of early motherhood

she ended up caring for the two of them. She desperately wanted it to be perfect and it was not.

I mean it's funny really. I think it's because he… The first year flies past and you do get to a point when you think they're six months old now and you think that they have completely moved on from that tiny weeny baby that's completely dependent on you into a six month old that is sitting up and gurgling. And I think it's at that point that you realise "Oh my God! I've like, I've missed the baby part of it!" Because all you do is panic – and you do, it's true. Everybody that I've spoken to. I mean when you are going through it you don't say anything to anybody you know. You say "Oh yes blah blah blah" it's only when… I mean all of us, everybody that, that had babies at the same time we were all exactly the same when they were six or seven weeks old and not probably coping particularly well. And it was only when they were six months old when we actually admitted to each other that it wasn't as easy as we had made out and that at times we hadn't got a <u>clue</u> what we were doing! [Laughs]
Yeah, just managing on a day-to-day, hour by hour basis. You know, you can't expect to do any better than that, you know given the situation i.e. having your first baby, the circumstances and your own abilities. You are <u>not</u> going to be perfect one hundred per cent of the time.
I mean it gets better because you just don't panic so much as they get older. But it's just, it's like this, this little baby is dropped on you and you haven't got a clue what you are doing. I mean you go to all these classes and you think "Oh well I'll do this and I'll do that" but you don't because you're panicking most of the time thinking "Oh my God what do I do now?" [Laughs] Because it doesn't matter what experience you've had with like other children or other people or what you've read. When you are faced with it you just do the best you can and it's not necessarily always your best. Or what's best for the baby. I think probably, I mean second time around, everybody says "Oh you're so much more relaxed". You know you just don't worry about silly things like, I don't know, like they'll cry out and you think "Oh my God that was like a pain cry!" I mean I can remember my dad holding him once and he like squealed and I said "Oh what have you done to him, what have you done to him?" And it was nothing, it was probably colic or something, but you completely panic. Because it is so new, and completely different from anything you've <u>ever</u> experienced before.
You've no idea!
Yeah! I mean I wish in a lot of ways people had been more honest about it. Because you go to all these classes and everybody tells you the positive sides of it and they'll probably say "The crying will get on your nerves and take time out blah blah blah" but they don't go into, not necessarily into depth, but about everything else that arises. And how you'll feel, and that, you know, there <u>will</u> be sheer panic, and yeah just accept it, you know, go with the flow. But people don't!
So do you think if people knew that it was going to be a kind of… A managing, a learning

55

as you go, a learn on the job kind of role, that that panic might not be so bad?
Yeah, I mean I felt so much better when I knew that other people felt the way I did. I mean I can remember like walking into Mothercare and seeing pictures of new born babies and filling-up thinking "God I made such a bad job of like the first few months" - and I didn't! I mean I breastfed him, I did everything I possibly could but I still felt I hadn't done enough. Because you think "I should have done this, I should have been doing that, I should be stimulating him more". You know, I mean I used to have everything, like baby gyms, rattles, I mean I was even sitting reading to him when he was a week old! But I still thought I should have been doing more. And I shouldn't have been. I probably shouldn't have been doing as much as I did! You know I probably did far too much and that was why I felt so bad in myself, but, but I think that's another thing. I think people ought to be told to like, you know, think "Bugger everybody else!" Just think of you and your baby but you don't. I mean I can remember filling the freezer up with all these meals that I'd made for Matt so that I hadn't got to go in the kitchen. Well, you know, within about a day I'm standing in there cooking Sunday dinners and silly things like that. And walking round breastfeeding Daniel whilst I'm doing it and silly things like that. And people will let you do it!
Yeah, that's it, yeah. I think that's it. You have to think about what you want to do, what you are capable of doing, and then only do that. Don't feel pressured into doing...
That's it! Your biggest pressure is from other people, like your mum, your auntie's and other folk. They all say "Oh well I did this and I did that" so you think "Oh well I'll do even more than you did". Which I did, I know I did! You know I… Crazy really! And you do regret that afterwards because you can't get that time back and you do feel guilty about it. I mean I don't so much now because you can see how he has turned out, but at the time you think you are doing so much damage to them. I mean I can always remember sitting in the rocking chair breastfeeding him at night. You know it should have been a really nice relaxing time when you are looking at each other and everything's perfect, but you're sitting there like you're breastfeeding and you're thinking "Oh I've got to do this I've got to do that"!
It's a bit like writing shopping lists whilst you're having sex! [Laughs] You are doing it and suddenly you realise you are and you think "What am I doing? I should be enjoying the sex!"
Yeah, dreadful! Or like breastfeeding and sitting and eating your tea at the same time, you know you should be enjoying the moment, and you're not you're sitting there shoving a sandwich in your mouth to nourish this baby! [Laughs]
{Julia}

The remaining three women had experiences that they felt matched up pretty well with their expectations. In Emma's case her imaginings of early motherhood were consistent despite the horror of the first month after Lotte's birth.

Their experience of early motherhood

I'd got a good idea of what was going to happen. But we didn't, not till later...
Was it about a month/6 week's delay (to bring her home from the hospital)?
Yeah, a month.
And was the reality the way that you expected it to be? I mean it can't all have been, but...
We've had a few problems with her, she doesn't sleep! [Laughs] But she did actually sleep quite early, slept through, and now she's not doing that anymore. But I think it was more or less what I expected it to be really.
And what about Neil, do you think it's more...?
He's from a big family, six, and he's the eldest, so he'd got a good idea. I think it's a lot more demanding, no not a lot more, but a bit more demanding than I thought.
Do you mean in terms of your time or...?
She's on the go all the time! My sister's little girl you see she's, when I was pregnant I used to watch her and she's just not as active as Lotte is at all.
So your niece, she could be left for a little while?
Yeah and my sister could get on with things but you can't, no way, she's constantly on the go all the time, she wants attention all the time as well. So it is a bit more demanding than I thought.
So is that the biggest thing that you would say is different from what you expected? I suppose the biggest in terms of having the most impact on your everyday life.
Oh my, I can't go anywhere without her now, by the time we've got in the car...!
And it's not just her, it's all her stuff too!
And the other thing is spare time as well. I don't have any anymore, not at all, not with working full-time, no. If she goes to bed early which is a total shock, then I think "Ooo!" I feel like I've won the lottery! [Laughs]
...
I think I'd got a really good idea really, I don't think I was under any kind of "It's not going to change my life" sort of syndrome. [Laughs]
Yeah but I've met a few...
Yeah, but I knew it was going to totally change.
{Emma}

Tanya tried to have a relaxed attitude to early motherhood, some things she did find difficult, like the lack of sleep particularly as she had no partner to help her, and to this day she continues to "take them as they come". I wondered if any resemblance in Katie to her father might have got Tanya down in those first few months.

And does she resemble her father?
I think she's tall like him, she's quite long, because I'm not, I'm a short arse so, she must

Nine Women, Nine Months, Nine Lives

take after him!
So am I, so...[Laughs]
She must take after him for that.
What about in her face, things like that, that wouldn't upset you if she looked like him?
Oh no, no...I'm quite lucky in that way because everybody thinks she looks like me.
Yeah, I think she looks like you, but then I...
But I don't see it. Yeah, exactly, nobody knows who the father is so yeah, I suppose you do see me.
I just wondered if you know, that would be upsetting for you really?
Oh no, no.
That wouldn't bother you at all?
No, everybody's different anyway, they've got their own features and that.
And what about the actual practicalities of motherhood? You know looking after a baby, regardless of whether you thought she was a boy or a girl, whether you would love her, or whether you would grow to love her, or things like that, had you considered them?
I knew it was going to be hard, well I thought it was going to be hard, and it was. And more demanding, because obviously night feeds, things like that. I mean towards the end I didn't get much sleep anyway, and I slept all day. But I mean I couldn't do that when I first had her, you see I slept when she slept, like they tell you to, forget everything else, just sleep when she's sleeping. [Laughs] So I did that, I mean I still do that now, if she has a nap in the afternoon I have a sleep as well, it's just like they say. Otherwise I mean, yeah, you know, housework, so what? Forget about it, yeah, I mean you have just got to do the best for your baby haven't you? I mean if you're tired, and when I'm tired I get snappy, and I don't like being snappy with her. So I'd rather have a kip when she has a kip and then I'm all right, you know, get my energy back up sort of thing. So when she wakes up you know full of life, I'm you know, I can cope with it, just let her get on with it. I suppose it was hard for the first, well it still is hard now but, not as hard. But then you had to get up in the night, change and then feed her.
And there was only you to do it then as well?
Yeah.
I suppose it must have been doubly hard?
Yeah, yeah it was, but I suppose I got used to it, it had to be done so I had to do it. At the end of the day that's the way you've got to think about it haven't you?
{Tanya}

In the last of this trio of realistic women, Sadie felt that motherhood in those first few months was as she had expected. This was undoubtedly helped by her recent experience of new motherhood with her friends, and also with her younger brothers and sisters.

Their experience of early motherhood

I've always had babies close to me so I was like used to (them) and I've always helped out. My friends have got babies, so I'd seen what they had to do, so I knew what I had to do. When I first had Alex I knew roughly how to do certain things, so I had an idea.
...
Was there anything that was better than you thought? Was there anything that was worse than you thought?
I don't know... Oh, night feeding.
Yeah?
Yeah, I didn't really expect that. Apart from that I think I knew about everything.
{Sadie}

So, some of their actual experiences did match up with their imaginings, some exceeded their expectations, and some fell below. One or two of them surprised me so it would be understandable if one or two of them surprised you. One thing that didn't surprise me was that the three women who had attempted to base their expectations upon the actual experiences of others coped better and enjoyed early motherhood more on the whole than those who were either unrealistically optimistic or overly pessimistic.

The highs and the lows

The nine women were asked to think back to the first few months after their baby's were born and tell me what was difficult in those early days, and what was the best thing about that time. The following experiences were reported to me as being difficult and as always the women who experienced these feelings are in brackets.
- Not being able to hold her baby or bring her home for a month after she was born as she was in special care {Emma}
- Night feeds – lack of sleep {Tanya, Helen, Rachel, Sadie}
- Crying at night – exhaustion {Helen, Claire}
- Feeling isolated and lonely {Sarah}
- Breastfeeding - painful {Ameena, Rachel}
- Re-organising your life and adjusting your body clock {Rachel}

Nine Women, Nine Months, Nine Lives

- Breastfeeding – leaking and feeling dirty {Rachel}
- Not feeling attractive - hair falling out and "your stomach was a great big blobby thing"{Rachel}
- Over sensitive and protective of the baby – difficult to be tactful {Julia}

The following are the nine women's best experiences from that time. They are listed in the same order that they appear in the last part of the book i.e. the full conversations that I had with them.

- Emma - Knowing that her daughter Lotte was going to live, "that was probably the best thing when they said to me "Oh no she'll, she'll pull through".
- Tanya - The peace and quiet when her daughter Katie was asleep, "but I do love you darling!"
- Helen – When her son Will started reacting to her, "when you said this or that he would smile or look at you or look for you".
- Claire – her daughter Hannah was so cute when she didn't cry, she first smiled when she was four and a half weeks old and "by the time she was six weeks she smiled all the time".
- Sarah – caring for and getting to know her son Jack, "I liked looking after him".
- Ameena – actually having her daughter Ayesha, "just holding her, it's just so peaceful, it's such a pleasure".
- Rachel – being the special person in her son Charlie's life, "I loved holding him close to me and hearing him breath, and watching him responding to me".
- Sadie – showing her son Alex off to people, "I actually had a baby!"
- Julia – feeling so close to her husband Matt and being a family with their son Daniel, "I can't ever remember a time when me and Matt were closer. It was an amazing feeling, the three of you being together, and what you had been through…I mean that's all we talked about all the time and it was lovely, really really nice."

Their experience of early motherhood

Their experience of their partner's involvement in early parenthood

Only one of the nine women did not have a partner. Tanya's partner was not involved in any aspect of their daughter's life apart from her conception and after his decision to leave her to it nor had she expected him to be. Four women had partners who were not really involved in early parenthood despite three of them having actively planned to be; Ameena's husband Yusuf; Rachel's partner James and Julia's husband Matt. The last of these four, Sadie's partner Paul, was not involved but then they had not talked about him being involved in a practical capacity and he rarely took any interest in his son. This was as she had expected it to be and she stated herself that this had in fact worked out "for the better".

Yusuf did not take any responsibility for their daughter Ayesha's physical care despite saying that they would share everything – "I'm going to be a dad as well". He helped out by playing with her whilst Ameena rested but this amount of involvement was not as she had expected. She felt that it had developed due to the situation at the time of her being at home and him working. She said that she had brought the subject up to make him feel guilty about not doing his promised fair share but thinks that on reflection it has worked out for the better.

OK, and so was he involved in changing her and things like that, night feeds?
No, he always saw that as a mother's role! [Laughs]
Right. So had you talked about who would do what?
Yes, no we hadn't talked as in the sense, I mean I always used to tell him "Look, whether it's a boy or a girl you have to get involved in nappy changing, giving the baby baths, pushing the push chair". Simple things like that, if she needs feeding you know, but he never has! [Laughs] He never has got involved in any of that! Only recently he has started, when, when I'm giving her a bath he'll join in and splash water at her and bring her toys. But, I think he's only ever had to change a nappy once when I had to go out, and I left her with him and she... I think it, no she didn't pooh otherwise he would have had to do it, it was something he tried, he thought "Right let me give it a go!" But ever since he's never changed a nappy. In the whole year only once! [Laughs]
...
So you had talked about it, and you had basically said that you would need him to help.

Nine Women, Nine Months, Nine Lives

So things like feeding, like at night, had you talked about that as being something you'd need him to help you with?
Yes, I mean he'll stay awake, like if she's up and at week-ends he'll say "Oh it's OK, you rest I'll take her downstairs and play with her."
OK so, that obviously didn't work out. You've ended up doing the majority, the lions share of the work. Would you say that was something you had discussed and said "Look it's easier for me to do it" or did it just happen?
It just happened.
Do you think it was a kind of natural division of labour that it worked out like that?
Yeah.
Do you think that was primarily because you were at home or, perhaps you feel more able to do it and Yusuf doesn't?
A bit of both really because I spend, I mean I took unpaid leave so I was off work for about 10 months, so I didn't feel I could turn round to him and say "Right Yusuf, the next nappy change is yours". I just got on with it really.
And was that OK? Or did you start to resent it towards the end?
No, it wasn't a problem.
So you didn't feel let down? That's all I'm really saying, that you discussed it would be one way, and it was actually different...
Yeah. So I mean we did discuss it and that was before Ayesha was born, he used to say "Oh don't worry we'll share everything out and I'm going to be a dad as well" and I think at that stage, at that point in time they look forward to it. They think "Oh wow!" you know, and then when the little one does arrive, it's such a shock to their system. It is quite tiring, it is a huge responsibility, and then working full-time 9 to 7. I mean, I mean personally, I don't mind changing her, feeding her and giving her a bath, so... It doesn't really bother me if he doesn't change a nappy or...
...
OK so would you say that on the whole that worked out for the better or for the worse? On reflection...?
For the better.
For the better, because if you enjoy doing those kind of things, and you're quite happy to do them...
I'm quite happy, but I do still nag him, you know put him through that guilt trip saying "Well you never did change her nappy!"
Well you know, it wouldn't really do him any harm to do things like that because you know... If you weren't around for any period of time, I mean God forbid if you were ill or something like that, your mum might not necessarily be able to be there for Ayesha.
Yeah, but I think that he does understand that if that were the case then he would have to pull his socks up and get on.
So he'd be capable of doing it?
Oh yeah definitely.

Their experience of early motherhood

But at the moment it's just not the way that you work?
Yeah, he just thinks "Oh Ameena is there, if I don't do it she's going to. The baby's not going to be left there". He does recognise his responsibilities, but he... [Laughs]
{Ameena}

James was very involved in his and Rachel's son Charlie's first week, after that he went back to work and the majority of the care involved in looking after a very young baby fell upon Rachel. They had been fairly open minded about the division of the baby's day-to-day care and Rachel thought that the situation evolved due to the circumstances of her being at home and him working, like Yusuf and Ameena. She too felt it had worked out for the better.

How much was James involved in the early days?
He had five days paternity leave, and... He did like change nappies and, but because he was at work most of the time until the evenings, I did most of those kinds of things, the night duties, really. I think that one of the things that I used to find frustrating was that at the weekends, he'd never know what to dress him in. I think it's still because I've done his food and sorted out all his clothes and things, I think he thinks that children just wear whatever - He'd be like "Oh I dunno!" [Laughs]
So in the beginning James was involved as much as you were, in that first week?
Yeah.
And then after that, when he'd gone back to work?
Me!
Was it just because of the change in the situation?
Yeah, it seemed for the best really. Yeah, because of the circumstances really. I think so. I think that, because I was at home, I was doing the shopping, the cleaning, the ironing, and you know just doing those kind of jobs.
...
OK, had you talked about who would do what? Had you thought about who would do nappy changing for example, in those early few weeks? Things would have changed and evolved once you had him, but before you did?
No, I think we'd just thought we'd try and see how it went.
...
So would you say that that has worked out?
Yeah, there are some roles that we have naturally taken on, like James will do the shopping, I'll do the washing of clothes. It was really an unsaid thing you know we never said "Oh I'm going to do this and you are going to do that".
{Rachel}

Julia and her husband Matt had "discussed everything". However, he was not as involved as they had planned, doing some tasks which suited him and not others. This was a source of much conflict as Julia felt that his behaviour was not as he had led her to expect. The rot set in early as Julia began to resent the chances she had given him to bond with Daniel in the first few weeks of parenthood. It definitely worked out for the worse. Like Ameena she wanted to make him feel guilty about broken promises.

You want everything as, as near perfect as possible, Matt had got three weeks off work and Matt was really worried that once he got back to work that he would have hardly anything to do with Daniel. So for them three weeks all I used to do was basically feed Daniel and then Matt used to sit and have all the cuddles and everything. And then Matt went back to work, and Matt would come home from work. It was like a really special time where we could have been bonding with Daniel and I didn't particularly. I mean I did bond but I didn't bond as I should have done because I gave that to Matt. So, so that he wouldn't feel left out, with hindsight that should have been a shared experience. So I missed out on that and it didn't work out in the end anyway. So, which, that, that took a lot of… Up until Daniel was about a year old I used to think about that and get really really upset.
…
You discussed it in quite some detail. And did it work out the way that you thought it would?
No! He did change him and what have you but as I say, every time he murmured it was "He needs feeding". And, so, that caused so many arguments in the middle of the night. He didn't necessarily need feeding, he probably needed his bottom changing or just needed…
To play, or perhaps just have some attention?
Yeah! That really got on my nerves. I mean the times I threatened to stop breastfeeding, I mean that was just pure spite, I wouldn't have done it because I enjoyed it, and it was obviously the best for Daniel. Yeah, silly things like that. And Matt, oh I don't know, no it just didn't work out the way… [Laughs]
But did you think it was useful that you had sat down and talked about it?
Yeah, yeah.
So that was a good thing, that you had actually contemplated what would be involved?
Yeah, you'd actually got fuel for an argument! [Laughs] "You said…" [Laughs]
{Julia}

The remaining four women's partners were all involved in their sons

Their experience of early motherhood

or daughters very early lives. Their involvement either being as much as the women had expected or better than they had expected.

Emma's partner Neil was very supportive of her throughout the time that Lotte was in hospital and indeed continued to be over the coming months. They had talked about who would do what for their baby, and decided to try and keep it as equal as possible. Despite Lotte's dramatic arrival into the world and her belated beginning to life at home with her family, Emma felt that early parenthood and her partner's involvement in it, once they had got Lotte home, had worked out as they had expected it to.

I think we'd decided we would try and split it. Because the original plan before anything was that I was going to go back to work about three months after I'd had her. And so we'd sort of got this plan that Neil would have her when he was at home and my mum would have her the rest of the time, it was all sorted, it was all planned. We'd decided we were going to split the night duty! [Laughs] Half-and-half where I would do it one night or perhaps the first feed or the second feed. We'd practically decided to split it really.
So you had talked about it and got it all...?
Oh yeah and when she came home that was...
It worked? What you'd sort of expected to be doing was what you were actually doing?
Mmmm, yeah.
To a lesser or greater extent obviously.
Yeah, no shocks!
No, no, I should think you'd had about enough of those anyway!
Yeah! [Laughs]
{Emma}

Helen looked to her husband Richard for a great deal of support in those early months with their new baby. He did not disappoint her. He was probably the father who was involved the most in his child's day-to-day care. They had not talked about the specifics of who would do what for their baby, keeping an open mind until he was born. Because Richard was so involved in his son's care, this meant that Helen could adjust to motherhood at her own and Will's pace, which she felt she very much needed to do. This meant returning to work as soon as possible. She felt that his support was better for her than her own mother's, and that it had worked out better for all of them than she had ever expected.

Nine Women, Nine Months, Nine Lives

And how much was Richard involved in those early days?
Totally, he did at least as much as I did. He was still working so I would try in the night to do the feeds because at that stage I could cover, but he was there as much as I was. He was very involved as well. He never, he never just left it to me, when he'd be away, I'd say OK I'd do it, and then when I was, it was him. Life's still the same, because with me, for half a week he has to do it.
Yeah, because you're not here (you're working).
So, we always knew that it would be. But I think it, I think it was probably… A shock to me that I had to do as much as half a week! [Laughs] Do you know what I mean? [Laughs] I was like "Well he said he'd be looking after this baby, why am I doing it?" [Laughs] I was just going to go back to work! I was like "Oh God, have I got to?" But yeah, he was the most help to me, more than my mum was; he was the most help, the most understanding. The most thoughtful, yeah, I was very lucky. And again, it's only when you listen to other people you're like, "Oh my God!" because you take it for granted… I didn't know and…
Well yeah; yeah, exactly.
So… Like I say, I was very lucky.
…
I mean we were at a party a few weeks ago and there were loads of guys saying that, and they all take the, this was a rugby tour party, and they all take the mickey out of Richard. But he's like… And I said to him, "Does it not ever bother you Richard, you know, you said you were going to give up work to help out?" He said "That's their problem, I've not got a problem with it". So at the party they were saying "He really does this because he wants to?" And I just said "Well what do you think, do you think his mum comes over and does it all?!"
Yeah, the magic fairy comes along and does it!
And yeah, he does go over there to eat [At his mum's] and stuff because he hasn't got time to cook a meal and do all the stuff. When there is two of you, one of you does it. But yeah, basically he's there, he does the same as I do if not more.
{Helen}

Tom and Claire did not really plan who would do what when their baby was born, like Richard and Helen they preferred to keep an open mind. They took it day by day and tried to talk over any problems that arose as soon as they could to try and resolve them. This flexibility was due in part to Claire having had a caesarean therefore necessitating Tom's participation in the majority of his daughter's care. Although Tom was very involved in Hannah's first few months, Claire suspects that their actual experiences of parenthood have put him off having any more

Their experience of early motherhood

children for now! Like Helen she felt that the early months had worked out better than she had anticipated it would.

Well he didn't have much choice really because he'd, we'd sort of, we came to a compromise where we just took it in turns, one got up and then the other one got up.
...
OK, so had you talked about who would do what?
No.
In the early days?
No, no, nothing. No it just kind of came that way
...
Oh she is such a good baby now, completely different, but as I say, it's still put Tom off wanting another just yet!
So what, did he want one quite quickly after Hannah?
Well when we'd, before I got pregnant, we were talking about having about four. And we were saying we'd have them, we did discuss whether we'd have them close together or... because I always said I wanted them about three or four years apart anyway but I wanted about four. He wanted a big family as well and he said "Oh I don't really mind what sort of gap" but... It's just come about that with her being the way she is... We probably will have one when she's about three or four so you're going to get a gap but I don't know whether we'll have four!
Well, you'll just have to see. I mean you know if you don't have four, would it matter?
No, no, I don't mind now, I'm so happy I've got her and she's great.
And do you think that, you say that you didn't talk about who was going to do what or whatever, do you think it worked out for the best in the end?
Yeah, yeah.
It wasn't a problem that you hadn't talked about it?
I often find that if you try and make plans they never work, I think you just... I mean some things you do have to plan obviously, I think it was just a case of see how it went. It was like with the birth, I didn't plan the birth I just wanted to see how it went and, it was taken out of my hands anyway but, I think it's always best to go in with an open mind and that's what we did. When she was born we just sort of... Whatever happened we just took it day by day and, you know, if something wasn't working we talked. We talk really well, you know, if there is a problem we discuss it.
{Claire}

The last of the four women who felt that their partners were involved at this time as much as they had hoped for, if not more so, was Sarah. Her partner Anthony had more experience with babies and children than her and consequently, like Helen, she relied on him quite a lot for advice. He was involved in his son's day-to-day care but they had not talked before in any detail about who would do what. He had the much-appreciated idea of her having a regular night off to catch up on lost sleep. His participation was as she had expected in those early weeks and months but she did wish that they had had more time together in Jack's first week.

So how much would you say your partner was involved in the early days?
Quite a lot, I mean I was grateful sort of when he came home from work! He used to leave early and then be back when it was dark. I was definitely pleased to see him! [Laughs] At night time he was brilliant, he would take him straight away because I was tired and getting grouchy by that time of night.
Did he manage to take any time off to be with you, when, just after you came home?
Not really, no, not really. Because I had him, I think he did have a couple of days off. Luckily I came out of hospital on the Thursday and he was at work on the Friday and then he was at home all weekend which was quite nice yeah… And on Friday nights he would be the one to get up. It was his idea that I should have one night were I could get some sleep which was great, because you know, he hadn't got to get up the next day and go to work so…
So you said that you didn't really know all that much about having children and what was involved, had you actually talked about who would do what…?
No.
So you hadn't talked about things like changing, the night feeds, bathing?
No, no I'd sort of jokingly said "you're going to have to show me because I don't know much". But no, we hadn't sat down and seriously talked about the night feeds and stuff like that. I think I just wanted to feel, I wanted to know that, well that I had the responsibility, I wanted him to be there, for him to help me and for him to back me up, I wanted him to know that that was how I was feeling really.
…
He was definitely willing to muck in and help. I don't think he, he never thought of taking over he never really criticised me you know "No don't do it like that, this is how you do it", you know nothing like that, he was never keen on changing nappies but then… [Laughs]
…
It would have been better I think if he hadn't gone straight to work so that we would have had a little bit more time together at home, but he had to go in. But I didn't, I would have liked him to have been there and I didn't resent it, it's just, well it had to be done. Especially when he was crying and I couldn't shut him up!
Yeah, that makes you feel awful! [Laughs] So do you think things worked out for the better or for the worst?
For the better really, because it was his idea that I should have a night off.

Their experience of early motherhood

Yeah that is a good idea.
Yeah it was his idea, and he didn't have to go to work the next day, I could just crash out and not have to do a thing, it was great!
{Sarah}

So the majority of their partners were involved in the care of their children. However, less than half of the women felt that their participation in the day-to-day tasks was as they had been led to believe would be the case. Only four out of the nine felt that their expectations were met and/or exceeded. The next chapter, amongst other topics for contemplation, looks at how each father's involvement continued throughout their baby's first year of life and the impact parenthood had had upon their relationship with their partner's.

Their experience of motherhood up to their baby's first Birthday:
To tell or not to tell your broody friends?

After the frenetic first few months of new parenthood, the remainder of the first year of their child's life seems calmer to most individuals. However, to others it seems just as busy with no definite end in sight. Regardless of how these nine women felt, every single woman was amazed by how much her life had changed upon having her first child. Not only had their lives changed but also they themselves had changed, for both good and bad, permanently and temporarily, as a result of their experiences of motherhood. This chapter describes these changes, the day-to-day effects these changes have had upon the women, how their partners have (or in some cases have not) changed and in what ways their relationships with their partners differ from before they became parents. And they do.

A life change

In response to the question *"How do you think your life has changed since you had your first child?"* the most common replies were along the lines of totally, completely, considerably and one hundred per cent. Or as Helen put it "Oh hardly at all!" This comment was heavily laced with sarcasm. Everything in their lives had been re-prioritised, including themselves and their partners - "Everything revolves around her… I just put her first in everything I do" (Tanya).

Putting the baby first was often born out of necessity not choice. Quite simply, it is very difficult to ignore the cries of a hungry/wet/tired/bored baby whether you are putting the dirty washing in the machine, having mind-blowing sex, or dropping them off at the child-minder's on the way to work. Those screams are designed to be attention grabbing and to make you respond to their needs. No matter how much you love your child you will feel like screaming yourself at some point. Frankly, you wouldn't be human if you didn't. Most of these women had felt like screaming in the past year including Emma – "Sometimes I could go out of the house and scream. Still do." Helen came up with an unusual solution to the problem; do read our conversation for enlightenment (I'll give you a clue – it involves a baby auction!)

The changes that these nine women had experienced in themselves and in their lives in the first year of motherhood are shown below and the women who reported having them are shown in brackets:

- Wanted to reduce or had reduced their working hours {Emma, Claire, Sarah, Ameena, Rachel, Julia}
- Found it difficult to go out individually {Emma, Helen, Tanya, Claire, Sarah, Ameena, Rachel, Sadie, Julia – All nine women!}
- Found it difficult to go out as a couple {Again all nine women!}
- Felt closer to their partner {Emma, Helen, Claire, Ameena, Rachel}
- Felt closer to their own mum {Emma, Ameena, Rachel, Sadie}
- Felt closer to their sister {Emma, Ameena}
- Less self-centered {Helen, Sarah, Ameena}
- More flexible {Helen}
- More organised {Helen, Rachel}
- More patient {Emma, Rachel, Sadie}
- More content {Sarah}

Their experience of motherhood up to their baby's first Birthday

- More relaxed {Emma, Helen}
- Less relaxed {Sadie}
- More responsible {Helen, Ameena}
- More restricted {Helen}
- More time pressured {Helen, Ameena, Rachel}
- More irritable {Rachel, Claire}
- Lost her memory {Helen}
- Lost her independence {Julia}
- Lost her self-identity {Julia}
- Lost a lot of confidence {Tanya, Ameena, Julia}
- Gained a lot of confidence {Sarah}
- Matured {Tanya, Ameena, Claire, Sadie}
- Physically aged {Claire}
- Worried more about money {Sarah}
- Worried less about herself {Sarah}
- Worried more in general – she worries about how much she is worrying! {Ameena}

As mentioned in the previous chapter regarding the side effects of the pregnancy and birth upon early motherhood, it is unlikely that you will experience all of these changes. If you are currently pregnant or have recently had your first baby, as I have said throughout, try not to worry too much about the length of the list, remember that these are nine women's collective experiences, it is unlikely that you will experience all of these changes. Nevertheless, you will experience some of them, which of them you experience will almost certainly be determined by your personality and the support you have from your partner, family, and friends.

Some of these changes were permanent and some of them temporary, for example, the loss of confidence reported by Ameena and Julia began to be restored when they went back to work. No doubt all of the women would like the feeling of closeness to their partner's to be a permanent change, however, Julia's has not been. As the two youngest women of the nine, Tanya and Sadie's maturity is a noticeable and permanent change, to the extent that Sadie finds it difficult to relax and "act daft" nowadays.

Some of the changes were spontaneous (becoming more content was for Sarah) whereas some changes had to be worked upon (becoming more patient had to be for Emma). Rachel has found that her personal experience of motherhood has helped her to be more empathic with her work as a Nursery teacher, more than likely a spontaneous change and almost certainly a permanent one.

I think also within my job, it's helped a lot too. You have more empathy for parents. I think whereas before you were very much on a professional level, whereas now there is a parental level. And you appreciate that they have concerns, not that you discussed it before, but you realised it was upsetting the child. Say a child is crying and you'll ask them "What's wrong?" and they'll say they want custard on their dinner, you know what I mean, you might think "Oh for goodness sake, what's the big deal?" But to them it's a big deal and upsetting their child. That kind of thing I think has altered in me, you know to understand a little more - parents with their children. When they drop their child off and they are crying, you <u>know</u> that if they go the child will be all right shortly after, but the parents can't do it. And you know sometimes when I've dropped Charlie off and he's cried and I've had to leave him, it upsets you for the whole day, do you know what I mean? You're left thinking "Is he all right?" Whereas before I'd be like "Oh will you make a decision, you either go or you stay!" I think you are not quite as impatient with parents, you know you realise that your child is the most important thing really and their happiness is paramount.
{Rachel}

Changes within themselves

The two areas of their lives, and the way that they responded to them, that seemed to change the most were with regards to work and to the time that they had to themselves for themselves without their child. A third major change involved that of their relationship with their partner, this is discussed in some depth in the next part of this chapter.

Deciding whether to go back to work was a quandary for most of these women - only Tanya, Sarah and Sadie were not employed in jobs that could offer them maternity leave and so they did not contemplate a return to their previous place of work. Some women were eager to return to work during their pregnancies, some were not, and some changed their

Their experience of motherhood up to their baby's first Birthday

minds about their career development entirely after they had had their child.

Those women who felt that they had a career to consider when they were deciding whether to go back to work after having their baby's included Emma (Regional Company Auditor), Helen (Flight Attendant), Ameena (Contracts Assistant for Social Services), Rachel (Nursery Teacher), and Julia (Care Worker for individuals' with challenging behaviours). Indeed, all of these women have returned to work, however, it has not been as straightforward as they had perhaps imagined for the last three out of the five.

For the first two out of the five, Emma and Helen, they have gone back to work full-time, and for the most part both of them feel that they have managed the transition from new mother to new working mother quite well. Emma found it hard at first to leave Lotte and returned to work later than she had planned to due to Lotte's ill health shortly after she was born. She feels that as Lotte stays with either her mum (who also looks after Emma's niece Abigail who is a year older than Lotte) or her partner, that Lotte doesn't miss out by having a working mum.

I wouldn't mind being at home a couple of days a week... Sort of doing three or three and a half days at work. But I think she benefits from being with her Dad on Monday and Tuesday, because they're so close, they really are. But then again you see, I have her every night and all day Saturday. And she obviously benefits from my mum and Abigail because my mum has Abigail as well, my niece, and she's learnt, you can see how she's learning off her. I don't think she misses anything from me working.
And do you think you miss anything about Lotte when you are working?
Yeah, some days I sit and I think "Oh I wonder what she's doing?" Especially when I first went back to work, I still do now but not as badly as I did when I first went back. Yeah I was like ringing every hour to see if she was all right! [Laughter] But now you know I'll just ring once a day or if she's teething then I'll definitely ring at least once.
{Emma}

Helen always knew that she would be returning to work full-time and had made plans with her husband Richard to go back when their son Will was three months old. As she would be staying away for three or four days a week a nursery would be looking after him during the day, and at

Nine Women, Nine Months, Nine Lives

night her partner, his parents, or her parents cared for him. This worked out really well which was very important for both Helen and Richard financially as he was starting up his own business at the time and she was the major bread winner, and for Helen as an individual to give her a break and build up her reserves for coping with her new life.

It's like I was desperate to get back to work... And that was my saving grace. As hard faced as it sounds, and I know it does sound hard faced but, that was my saving. Because I got, all right sleeps still messed up [with regularly flying across time zones] but I got one full nights sleep a week. So I mean that was great, but it was hard for Richard because he was still here. Yeah, it was the best thing.
...
Yeah it worked out to be the best situation that we could have.... Had Richard gone back to work and I'd stayed at home like full-time, that would have been madness. There was absolutely no point. And as much as you know, the people in their fifties and sixties think that that's what you should do, not all people, but a lot of people do, and a lot of people say "Oh are you going back to work? So that's you not working anymore, is it?" Well, no. Because, you know, I've worked long enough that I've worked up to a good level of salary.
Yeah exactly, and you get used to it.
Oh yeah! I have never, ever, and I'm sure you've not, been in a situation where I've ever had to say to Richard "Look, can I have this?" [Laughs] And that would needle me so much. Really, that's, that is another reason why I was desperate to get back to work, I did not like having to say, and it was no problem to Richard at all, but it...
But if that was how you felt and you felt so strongly...
Yeah, so... No it couldn't have worked any other way. I could <u>not</u> have stayed at home. I couldn't have let Richard support everything, it would have been worse. While they're working on a garden the other guy would be off building and doing other stuff, and then they wouldn't have been paid until three months later. We couldn't survive on that, we'd have got by but that would have been it. And that's reality. I mean hopefully in time things will work out but... And I think, I do think, that I am better towards Will for being away.
Yes, yeah.
And I say that without a doubt. I think I would be an awful person. I don't know what kind of state I would be in if I had to be here all the time. Get away, get a break, come back, and I can deal with the situation. And Richard and I have always been used to us living like that anyway so, he's got to fit in [Will].
{Helen}

Moving on to the experiences of the three out of the five "career

Their experience of motherhood up to their baby's first Birthday

women" who found returning to work less straightforward than they had imagined; when I saw Ameena she had been back at work for two and a half months having intended to have gone back to work much sooner than when Ayesha was nearly ten months old. She wanted to return to work for herself, not for financial reasons, and felt proud of the fact that she was a working mum. However, due to a combination of factors such as her daughter Ayesha developing eczema and continuing to breastfeed, Ameena decided to take extended maternity leave and went back to work initially for five mornings a week and then changed this to three full days. She was contemplating increasing her hours by one extra day a week because she found that she spent a lot of her time at work worrying about Ayesha, and a lot of her time at home worrying about work. She felt as though she never managed to finish anything to the best of her ability. She was trying to squeeze a full weeks work into three days and still look after her child as much as possible. Her own mother had Ayesha both during the day and sometimes overnight and Ameena felt jealous of the close bond between grandmother and granddaughter that developed during the time she was at work. Since returning to work her husband still did not help out at home, and when he suggested getting a cleaner Ameena dismissed the idea saying that she wanted to clean her own home and look after her own family. Despite her belief that going back to work was helping her to increase her confidence, it was also exhausting as very little had changed at home. The strain was beginning to show.

She wanted to have no regrets and I urged her to spend some time identifying her priorities and to seek the support she felt she needed to ensure that she didn't have any regrets. Like many women she missed her baby when she was at work but knew that she needed some time away from her daughter in which she could be "Ameena" first and foremost and "Ayesha's mum" second.

I enjoy being at work but as I say my mind is always with her. Is she OK? I wonder if she's had anything to eat and…
She stays with your mum?
Yeah, she stays with my mum. And my mums brilliant, she runs around after her, I mean when she's exercising this one is giggling, they, they just get on like a house on fire. So

in that respect, that's not the reason why I worry. But if I did have to leave her with a child minder I would never have gone back to work. But because mum's there and she's babysitting for me, she's happy with that arrangement, this one's happy so no qualms about that. But, it's like, well, am I losing out? When I'm 60 years old, old and grey, sitting there on my rocking chair will I be…?
Looking after your granddaughter?!
Yeah, hopefully! [Laughs] Will I be sitting there thinking "What did I miss out on?" and "I shouldn't have gone back to work!" and "Why did I go back?" Will I be sitting there regretting…
{Ameena}

Rachel went back to her work as a nursery teacher very reluctantly, much to her surprise. As mentioned previously, her experiences as a mother enabled her to now operate on not only a professional level but also now on a more empathic "parental level". She had thought that she would not enjoy being at home with her baby but in fact hated being apart from him when she did have to go back to work full-time for financial reasons. Initially she was still doing the majority of the domestic chores and the child-care when she returned to work. However, like Ameena, the strain began to show and after "discussions" with her partner, they decided to get a cleaner and have now split the domestic tasks evenly as *both* of them are now working full-time with a young son to consider. In addition she has decided that she would like to have one day for herself and Charlie to be together and is trying to reduce her working hours to four days a week. This way she feels she would not be missing out on Charlie growing up and would feel less guilty for going back to work.

I think that, because I was at home, I was doing the shopping, the cleaning, the ironing, and you know just doing those kind of jobs. And then when I went back to work, things like that didn't get done and caused a bit of conflict, especially because my mum is in [Another village 8 miles away] and she does the child-care. So that's quite a big detour as well, to go over there and then have to go back into the city, and trying to get into work early, what with being a teacher. Before I had him I used to get in at eight and now I don't get in until half past eight.
…
We've rearranged it now so that he goes to my mums on Wednesdays and Thursdays and he (James) picks him up, so that's better. You see I always have a staff meeting after work so I don't leave work until twenty to six, so by the time I've been to mum's house it'll be

Their experience of motherhood up to their baby's first Birthday

half past six when we get home. You see I can't just go and pick him up I always have to find out what's he been doing in the day, what he's eaten, you know, find out, notice the transitions... So you know that has helped, having had a bit of a heart-to-heart about what was working and what wasn't, that it needs to be more of an equal split really. And this term's been a lot better, it's worked better.
{Rachel}

The last of the trio of women who found going back to work not as they had expected was Julia, she went back to work nine weeks after the birth for financial reasons. She also worked week-ends and had the additional strain of her husband having had an immobilising operation when their son Daniel was seven weeks old, in effect leaving her feeling as though she had two babies to look after. She had thought she would want to go back to work part-time but once her son was born and she had to go back to work she found it very difficult to leave him.

Yeah, it was a dreadful time really. And I really really, the last thing I wanted to do was go back to work, but I had to. Got no choice.
Out of necessity.
And it was the last thing that I really really wanted to do. You see that caused a lot of arguments as well. It was the worst possible time he could have done it. You know what with having a nine-week-old baby. And to try to look after him, trying to look after a baby, plus go to work, plus get somewhere, because I'd have to take Daniel somewhere to be looked after...
So there was all the extra hassle involved in sorting that lot out as well?
Yeah, and timing sleep as well. You can't always necessarily... "Right I'll get the baby here for nine o'clock" - well the baby's asleep, you've got to wake the baby up and you know, which causes anxiety to the baby. No, I hated it, hated every minute of it.
{Julia}

Of the remaining four women, Sadie had been working in a factory in the early part of her pregnancy but had left as she became too tired from the physical nature of the job and would not have qualified for maternity leave anyway. She had not returned to work since having Alex as she became pregnant with her second child Nathan when Alex was only three months old. She had intended to return to work or to college, and hopes to still do so when her youngest son is about one year old (when Alex will be two).

Similarly, Tanya had been working as a part-time sales assistant during her pregnancy and did not qualify for maternity leave. She would like to go back to work but feels that it would be difficult to strike a balance between spending time with Katie and finding a job that paid more than her benefits and the child-care costs involved in looking after Katie whilst she worked. She was exploring the possibility of doing an evening course to widen her skills when I saw her when Katie was one year old.

I still hope to go back, when she is older. I mean I could go back now and do a part-time job because my dad said that he would have her in the afternoons because he works mornings. Which would be lovely but it means, but obviously I would have to earn preferably more than what I get for my benefit, so...
Exactly, otherwise...
Yeah, otherwise if I don't then I am losing out, and in the end it just wouldn't be worth it. I mean, I don't want to go back yet, give it another while, a year or so I suppose.
{Tanya}

Sarah also had a job that did not enable her to get paid maternity leave, and as the job was quite a physical one (she worked with horses) she too gave it up whilst she was pregnant. She has returned to work part-time but now works in the evenings whilst her partner Anthony looks after their son Jack. She feels that she has adjusted well to working part-time but finds it difficult not seeing her partner very much as he works in the days whilst she works in the evenings.

I work in the evenings and it sometimes feels like we barely spend any time together, we don't sit down and talk like we should. He leaves for work at six in the morning whilst I'm asleep, and then when he comes home I go off to work and when I get back in again he's asleep so...
{Sarah}

As the final woman out of the nine to be described with regards to returning to work, Claire is unique as she and her husband Tom have their own catering business (a chip van). Like the three women described above who did not qualify for maternity leave, nor did Claire as a self-

Their experience of motherhood up to their baby's first Birthday

employed person. She went back to work when Hannah was six weeks old, which she now thinks was too soon, and works four evenings a week rather than five evenings and one lunchtime as she had whilst expecting Hannah. When she is at work her mum has Hannah either at her house or she comes to Claire and Tom's home. She feels like she is managing to balance work and home now that Hannah is older but finds it difficult to maintain her relationship with her husband as he works every evening either with or without her.

> But no, we don't really get that much time to sort of, just the two of us, and it doesn't help with the hours that he works. You know like most couples they work during the day and then they've got the evening, we don't really have that.
> {Claire}

The next major area of change that was identified from the conversations with these women was the (lack of) time for themselves. It was very thin on the ground for the entirety of the first year. Many women were amazed at how much spare time, on reflection, they had had before having a baby, and how much of that spare time they had wasted. Time was now pressured and precious. Any time they had away from the baby wasn't so much spontaneous spare time, as it had been previously, but planned and organised "time for me". After all someone had to look after the baby whilst they did whatever it was that they wanted to do. If they weren't happy that their child was being well taken care of then they were not having a relaxing break themselves.

Sarah managed to have some time for herself, when either her mum or her partner could have Jack, which was usually when she took the dog out for a good long walk. Although it was not a regular part of her routine to have some time for herself, she looked forward to "just knowing that I haven't got that responsibility for that short time". Sadie had time for herself only because her mum had Alex in order for her to have a rest; it did not happen very often and only when her mum offered to babysit. Despite Sadie being pregnant with their second child and her partner Paul not working, the majority of the child-care fell to Sadie. As a single mother Tanya had time for herself every evening when Katie went to bed.

Nine Women, Nine Months, Nine Lives

Living on her own proved to be a double-edged sword as she had lots of time on her own but was limited to staying at home with her daughter in her time for herself as no-one could easily keep an eye on Katie whilst she went out to say, an evening class. However, she had recently begun to organise a regular Saturday night out for herself and her daughter – Katie went to stay at Tanya's mum's over-night and Tanya went out with her friends.

I couldn't live without my Saturday nights, I don't know how I would be able to cope!
And how long have you had this Saturday night arrangement with your mum, has that always been in place?
No, she always said from the start that she would have her once a week. When I was at home I used to go out Friday nights with my dad, not with my dad all the time but, I used to go out with my dad occasionally because he goes out Friday nights. But I used to go out with my friends on a Friday as well. But since I've moved in here, it, it started off once a week and then they'd be doing things on a Saturday so I wouldn't go out, and I'd miss going out. And then, I'd take it, I'd not take it out on her but I'd be, I wouldn't be myself because I hadn't been out. And then just recently it's gone back to Saturday nights, it's just like a routine now she goes to stay with grandma. Grandma picks her up about four o'clock Saturday and takes her back to her house and then she comes and picks me up too, because I go round there for Sunday lunch, so, it's nice, I get a lie in as well.
{Tanya}

Helen was a unique individual in this group of women as her job involved her routinely staying away from home for three or four nights a week. When she was away from home and had a night off (Helen worked on the long haul flights and often worked through the night) then she could relax and either stay in and catch up on her sleep or go out with her colleagues – "nice things that I took for granted before". However, when she was at home, it was quite a different story.

So, loads of times when I'm away, but I don't find I really have very much time at all to myself when I'm at home. But that's, you know, that's life.
That's the way it is.
You've got to keep doing washing, you've got to eat properly, and there's always stuff that needs doing. I take care of him full-time when Richard's working.
…

Their experience of motherhood up to their baby's first Birthday

You don't have time to do anything else, and there just isn't any time left over. You are completely dictated to by your child. I mean like in conversations, with other people, you're not used to having to try and talk about stuff other than the baby!
Yeah you know "What have you been doing?" Well, what have you been doing?!
Exactly!
I mean astronauts come back from space and they...
They're molly coddled! [Laughs]
Yeah and they're put in a special room and molly coddled, and yeah "You'll be all right in a few days time, and we'll get you sorted, and get rid of the bends or whatever, and then you can come back when you've adjusted"!
Yeah, exactly!
You get none of that when you've had a baby!
{Helen}

The next three women, Claire, Emma and Ameena, recognised their need to have some time for themselves but found it difficult to relax and have time for themselves at home because they felt that their husbands or partners would come home and find them doing nothing and assume that they had been doing nothing all day! None of their husbands or partners had *ever* said anything, even jokingly, about them being lazy. In fact Emma's partner Neil had said to her after having looked after Lotte all day on his own "oh, I don't know how you cope, she's been on the go all the time". This self-inflicted guilt only served to make the time the women had for themselves even more of a rarity, and when they did make time for themselves to relax they were less likely to enjoy it. In Ameena's case it was strongly linked to her need to feel that she was able to "have-it-all" as a working mum. If you read our conversation in full you'll see that having it all often means putting yourself last in everything you do. Obviously this is not conducive to being a happy person. I encouraged Ameena to look at the two extremes of her situation and to identify what was important for her.

You need to sit down and think about what things are important to <u>you</u>, and kind of rank them for what is the most important thing for now. It's like you say, when you are 60 and you look back, would you rather look back and think I had a clean and tidy house and went to work full-time and I saw my daughter on the week-ends and she ran towards her nanny and not towards me? Or would you rather say, I worked part-time and thought

Nine Women, Nine Months, Nine Lives

stuff the house and the cleaning, we had take-aways, we had a good life, we enjoyed the weekends because we spent time together as a family? You know, you've got to look at the extremes of the situation, yeah, you won't get to one or other of the extremes but you've got to work out where the in between is that will work best for you.
{Ameena (Sandra speaking)}

So like some days he's out all day, just comes back for a few hours and stuff like that. Say I've been cleaning, I'll sit down for five minutes have a cup of tea and watch telly, he'll always come home then! [Laughs] Always! He never says anything, but I feel guilty because I've sat down and watched telly, that's how I feel. Even though I've probably only just sat down and turned the telly on!
Well he's just come back in from work so he's stopped work too!
I know but you get, you can guarantee that just as I have sat down with my cup of tea he's come home. You know there are times where I've been doing things and I think "Oh I'll just carry on and do a tiny bit more - he should be home in a minute!" And half an hour later I think to myself I could have sat down and had a cup of tea and he wouldn't of known! [Laughs] Oh and it's so stupid – I shouldn't feel like that! I mean there's absolutely nothing from him to suggest that he thinks that, it's just the way I am.
{Claire}

The remaining two women to be discussed both felt that all their time, when not working, should be spent with their sons'. Rachel had to cope with children all day from 6.30 in the morning, when she got up to feed Charlie, until nine at night, when he went to bed. Work as a nursery teacher was "a bit like a busman's holiday!" She did try to go swimming once a week to have some time for herself, but she did not always manage it.

Other things crop up don't they Charlie? So... I kind of feel guilty about that too. That you know, I'm doing it for me, (a) to lose weight and (b) to get some exercise. I find I'm watching the clock, using up my time for Charlie.
...
I just pine away, I want to be with Charlie, I feel like I should be with Charlie. I feel that I only really see him at the end of the day and I really don't like that. So my time is for Charlie really. I think it's that you put Charlie first in everything you do.
...
It's like when you come home and you don't put your feet up, you play with Charlie. So he has a sort of quality, play time. Don't we, we play with you! And... I think it's being organised. I think it's, I feel as though at work I do my preparation time whenever, now

Their experience of motherhood up to their baby's first Birthday

everything seems to be to a schedule and everything is precious.
{Rachel}

Julia admits that she was very bad at making time for herself, she like all the other women realised that it was important for her sanity, but still felt torn between her son and herself. Often she would also feel so tired that she could not be bothered to go out or even do "silly things like sitting down and painting your toe nails!" Like Rachel she wanted to do some swimming and aqua-aerobics but would more often than not end up not going and feel guilty about it. Part of the problem was also their financial situation. Julia's husband was working evening shifts for the majority of their son Daniel's first year so she would have to rely upon a babysitter if she wanted to go out in the evening, a non-affordable added expense to whatever it was that she wanted to do.

A lot of it you see is financial as well you know, if you do go out it involves money. And I tend to think "Well if I go there that's like thirty or forty pounds, what can I buy for Daniel for that?" Which is dreadful! I mean I'm sure I'll get better as he gets older, I'm getting better now. Things are settling down now more financially wise with you know, we're more comfortable than we were when Daniel was first born.
{Julia}

You can see from some of these women's experiences that returning to work and having some time for themselves were closely linked. Nearly all of the women who had returned to work mentioned at some point in our conversations that going to work provided them with a welcome break from their child and the rather repetitive routine of caring for them. You may have also noticed that how easily they returned to work, or had time for themselves, was influenced by the support they received from their partners. In the final part of this chapter we explore how their partners, and their relationship with them had changed, which they almost all had, in the time since their child had been born.

Their relationship with their partner's

As mentioned previously, only one woman out of the nine did not have a partner, therefore, there will be no references made to Tanya in this

85

part of the chapter. The remaining eight women all thought that their partners had changed over the course of the first year of parenthood, as had they themselves. However, a pattern seemed to emerge such that any changes in their partners seemed (to the women) to have spontaneously happened without them having to make any effort. This was contrary to the women's perception of the changes that they themselves had experienced in the last year which they considered, on the whole, to have taken quite some effort. For example, becoming more patient had been an uphill struggle for most of them!

Many of them said that they felt their husbands or partners had become more loving and openly affectionate towards them, and nearly all of the women thought that they had mellowed and matured. Despite these really quite noticeable changes in themselves and their partner's it was very rare for them to say anything to each other about the ways they had developed and changed. A few of them made a joke out of it but none of them had felt the need to discuss it. This suggests that many of these changes were gradual and welcome on both sides of the relationship.

He's actually a bit more loving, a bit more open with his affections yeah and he's absolutely brilliant with Lotte. Yeah he's sort of mellowed a bit, you know, if that's the right thing to say, yeah he's calmed down a lot.
...
Do you think him mellowing has been a conscious effort or do you think it's just happened?
No I think it's just happened, it's just happened. I don't think he's thought about it, he's just got on with it really.
...
He's started getting more homely now, he's started doing things around the house. [Rolls eyes and grimaces]
Oh no! [Laughter] What, putting up shelves and things?
Gardening, yeah, he used to do a bit before but now he's saying things like "When she plays out in the garden we'll have to do this and that". Bought a tool kit! [Laughs]
Does he know how to use it?
[Laughs] Put the stair gate up which I thought I'd get my dad to do, and he has actually done odd jobby bits now and then! [Laughter] But yeah, more sort of homely.
Well he's got a home and a family now.
That's right. [Pride in voice]
{Emma}

Their experience of motherhood up to their baby's first Birthday

I think he understands a lot more... Before, as long as we could have a holiday away every year and escape for a bit, then that was good, and you know, do up the house in between. But now he looks at the bigger picture of like, what's the situation going to be in five years time, ten years time, you know, even when he´s retied, and he never looked at that before <u>ever</u>.
{Helen}

I think he's matured, really <u>really</u> matured.
Are you surprised about that?
No, no.
You look surprised!
No, I didn't expect it. Not that he was, not that he was immature, it's just really changed him, having a baby.
...
OK, and do you talk to him about how you think he's changed? Does he ever say to you that he thinks that you've changed or...?
No not really.
Don't you ever look back and think "Cor weren't things different before we had Hannah?!"
Oh yeah, we say that, yeah we say that!
{Claire}

And do you talk about how you have changed...?
Generally in a jokey sort of way! [Laughter] I don't think we're that aware, we haven't sat down and thought about how we've changed, I think we're both aware that we have changed.
{Sarah}

So do you talk about how you have changed as individuals? Does he ever say you know...?
No, no!
Do you think that you need to?
Yeah, I think that's one thing that we are both failing to do... I'd like to say to him more "Yusuf you're so special, you're so nice" but I can't! [Laughs] No we never talk about positive changes to each other, about each other. I'd like to sometimes. I think I'll tell him he's special tonight.
He'll probably look at you like you're mad! [Laughter]
Yeah!
He'll probably think what has she broken? Has she crashed the car?! [Laughs]
Yeah [Laughs]
Yeah give it a go, If it's something you think might make a difference, then yeah...

87

Especially when you've gone through an arranged or introductory marriage, you think "Oh God, is it going to work?" and...
Mmm, it must be very difficult.
I mean they say that you grow to like each other, you grow to love each other. But you always have that thought at the back of your mind, when you do know him after about four years time, that you are going to get fed up of him or bored of him. You develop that relationship, that understanding, a lot through respect and caring for each other. Yeah I think more than anything it's, it's the caring.
{Ameena}

I think we have a different perspective. I think James seems more keen on the house, he's often in the garden. I think that the practicalities are more his... But anyway I think he's got more mature, he's happy to play together with Charlie at night times. I think, you know, we're both grown ups now, do you know what I mean?! [Laughs]
{Rachel}

He's probably not as happy go lucky as he was. You know he's...
More responsible?
Yeah, yeah. Whether that's a good thing I don't know. He takes things more seriously whereas you know, he was... Life's more serious to him now, whether he wants it to be or not. Things are.
...
OK, and do you talk to Matt about the way that you feel that you've changed and perhaps that you think he has changed?
Yeah, yeah. We have talked about it.
Is that just something that crops up and you laugh about it? You know like "God look at us! When you think..."
No, it has been when in absolute desperation you'll say "Ooh! I can't do this that and the other" and you have a real downer. I mean sometimes you do laugh about things, you know things that you do. But most of the time it's not, it's the other way round unfortunately.
Is that for him as well as for you?
Matt never really comments about things like that.
{Julia}

The two slightly unusual cases with regards to how their partners had changed were Sadie and Sarah. Sadie felt that her partner Paul had not changed as much as her and felt quite resentful about that. Sarah thought that her partner Anthony tried to hide just how much he had changed as his behaviour in private was different to his behaviour in public. On the

Their experience of motherhood up to their baby's first Birthday

whole the women perceived that their husband's or partner's had adapted to parenthood really quite well.

OK. And do you think that your partner has changed? Has Paul changed?
No! [Shakes head vigorously]
No? You don't think he's changed at all?
No.
You don't think so, not at all? You don't think he's perhaps got a bit more patient?
Yeah maybe a bit more. He's got quite good with Alex, yeah he's good with Alex, he's got time for Alex.
...
So he must have changed a little bit because if he's spending more time... If you think in terms of the whole year?
He's changed a bit. [Said with reluctance]
But not as much as you?
No, not as much as me.
And have you ever spoken to him about the fact that you have changed, that you feel like you're that bit sort of more mature, like you said?
No, no.
No... Does he ever pass comment, said anything, even jokingly, you know like "You're old for your age" or something?
He says I'm a bit boring now... But if you think about it I've been pregnant for nearly two years!
Yeah! [Laughter]
Apart from that he hasn't said anything.
{Sadie}

And how do you think your partner has changed? Do you think he has?
He tried not to let it.
Really?
Yeah, I think so. Especially with other people. When he is at home he loves Jack to bits and will sit and play with him, yeah, but when other people are around he tends to be a bit more reserved! [Laughs] He still goes out with his friends, plays football on a Saturday, because I wouldn't stop him. [Laughs] No, and he knows that I wouldn't stop him from going football training with his mates or whatever, you know he likes to keep it, I suppose it's just his way of, you know of keeping that side as it was.
{Sarah}

As the two individuals in the relationship had changed, it would seem reasonable to predict that the relationship itself would have changed.

Instead of simply being lovers they were now parents as well and that "little" bit more dependent and reliant upon each other. Indeed, they now had a very big mutual interest: the happiness and health of their child. Their priority may have become the welfare of their child but their next priority could most usefully be the maintenance of their own relationship as a couple. Just as having time for themselves was identified by the women as something they knew they needed and wanted, time together as a couple was also a very real need too. Unfortunately, like the conflict they felt between caring for the child and caring for themselves, the women quite often felt torn between their partner and their baby. They spent the vast majority of their time being a mother and as much as they longed for time alone with their partner, the switch to becoming his lover wasn't always an automatic one. However in general, as their child got older and their lives became more settled, it was easier to balance their own, their partner's, and their child's needs.

As in the previous discussion of how the women felt that their partners had changed, it was rare for them to talk about how they had changed as a couple, again even by making a joke of it. All of the women described feeling closer to their partners or husbands. Only Julia and Matt's closeness seemed to be short-lived as their relationship steadily deteriorated over the course of the year. Reading through our conversation it is possible to suggest that a likely reason for this decline was that they did not spend any real time together as a couple, primarily due to a clash in the hours that they worked, such that they hardly saw each other. Julia described how when they did have some time together that they spent it as a family and that there was enormous pressure to enjoy themselves – smile or else!

After a recent heart-to-heart, and remembering that Julia's son Daniel is approximately nine months older than the rest of the children in this book (i.e. the heart-to-heart took place after her son's first birthday and therefore outside the perimeters of this chapter), her husband has changed his shift so that they can try and rebuild their very nearly defunct marriage. The fact remains that during the first year of Daniel's life his parent's did not have a good relationship. The recent turn around due to

Their experience of motherhood up to their baby's first Birthday

them trying to maintain their relationship as lovers by spending time together without him provides evidence to support the importance of this need as felt by the majority of the women in this book and their partner's alike. Neglect your partner at your peril, or he may begin to neglect you. It is worth making time for yourselves as a couple even if it is difficult to do so.

OK, now I've asked you about time for yourself, do you and Matt try and spend time together without Daniel? Even if it's just sitting here watching a video, having a quite evening in.
Well, it is difficult what with Matt not being here.
Has it become easier what with Matt changing his shifts?
Yeah, yeah.
How long has it been since he has changed his shifts?
Only three weeks, and he had a weeks holiday before that, so only four weeks really that he's not been on this silly shift. But yeah we've, we've been to the cinema and you know just sitting outside, because you know the weather's been so nice and with a bottle of wine and what have you. And Daniel has been at Matt's mums or my mum's and... We've got things coming up which we are going to on our own so...
That's good, yeah that is good. That's an improvement isn't it? So give it a while and see what happens...
Yeah, yeah. And just the fact that Matt, that Matt's here at night means that I can go out on my own, and Matt can you know, (go to) football training or just nip round and see a friend, which neither of us could do before.
They are more sociable hours. Well they're not really more sociable hours are they, doing nights? [Laughs] But it is more sociable for the two of you, to lead fairly independent lives. I mean like you said earlier, every moment that you had then you had to spend together because it was all you had.
Yeah, it was very <u>very</u> stressful as well. Because...
It's a lot of pressure?
You know, I'm forever trying to organise things to do together as a family. I mean I'm terrible, I try so hard to have things perfect that it always ended up backfiring. Because you're both tired... you are so desperate to make things right, and because you're tired and you are trying to cram so much in it just doesn't work.
{Julia}

The other seven women had relationships that seem to have adjusted well, on the whole, to parenthood. This includes Emma, Helen and Rachel who were not expecting to become mothers. In particular, Emma and her partner Neil had a good relationship over the year as a whole, despite for the first few months of parenthood having had the cloud of their daughter's ill health hovering overhead throughout. Of the remaining four couples, a more recent development that may have negatively influenced her relationship with her partner was Claire's poor physical health. About nine months after having Hannah, Claire discovered that she had endometriosis and had to undergo somewhat unsuccessful abdominal surgery shortly afterwards. Her partner Tom supported her throughout this time.

We're a lot closer than we were, we were close before but you know there's that sort of like completeness really.
And do you talk about how your relationship has changed?
Not really, no.
Do you feel that you want to talk about it?
I don't think, you just, we just get on with, it's not, we know it's changed, and we've accepted it's changed but it's not…
You feel he knows it's changed as well so you don't need to say it and flag it up and say "Look isn't this great!"
Not at all. We're both aware of it.
And both pleased about it?
Yeah, we're a lot closer.
…
We do try, yeah definitely. You need a, I know it sounds silly but you need a break, you need a break so you can be together, you catch up on things that you haven't talked about in a long while.
Yeah I mean she's only been around a year!
Yeah, but, I don't know everything about what he's doing anymore at work and he certainly doesn't know everything about my work. And yet before we knew exactly what we were doing and he knew everything about what I'd been doing and that doesn't happen any more. But we do try and catch up.
Do you feel like you want to know about things like that?
Yeah because then I don't feel like I'm neglecting Neil and everything's not just focused on Lotte, because I think you have got to spend time together.
Do you think he feels the same?
Yeah, yeah I do.
{Emma}

Their experience of motherhood up to their baby's first Birthday

So your relationship must have changed, I mean you say you had half-expected things to be more strained?
Yeah, I did. I really did. I was just very negative about the whole thing. I knew it'd be a stress, I thought it'd be really bad, but... [Laughs] So yeah things have definitely changed. As much as I had just got married six months before finding out, I felt pretty secure anyway, but now I feel completely secure, again that might be naive but that's the way I feel. I do feel more confidant that we can do this on a larger scale.
...
So do you get much time to spend together, just the two of you? Like in the evening if he goes to bed early
Yeah, we do in the evenings. At the weekends it hasn't been so good, but when we do have time together we make the most of it and we've started to go out, which is better than we used to do.
{Helen}

I think that the only thing that we miss is the fact that we can't do things when we want to do them. That's the only really difficult thing, like sometimes you think "Oh wouldn't it be nice just to go out for a meal" but then, if you want to go out for a meal you've got to arrange cover (for the chip van). I mean most times as I say my mum will have her, but sometimes you don't want to burden people all the time so we don't go out. I mean we don't really mind, but like I say, the odd time, you just think "Oh yeah, it'd be nice if we could".
...
So your relationship has changed because of Hannah, and you feel like you can be less spontaneous?
Yeah, I think also... I've not been very well, I've got endometriosis.
Oh no.
Yeah, I've already had surgery, in January, and that's put a huge strain on the relationship as well, which doesn't help. I think that's what has really made a lot of difference to us both.
...
So it's gone from bad to worse really. From having a rough pregnancy to having a caesarean, then finding out I had this. I must admit my husband has been absolutely brilliant really.
That must have been really hard.
Yeah, I mean it's a lot better since I've had the surgery but it's just a case of, they could only take so much away and, it still hurts a bit. But not to worry, I'll just have to wait and see how things go.
...
OK and do you try and make time for the two of you to spend time together without Hannah? You said that you've got people who can babysit and things like that.

Nine Women, Nine Months, Nine Lives

Not really no. I mean, Saturday night, we get a take away and a video and hope that she goes to bed. But just lately she'll just sit and play but she won't bother you and you can just sit and watch the video... But no, we don't really get that much time to sort of, just the two of us, and it doesn't help with the hours that he works.
{Claire}

So have you changed as a couple? Your relationship, has it developed into something...?
Well it's a lot steadier... I mean we don't, well we used to have silly little arguments, things like that, but we don't so much now. I think we're more on a level, certainly, with things.
So, what do you mean by you're more on a level?
We used to have a lot more differences of opinion or you know I'd want to do something and he'd want to do something else. Just wanting different things whereas now we're much more compatible.
Do you agree with each other more or do you just agree to disagree?
A bit of both really! We certainly do agree more, but instead of getting into an argument we tend to just walk away now, when we can see that we're definitely going to have a row we just don't. We certainly don't argue as much.
...
Do you try and make time to spend together without Jack?
We don't really, no. I think perhaps we should do. I think that we should spend more time together, not that I don't want Jack with us, but...
No of course not.
Just for us to be together on our own... I feel that we should spend more time together.
{Sarah}

And do you try and make time for yourselves as a couple? I mean for instance with Ayesha if she does fall asleep in the evening?
Yes, yes we do, initially it was... Yeah, yeah we do.
And do you manage it quite often?
Yeah, now, now... When she was depending heavily on breastfeeding it was very difficult because she was, every, about every half an hour every hour she was so demanding that, but now with that change, it's a lot better.
So it's a lot easier now?
Yeah, it's a lot easier now.
{Ameena}

And do you try and make time for the two of you to be together? Like going out for a meal in the evening?
No.
Perhaps putting a video on when Charlie is in bed, or sitting down together?

Their experience of motherhood up to their baby's first Birthday

No, no. I think that now Charlie is going to bed that little bit earlier, we do actually have a bit longer to sit and talk. It's easier now that he goes to bed that bit earlier, and that's just, and he's slept through on eight times out of fourteen – haven't you? Yes! So that means we're not quite so shattered!
…
So would you say that is something you are trying to move towards now with Charlie going to bed earlier?
Not really! [Laughs] I think you know… You suggest it more that we should do more just the two of us don't you? [Addressing James]
James: Mmm. But we survive!
Survival's about the best way to put it yeah!
Also I think it will be easier when I'm working just the four days, when I've got a whole day of Charlie to myself really.
Yeah, and perhaps then you won't feel quite so reluctant to leave him, not necessarily over-night, but for an evening to start with.
Yeah, I think it might be better when I've had the seven or eight weeks in the summer, you know had him solidly, then I'll perhaps be able to do that more.
{Rachel}

And would you say that your relationship has changed? From what it was before you had Alex?
Yeah.
And in what way would you say it has changed, both good and bad?
Well I can't really go out gallivanting like I used to, he goes out with his mates, I used to go out with him, but not now.
So… Is there anything that you would say has changed for the better, do you feel closer to him?
Yeah, yeah I do feel closer to him
Is that because now you've got two children whereas…?
Yeah, yeah definitely.
{Sadie}

This chapter completes these women's journeys to their child's first birthday. Some of what you have read may have surprised you, hopefully it will not have shocked you too much, if at all. Remember that the quotes that are included in the text are drawn from the conversations that I had with the women. If you are curious about a particular individual's experiences because they are so similar to your own, or equally possibly, so different from your own, do read their experiences in full.

Let us now look towards the future. As I have said to some of the

Nine Women, Nine Months, Nine Lives

many women I have come into contact with over the years, not just the nine women in this book, *you have changed, you are changing, and you will continue to change.* If you want to change in a particular way, now is a good time to start thinking about how you can make it happen.

Their immediate future:
Will you have time for one?!

All but one of the nine women said that they very rarely had time to stop and think about the future, as they were so busy managing their lives on a day-to-day basis. Interestingly, the one woman (Ameena) who had thought about the future commented that she rarely had time to think about the past. It is of course important to reflect on what has happened and how one has coped with life, in order to have a realistic idea of what the future might hold, and whether one is capable of dealing with the banana skins that life often leaves in one's path. If you can do this then you are more likely to have a contented life. However, it is not always possible when you have a diddy-demanding-darling to deal with.

Hopes for the coming year

Every single woman could think of at least one thing that they hoped to achieve in the coming twelve months. They were all confident they could achieve them too. The most common hopes for the coming year are shown below and the women who reported having them are shown in brackets:

- Continue being happy as a family {Emma, Helen, Rachel}
- Change their own work to become more compatible with family life {Helen, Sarah, Ameena, Rachel}
- Have a holiday – with or without their child {Claire, Tanya}
- Continue to be a good mum {Tanya, Ameena, Sarah, Claire}
- Make more time for themselves {Rachel, Sadie, Claire, Ameena, Julia}
- Do more things as a couple {Helen, Claire, Sarah, Rachel}
- Do more things as a family {Helen, Claire, Sarah, Rachel}

Three women had particularly individual and personal hopes for the future. Julia wanted to give her marriage one last chance so that her own, her husband's and her son's lives could become more settled and "normal" – whether they separated or remained together she felt she just needed to know one way or another. Emma wanted the ordeal with her daughter Lotte's birth to be finally over. She felt that a sense of closure to the birth and the first few fraught weeks of her life would only be achieved when Lotte was discharged from the hospital by her Paediatrician as having a clean bill of health. And finally, Claire wanted the problem with her physical health, endometriosis, to be resolved so that she could start to look beyond that to the future. Depending on the treatment course she decided to have and the possible side effects, she would know whether to feel more positive about the possibility of having or not being able to have, another child. The idea of being barren at 26 was not appealing for either her or her husband Tom.

Julia's hopes

OK, now your immediate future, so the next twelve months. What do you hope to achieve this year? Have you some kind of goal in mind, either a personal goal for yourself, or like you said earlier, a career goal or not hating computers? Something like that...
I think to get back on an even keel in every aspect. For me and Matt to try and definitely get on better or get something sorted out one way or another, do you know what I mean? Things need sorting one way or the other. [Currently contemplating separation]
Mmm. You need to know, you need to be sure?
Yeah, yeah! For me to be my own person again to a certain extent... To definitely be me

Their immediate future

again. I think career-wise I'm not interested! [Laughs] I'll be quite honest with you. I mean in the next twelve months Daniel will be going to playgroup and I've got somebody coming next week about him going to a crèche, just for a couple of hours just to break him in, before he goes to playgroup and he's...
Yeah, good idea.
I mean I'm quite happy for him to be here all the time but I think it would be good for Daniel to go because he is quite a sociable little person, I think he'll enjoy going. Without me as well, I mean we go to lots of things, but everything is with me.
What so that he's always got somebody to run to if it's...?
Yeah, yeah to do that and for Daniel to settle in well. Yeah, just to really get back, to have a little bit more normality in life again. Because things have been so much up in the air over the last fourteen or fifteen months it's been silly really, so...
So when you say normality, do you mean sort of, a little bit like how life was before you had Daniel?
Yeah, a little bit like everybody else's life as well, you know, family life, you do spend time together as a family. That one doesn't walk in the door and the other one walks out... So you know, hopefully Matt will come back to the fold a bit now, and we'll be together.
Yeah, at least he's trying. At least, you know, whatever happens from this point on at least you are making a go of it now. And you know, you may get to a point in time when you think "I've done the best I can and it's either worked out fantastically, or, we've got to a point where we have explored every avenue thoroughly and it just isn't going to happen". At least you have, I don't know, what would be the word, well you wouldn't have a guilty conscience about it. You can feel quite, not reassured, but quite comfortable knowing that you did try.
That's it, yeah.
See how it goes, give it six months or so and see what happens.
Yeah, I mean we had a bit of disagreement last night. And I think it's because there has been so much damage done and there is a lot of repairing to do. And Matt, I mean Matt has made an effort, we're both really trying hard. And Matt will say you know "I've made so much effort over the last couple of weeks!" And I've had to say "Matt things can't be mended in just a couple of weeks, there's been so much damage done, that there is a hell of a lot of repairing to do, it can't just be repaired in a couple of weeks!" And that's what Matt finds difficult, he thinks, you know, he's been really good and kept his calm and ignored me when I've been nasty, you know for a week, and he thinks "Well that's it now I can go back to like if I'm tired being a bit niggly". And you can't, you've got to constantly make an effort. I mean obviously you do revert back, but you've both constantly got to make the effort, and things just can't be repaired in a couple of weeks.
But things become... You remember them less quickly as time goes on. The, the sort of the feeling of "My God! When Daniel was a new born baby I didn't do the best for him because I did this that and the other and I didn't do that", you know, that doesn't jump to mind as quickly now as it did then?
No, no it doesn't.

99

Nine Women, Nine Months, Nine Lives

And the same thing will happen. I mean if you could repair your marriage by a quick fix, it would show there would be something very wrong with it to start with. You know if all it took was a bit of Super-glue and fingers crossed... The deeper the bond is, the deeper down you've got to enmesh it and build it up again.
Yeah! I think that, I think that's Matt's problem, Matt thinks it can be fixed straight away.
You can't just surface repair it.
No, no.
But at least you are both trying and maintaining it. You are both going to slip, you are both going to lose your temper with each other and that is perfectly normal. Everybody argues. Some subjects you can agree to disagree on, and some subjects are just far too important for you that you just can't. Unfortunately when you are feeling the least rational you could possibly ever feel is when you need to be the most rational you could ever be! [Laughs]
Yeah! [Laughs] But as I say, all we can do is try.
Yeah, that's it. I really do think it's great that you are trying.
It's so, it would be the easiest thing in the world to walk away from. Because you do feel unhappy and you do think "God I can't go through life feeling like this all the time". But, there's so many other things that come into the equation, you know, like how would it effect, it's easy to walk away, but how would that effect Daniel? I mean everything would be a complete upheaval for him, and you know even at this age, they know, they know things aren't, they're not silly.
No, no, they do know, for sure.
Yeah, (we'll) keep trying anyway.
{Julia}

Emma's hopes

The future! We'll say your immediate future so the next 12 months. What would you say you hope to achieve in the next year? What are your hopes for the next year?
With Lotte that she gets discharged from Hospital in May [Laughs]. That's my main hope really... and just to continue being as happy as we are now really because I think we've got everything sussed really.
Just continue to build?
Yeah, for Neil to move closer to home really (with work). [Laughs] That's a hope, which he is hoping to do actually.
Yeah? Is that in the near future?
Hopefully. He wants to as well which makes a big difference.
What about you reducing your hours?
Yeah, that's going to be in about a year.
So that's something you'd hope to do within the year?
Yeah.

Their immediate future

But realistically you think...
Yeah it might be a bit longer.
OK so do you think you'll be able to achieve it? Do you think Lotte will be discharged in May?
At the back of my mind I think so but I don't want to say yes just in case it doesn't happen. They were really pleased with her, I haven't seen them since, she's been back in November and they were very pleased with her then and on the letter I had back they put on it that they want to see her again at 18 months for a possible discharge. So I've got that in the back of my mind that it's going to happen but I don't want to sort of say it's definitely going to happen and then me getting upset because something's not quite right.
So what difference will it make, do you think, if she is discharged, is that like she's been given a clean bill of health?
Yeah, yeah, basically that's what they've said to me. They're not checking her lungs or anything like that, it's developmental and at the back of my mind I keep thinking "Is something wrong?" And until they turn round to me and say "No she's fine you know she's doing what she should be doing, blah blah blah" I don't think I'll ever be a hundred percent happy, it just doesn't seem to be, it doesn't feel like it's finished. You know like, most people when they come home they think that's it really apart from health visitors and that, but I feel like I'm still attached to them somehow! [Laughs] You know, yeah, they've said to me yeah she's fine, but I still feel like I am still there.
So that will make a big difference then?
Yeah.
And if that doesn't happen in May, when do you think it will happen, do you have another appointment?
No, no they usually say every three months but I only go every 6 because she did quite well, so they said they wouldn't see me in three months but in 6 months which takes me to May.
{Emma}

Claire's hopes

OK the last chunk is your immediate future, so the next twelve months. What do you hope to achieve this year?
To feel better! [Laughs] Yeah.
Physically?
Mentally. I think I'm mentally worn down really. I think of everything, you feel like you're just getting back on your feet and something else comes along and you get knocked down. So I think I'm, I think I'm mentally worn out. You know like I just need a holiday.
You need a break?

Nine Women, Nine Months, Nine Lives

Yeah. I just want to be better again, and just think about, like the future, but at the moment... I mean I know it's not like cancer or anything where you know you are going to die. But you still feel that because you're ill, you still feel that you can't sort of get on with your life.
Is there ever, I mean you say that you like, that you've got pains and things like that, does that stop you from doing things?
Not, not really. It's because you don't feel well you don't want to go places.
Yeah yeah, that is difficult. [Telephone rings – it is Tom and she has a brief conversation with him]
He says "Are you going to tell me about it later?!"
Does he think it's a conspiracy?!
I must admit when these [Preparing for Parenthood] classes first, you know because it was like, it was like concentrated on postnatal depression, he was saying "Oh you know you shouldn't go to these classes because you'll end up getting postnatal depression!" [Laughs and rolls her eyes]
Oh right! [Laughs and shakes head] OK, well you said that one of the things that you hope to achieve this year is a holiday, maybe abroad? Do you want to go on holiday with Hannah, or a short break away with just Tom?
Oh no with Hannah, definitely.
Yeah?
I don't think that getting away from her personally would make me feel any better. I think it's just because of everything that has been going on and like this it's just brought me down, but... She's so much better now, it's not really her that gets me down, it's just, you know, life! [Laughs]
[Laughs] Life yeah. OK, and of the things that you hope to achieve this year, to mentally feel better, do you think you can achieve it? And if so, how?
To be honest with you I've not really, not really thought about it!
What, the future or...?
Yeah! I mean the only thing that I have really thought about is just getting better, and I've not really thought about that particularly, a lot. But no I've not really looked into the future and thought "Ooo" you know. I mean, not twelve months, I mean we have sort of said, that in a couple of years we'll think about trying for a baby, if everything's sorted out, but that's about the only thing we've ever really discussed. No, I can't say that I've looked into the future and...
And yet you seem very certain of what you want to do in the next 12 months - to feel better mentally.
Yeah, yeah, that's...
It was an instant reaction.
Yeah that's probably the only thing because that is what is bothering me at the moment. I just want to be well. I just want it to be over and done with.
{Claire}

102

Their immediate future

These three examples involve the three things that most people (with a young child) tend to hold dearest: their relationship with their partner, their child's health, and their own health. The order that they are presented in here does not necessarily reflect an accepted order of importance, this was simply the order in which I recalled these women's unique experiences. Read into that what you will about my own priorities!

On a lighter note, Sadie's immediate reaction to being asked what she hoped to achieve in the coming year was "Not to get pregnant!" and was said with *real* feeling. On the other hand, Ameena hoped to conceive before the end of the coming twelve months as she cheekily said that her husband was "not getting any younger!"

Unlike in the previous chapter, when I outlined as a list the changes that these nine women had experienced in themselves and in their lives in the first year of motherhood, it is possible that you will aspire to some of these hopes for the next twelve months. As always, do remember that these are nine women's collective thoughts, so it is unlikely that you will hope to experience, or indeed actually experience, all of these things. Nevertheless, you will experience some of them, which of them you experience will quite probably be determined by the type of person you are and your individual circumstances.

As an aside, the interviews about the second year of their experiences of motherhood are currently being completed. Therefore a comparison between the nine women's expectations as recorded here and the achievements they will have actually managed will be possible. These will be outlined in the next book of the series which will describe their experiences as the mothers' of toddlers.

Building upon their new experiences

As was outlined in the introduction to this chapter one of the most effective ways of having a contented life is to realise what we are good at and what we are bad at. Sorting out what we are capable of coping with means being honest with ourselves, for example, about what we like about ourselves and feel proud of, and equally what we wish we could change about ourselves or improve upon. These beliefs are most usefully based upon our previous experiences. If we can build upon a realistic appraisal of ourselves, based on our experiences, then the contented life that we all to a greater or lesser degree strive for will be closer to being within our grasp.

The next part of the chapter contains the nine women's responses to the following two questions: *"What have you learnt about yourself in the past year that you would like to develop next year?"* And *"What have you learnt about yourself in the past year that you would like to change next year?"* Their responses are listed in the same order that they appear in the last part of the book i.e. the full conversations that I had with them.

To be developed…

- Emma – to continue to "take each day as it comes" and to attempt to be structured but remain flexible and realistic.
- Tanya – to continue being responsible and regaining her independence and developing her daughter's independence.
- Helen – to continue to take each day as it comes but try to be more realistic about her own limitations, "to realise that there really are some things that I can't do".
- Claire – to continue to try to regain some of her own independence and "to be more positive!"
- Sarah – to be a bit more organised, take more time out for herself, "definitely me being more positive and just keep being a good mum!"
- Ameena – to continue to think about what her priorities are, decide what they are and structure her life accordingly.
- Rachel – to have more time for herself, be even more tolerant of Charlie and continue to build her career.
- Sadie – to have more time for herself, "I didn't have enough time for myself, I had to make sure that he was, that I was there for them

Their immediate future

first, and then Paul, never myself".
- Julia – "I need to develop my tactfulness, definitely".

To be changed...

- Emma – "I'd like to lose weight!"
- Tanya – "I need to be more flexible."
- Helen – to not get so frustrated with her situation i.e. that she had a baby when she had not thought she wanted one, "It's probably the hardest thing I've had to do in my life. Full stop."
- Claire – to realise her own limitations and act upon them, "I'm only human!"
- Sarah – to have more social contact with other mums and plan her future, for example, go back to work full-time. "I think I ought perhaps to start looking at the side of getting him involved (in a playgroup), and I'd be making some effort towards getting out and meeting people too".
- Ameena – to worry less about everything! "I want to be less stressed, I don't want to worry as much as I do."
- Rachel – to lose weight, "I would actually like to find more time to do keep fit but I hate the gym and I hate swimming"!
- Sadie – to put herself first occasionally and "to feel good in myself, because I always feel down".
- Julia – to have patience with others, not just Daniel.

As you can see there is a great variety in the type of things that these nine women felt good and bad about themselves for. From the desire to lose weight, to being patient, to getting a little bit of their freedom and independence back again. They have all changed and recognise that they will continue to change over the coming year. The changes that take place within your child are often more obvious to you than the changes that take place within yourself. Because you are not looking for them, and perhaps do not notice them as much, does not make them any the less important. As your child grows and develops, so too do you.

Concluding thoughts

As I mentioned at the beginning of the book, many women feel as if they do not really know what to expect when they have a baby. When they ask people about their experiences they often only hear "horror stories" or that the world became rose coloured and glowing the moment the umbilical cord was cut. The truth lies in the vast expanse in between. This book is here to provide you with some of that in between, nine women's actual experiences of pregnancy and the first year of motherhood. The conspiracy theory of motherhood as described by Claire and Julia below has no useful place in life and is included here to illustrate the extreme frustration that can result from a lack of realism.

Do you know what I saw once on a film, it was about teenage mums who were still at school having babies, and they, they made it look so easy! And like you see all these single mothers that are walking round the streets and stuff and they just make having a baby look so easy!
How do you mean?
Well, they've got these little babies in their prams and they're so good and quiet, so well behaved. It was ages before I could go shopping with her. I used to have to take her in the rock-a-bye car seats, and I had to have someone else with me. I had to put her in the trolley and then have my own trolley for the shopping. And when she was a bit older I used to sit her in the seats (on the trolleys) and she used to hate it, she used to scream and scream, I couldn't take her. I used to dread having to go shopping even if somebody

was with me. Because she'd scream and scream, I used to have to carry her around and she used to get so heavy. And then now, she will actually sit in the, in the seat bit, and she's fine now! I used to dread it, oh for months, whenever we went shopping.

Yeah, yeah. If you knew how many times I had heard girls say that to me! You've no idea! Everybody seems to have this idea that other people are making it look easy! There's a conspiracy going on! "How is everybody else doing this and I'm not?!"

I know, where does it come from, where did this idea of a perfect mother and everything, where did it come from? [Quite angry]

It's basically insecurity. It's just you know, everybody thinks "I must be doing something different or wrong".

Well, I had realised that to be honest with you because after I'd spoken to this girl [A neighbour with a little boy who is three weeks younger than Hannah], and it's funny, we'll start talking, and I don't know, things I've gone through, she's gone through, you just think, well it's not just me!

No, no it's not! But everybody goes through it differently. Some bits that you found easy other people will have found horrendous. You know, it's swings and roundabouts.
{Claire}

OK well that's it for the questions that I have. I don't know if you can think of any experience that you've had, right from the word go - from wanting to get pregnant, from trying to get pregnant, right the way through to Daniel's second birthday, to waking up this morning - anything else?

Not really, only I really do think that people should be more honest about it all. About everything. I mean I don't think that anything's, like the absolute joy of it all, but also like the downfalls of it. And that, as I say, the only thing that anybody ever mentions is in the pregnancy morning sickness. That's the worst thing you can probably think of in your pregnancy and then when a baby's born it cries a lot. And that's all that's ever mentioned to you. Not anything else. So I wish that people were more honest about it and that everybody, to explain that everybody feels like it, it's not just you!

You're not the odd one out.

Yeah, I mean I can remember when Daniel got to six months and I thought "Oh this is a breeze now". I mean it was, from about six months he was an absolute pleasure! Up until that, I think, it's just like such a mixture of emotions, and you panic, you're so overprotective, so sensitive. I think if just somebody explained to you that you are going to be, at some point, that you will be like that, you know you will be oversensitive and that's fine. That's not a problem that's what every new mum goes through. I think you would accept it better. I think I definitely would have done.

Yeah?

Yeah, like what I said about not sleeping. I mean that was a massive problem and I had panic attacks worrying myself stupid about not sleeping. And then as soon as somebody else says "Oh yeah, at a quarter to five I was decorating" – fine! It wasn't a problem any

Concluding thoughts

more. I just didn't sleep!
[Laughs] Yeah!
But you know, I could cope with it, I went and got loads of books. I went to my dads and got loads of books. And I was like "Right, I've got my pile of books" and I would actually sit down in the day and think "Right tonight when I'm not sleeping I'll do my patio doors, I'll do some cooking for the freezer, I'll...!" I mean I used to go and sit in Daniel's bedroom, I used to get a book, I can remember reading, being that desperate and reading an autobiography on Brian Clough! [Laughs]
[Laughs] Oh my God!
I can actually remember sitting in Daniel's nursery in his rocking chair with my feet up on the cot reading this Brian Clough book, yeah! But once you accept it, it's fine, it's not a problem. You just adapt your life to not sleeping.
Yeah that's it.
Yeah, you know, it's not a problem then. I think if people just said you are going to be silly and stupid and hormonal and then when it had cropped up... And like to tell other people, I mean like parents, parents forget what you were like. I mean my mum, I can always remember my mum before I was pregnant saying to me "If you ever feel down just let somebody know, let me know because you might feel like you've got postnatal depression". Well, once I'd had Daniel, people had forgotten about postnatal depression and I could have been quite easily suffering with it!
Yeah, yeah that's it.
But you see Daniel was there then and I didn't matter. Do you know what I'm saying? I wasn't priority any more. When you are pregnant, and especially if you are the first in the family, you are priority and you know you are extra special but as soon as this baby is born that attention is taken from you. And I don't mean that in a, like a jealous way or...
No, but it is, it is an effect, it does happen.
And I know that if I got pregnant again, it would be completely different.
Yeah, yeah, a second pregnancy. Definitely.
Yeah, I think it would have been so much easier to cope with if I had known that other people feel like that. And as I say all the mums who had children round about that period, all felt exactly the same. But you don't say anything because you'd feel such a failure.
{Julia}

So, for these nine women, nine months changed their lives. Some of them had instigated that change, some of them had not. They all survived their child's first year, but for some it was much more of a mixture of positive experiences and negative experiences than they had expected or anticipated. Some of their thoughts about the changes to themselves and their lives are shown below. Beneath them are the thoughts and experiences of having a first baby from another woman, not one of the nine. I contacted her in her capacity as a commissioning editor with the idea for this book to ask her whether she would be interested in publishing this work. She offered to tell me her experiences and extracts from the emails she sent to me (and my replies to her) are included here.

I think sometimes you have to change, sometimes you don't want to but you have to.
{Ameena}

Yeah but as I say, your priorities completely change. I think, I personally think they should do. I think there's something desperately wrong if your priorities don't change. I seriously think you would need to have a really good re-think of your life if things don't change. Because things <u>do</u> need to change.
Had you any idea how they would change?
Oh God no! [Laughs]
Do you think if somebody had told you how they would change you would still have gone ahead and had him?
Yeah I think you would. I mean, I do, yeah.
So you don't think that being forewarned would be too terrifying?
No, because there are so many pluses from it. I mean you, you talk about the down sides of it but like there are so many positives, there really are.
{Julia}

Yes, so a major change, although a reluctant one, it is a positive one! [Laughs]
{Helen}

Dear Sandra,
I've been reading your proposal and I must say that as a mother who went through rather bad postnatal depression (albeit 20 years ago now) it is both interesting and a project to be encouraged. Unfortunately, I don't think XXXXX is the right publisher for you.
I must stress that I personally think it's a great topic. Looking back, one of the biggest factors in my depression was to do with not being able to fulfil the expectations I had both in the actual delivery room and when the baby and I went home. However, most of those expectations were very much influenced by "doing woman", i.e. trying to be what society deemed I should be as a mother rather than anything to do with factual information from medical sources. So typically, when I didn't feel overflowing with love for my baby and resented the time he took up, I felt guilty and inadequate.
I'm not trying to say that the sort of book you want to write won't help because I think

Concluding thoughts

that simply by making it more common knowledge that motherhood CAN be like this should help to either change women's expectations or society's or both. But I also think that society and women's role within it has an awful lot of blame to answer for.
Sue.

Hi Sue,
Thanks for your encouraging comments. I'm glad that you also think there is a place for a book that tells the <u>whole</u> story. Dare I ask if you sought help for your feelings after having your son?! Did you even know you might not always feel 'blooming marvelous' as a new mum? Hopefully more women will feel less guilty and other women will stop setting them up for a fall when my book gets out there. Optimism springs eternal!
Sandra.

Hi again!
Yes, I'm sure it would've helped to have known more. I didn't seek help for 2 reasons. First, because I realised the GP would just send me home with Valium or something and second, because I really believed it was my own inability to cope that was the problem and I couldn't see what could be done to make me more worthy of the name "mother". I used to torture myself with the thought that women had twins, yet I couldn't manage one healthy baby. That my Mum lived in a house with no bathroom, no running hot water, fridge, etc yet coped with 2 babies only 15 months apart and here I was with a washing machine and all mod cons and still a failure.
I was very depressed for about 6 months. I seriously considered suicide, but couldn't think how I could do it painlessly enough. I kept wishing we had a garage, so I could sit in it with the car engine running. Luckily, I hadn't heard about the trick of running a tube from the exhaust to the car interior. I also felt that it was my duty to make sure the baby was OK, since I'd deliberately conceived and I wasn't convinced his father would cope at all. My family were all over 100 miles away and wouldn't have been able to very easily step in for various reasons, either. So I told myself I'd made my bed and would have to lie on it for a bit longer at least.
When he was about 6 months old, I saw a card in the local newsagent advertising a mother and baby group in a local church hall. I knew I was desperately lonely; I used to look forward to talking to the checkout girl at the local supermarket, so I plucked up courage and went along. There I met other Mums and found out that their babes weren't perfect either, so began the long road to recovery. I think the worst of it was over after 12 months and I'm sure it has made me a stronger person now, but I wouldn't want anyone to go through that.
I think the baby's personality is also a factor. This one was and still is "awkward born" as Mother would say, whereas his younger brother (yes, eventually I did it again) is about 100 times an easier person to deal with. I never experienced the joy of motherhood until the younger one came along. Some babies cry a lot and resist physical comforting and

Nine Women, Nine Months, Nine Lives

that's extremely unrewarding - especially when you're determined to breastfeed on demand. I also now know that a vicious cycle can be set up with a depressed mother and baby. I saw a documentary about it on TV only a few years ago and I was in tears because it mirrored so closely my own experience with Nick.

Basically, I think I've learned to take control of my life rather than vice versa and not live by other people's rules, only my own.

Sue.

Nearly every woman who has had a child has her own unique story to tell about that experience. You will have one too. If you are reading this whilst you are pregnant, I hope it will be a very happy one.

Acknowledgements

Quite simply, this book would not have been possible without the contributions of the nine women. I would like to thank them all and their families for their irreplaceable and immeasurably valuable participation. Thank you.

On a more personal note, to all those good friends and family that I love dearly, and especially to my darling boy for his belief in me and his unswerving and much appreciated support.

Nine Women, Nine Months, Nine Lives

Index

A

Age
    Biological Clock 19
    Maturity 14, 73, 86, 87, 88, 89
    Mellowing 86
    Thirty Years Old 12, 19, 85
    Young 19, 20, 24, 37, 48, 50, 63, 78, 103
Alex 5, 15, 59, 60, 79, 81, 89, 95
Ameena (See Yusuf and Ayesha) . . . .
    5, 9, 24, 25, 26, 27, 28, 29, 32, 36, 40, 41, 42, 46, 47, 48, 51, 53, 54, 59, 60, 61, 63,
               64, 72, 73, 75, 77, 78, 83, 84, 88, 94, 97, 98, 103, 104, 105, 110
Anger 16, 52
Antenatal Classes 29, 32, 38
    National Childbirth Trust 32, 39
    Parentcraft 29, 32, 38, 39, 43, 51, 55, 102
Anthony 4, 12, 39, 40, 41, 67, 80, 88
Anxiety 7, 10, 12, 27, 33, 79
Assisted Delivery 33
    Ventouse and Forceps 30, 33, 37, 43, 46
Asthma
    Baby 53
Avoidance 27, 28, 46, 48, 50
Ayesha 5, 36, 53, 54, 60, 61, 62, 77, 94

B

Bathing the Baby 41, 61
Benefits 2, 15, 75, 80
Maintenance 15, 90
Bills 15
Birth
    Contractions 28, 29, 30, 31, 33, 43
    Episiotomy 29, 46
    Labour 24, 28, 29, 30, 31, 32, 33, 41, 42, 43, 62
    Stitches 29, 30, 47
Bond
    Baby and Parent 48, 49, 64, 77, 100
Breathing Problems
    Baby 3, 34

115

C

Caesarean Section. 4, 30
    Emergency Caesarean Section 4, 30
Career/Work. . . . .
    1, 3, 4, 5, 9, 10, 11, 17, 18, 20, 21, 32, 38, 42, 43, 48, 51, 53, 54, 56, 62, 63, 64, 65,
    66, 67, 68, 69, 72, 73, 74, 75, 76, 77, 78, 79, 80, 81, 82, 83, 84, 85, 88, 91, 92, 98,
                                                                                                                              100, 104, 105, 110
    Career Woman 3, 10
    Employers 11
    Maternity Leave 74, 77, 79, 80
Change . . . .
    1, 3, 4, 7, 9, 11, 14, 18, 19, 20, 21, 38, 40, 43, 48, 57, 58, 61, 62, 63, 64, 71, 72, 73,
    74, 77, 81, 85, 86, 87, 88, 89, 90, 91, 92, 93, 94, 95, 96, 103, 104, 105, 109, 110, 111
    Gradual 86
    Permanent 71, 73
    Spontaneous. 74, 81, 93
    Temporary 3
Chaos. 52
Charlie. 5, 60, 63, 74, 78, 84, 88, 95, 104
Child Care 78, 80, 81
    Babysitter. 85
    Child Minder 78
    Nursery. 75, 78, 84, 109
Claire (See Tom and Hannah). . . . .
    4, 8, 24, 25, 26, 29, 30, 31, 36, 40, 46, 47, 48, 51, 52, 59, 60, 66, 67, 72, 73, 80, 81,
        83, 84, 87, 92, 94, 98, 101, 102, 104, 105, 107, 108
Colic. 52, 53, 55
Commitment. 45
Common Sense. 50, 51
Communication . . . .
    10, 17, 19, 21, 28, 37, 38, 39, 40, 60, 61, 62, 63, 64, 65, 66,67, 68,
        80, 83, 87, 88, 90, 92, 95, 108, 110, 111
Concern
    The usual concerns 11, 33, 38, 46, 74
Confidence 4, 47, 73, 77
Conflict. 4, 5, 50, 64, 78, 90
Confusion. 10
Contentment 72, 74, 97, 103, 104
Contraception 9
    The Pill. 8, 16, 17, 18, 20

Index

Control 26, 33, 112
    Out of control. 33
Coping 21, 27, 28, 33, 41, 42, 51, 55, 58, 59, 76, 82, 83, 84, 97, 103, 109, 111
Crying
    Mother and Baby 35, 36, 49, 52, 53, 55, 60, 68, 74, 111
Culture
    Cultural perceptions. 36
Curious. 38, 95

D

Daniel 5, 54, 56, 60, 64, 79, 85, 90, 91, 99, 100, 105, 108, 109
Daughters. . . . .
        3, 4, 5, 13, 27, 34, 36, 40, 41, 42, 46, 48, 57, 58, 60, 61, 66, 77, 82, 83,
        92, 98, 108, 111
Day to Day Care. 3, 21, 45, 51, 55, 63, 65, 68, 69, 71, 97
Decision
    To have the baby . . . .
        4, 5, 7, 8, 9, 10, 11, 12, 15,16, 18, 19, 20, 28, 30, 33, 39,40, 54,
        61, 65, 74, 77, 78, 98
Dependence 47, 55, 90
Disappointment
    Feelings of 27, 38, 43
Discomfort. 40
Distress. 30, 33, 34, 41
Doctor Care. 13, 19, 20, 30, 54
Due Date 28, 32
    Induction. 28, 30, 32, 33, 37, 41, 46
    Overdue. 54

E

Eczema
    Baby. 53, 54, 77
Embarrassment. 26, 39
Emma (See Neil and Lotte) . . . .
        3, 10, 11, 23, 25, 26, 27, 33, 34, 35, 38, 39, 40, 41, 46, 48,
        56, 57, 59, 60, 65, 72, 73, 74, 75, 83, 86, 91, 92, 98, 100, 101, 104, 105

117

Emotional Aspects 18, 23, 25, 38, 39, 40, 41, 42, 45, 50
Emotions
   Mixed Emotions 3, 11, 33, 45, 108
   Mood Swings. 37
Enjoyment 3, 25, 29, 48, 50, 59, 62, 64, 77, 78, 83, 90, 99
Excitement 12, 33, 43, 49
Exhaustion/Tiredness . . . .
   6, 30, 31, 32, 35, 36, 43, 46, 48, 49, 50, 53, 54, 58, 59, 62, 68, 72, 77, 79, 85, 91, 99
Expectations. . . . .
       3, 5, 12, 23, 24, 25, 27, 30, 31, 33, 38, 40,43, 45, 47, 48, 49, 52, 53, 54, 56,
                57, 58, 59, 61, 65, 67, 68, 69, 79, 103, 109, 110, 111
   Realistic Expectations 25
Experiences
   Actual Experiences 3, 22, 25, 27, 47, 59, 66, 107
   Negative 18, 26, 27, 31, 48, 49, 93, 109
   Positive. 7, 9, 11, 13, 21, 24, 27, 33, 39, 48, 55, 87, 98, 104, 109, 110
   Variety of Experiences 27

F

Family . . . .
      2, 3, 4, 5, 8, 10, 11, 12, 24, 28, 38, 49, 53, 54, 57, 60, 65, 67, 73, 77, 83, 86,
                        90, 91, 98, 99, 109, 111, 113
Fatherhood
   Becoming a Father 4, 13, 14, 57, 58, 65, 111
Feeding
   Bottle. 49, 50
   Breast. 35
      Comfort feeding. 49
   Night Feeds 58, 59, 61, 68
Feelings
   Floaty. 24, 48
   Lovely. 24, 28, 32, 36, 48, 60, 80
   Magical 35
Flexibility. 43, 66
Friends. 2, 8, 10, 15, 16, 17, 19, 20, 48, 49, 53, 58, 59, 71, 73, 82, 89, 91, 113
   Best Friends 10, 19, 20
Frustration. 16, 45, 50, 52, 105, 107
Future, the 2, 5, 9, 20, 24, 37, 38, 43, 47, 48, 96, 97, 98, 100, 101, 102, 105

Index

G

Guilt 39, 53, 54, 56, 61, 62, 64, 78, 83, 84, 85, 99, 110, 111

H

Hannah 4, 8, 60, 66, 67, 80, 81, 87, 92, 93, 94, 102, 108
Happiness. . . . .
    8, 9, 10, 12, 13, 14, 35, 36, 37, 53, 62, 67, 74,78, 81, 83, 88, 90, 98, 99, 100, 101, 112
    Laughter. 29, 36, 42, 88
Heartache. 7
Helen (See Richard and Will). . . . .
    4, 9, 10, 16, 22, 23, 25, 26, 28, 31, 32, 35, 38, 39, 42, 46, 47, 48, 50, 51, 59, 60, 65, 66, 67, 72, 73, 75, 76, 82, 83, 87, 91, 93, 98, 104, 105, 110
Hindsight 2, 10, 64
Holding the Baby 17, 30, 31, 32, 34, 35, 36, 42, 46, 47, 55, 59, 60, 97, 103
Honesty 17, 27, 34, 55, 99, 102, 104, 108
Honeymoon 8
Hopes and Fears. . . . .
    9, 10, 15, 16, 20, 23, 27, 28, 29, 31, 34, 35, 38, 40,41, 42, 43, 48, 79, 80, 94, 97, 98, 100, 101, 102, 103, 112
Horror Stories. 26, 27, 107
Hospital 3, 29, 32, 34, 38, 39, 41, 43, 57, 65, 68, 98
    Hospital Tour. 38
Housework 58, 63, 77, 78, 83, 84

I

Inadequacy
    Feelings of. 2, 33, 110
Independence 73, 91, 104, 105
Infertility 98
    Endometriosis. 92, 93, 98
    Fertility Treatment 5, 7, 25
Information 2, 27, 28, 48, 50, 110
    Books and Magazines . . . .
        1, 2, 3, 6, 27, 47, 60, 90, 91, 96, 103, 104, 107, 109, 110, 111, 113
Instinct 49
Isolation 48, 52, 59

119

Nine Women, Nine Months, Nine Lives

J

Jack 4, 52, 60, 68, 80, 81, 89, 94
James 5, 11, 12, 32, 39, 43, 49, 61, 63, 78, 88, 95
Julia (See Matt and Daniel) . . . .
        5, 6, 7, 8, 23, 24, 25, 26, 27, 28, 29, 32,35, 38, 42, 43, 46, 47, 48, 51, 54,
        56, 60, 61, 64, 72, 73, 75,79, 85, 88, 90, 91, 98, 100, 105, 107, 109, 110

K

Katie 4, 14, 36, 38, 42, 57, 60, 80, 81, 82

L

Leicester General Hospital 1
Living Together 11, 12, 13, 15, 21
Lonely 59, 111
Lotte 3, 34, 41, 48, 56, 57, 60, 65, 75, 83, 86, 92, 98, 100, 101
Love 5, 49, 58, 60, 72, 88, 110, 113
    Loved 5, 24, 35, 60
    Loving 86

M

Marriage 4, 5, 7, 8, 9, 18, 21, 22, 24, 88, 90, 93, 98, 100
Matt 5, 8, 29, 38, 42, 43, 54, 56, 60, 61, 64, 88, 90, 91, 98, 99, 100
Midwifery Care 29, 31, 32, 37
Money/Finances 15, 73, 76, 77, 78, 79, 85
Morning Sickness 17, 24, 31, 108
Mother and Baby Groups 48
Motherhood . . . .
        1, 4, 5, 9, 22, 45, 46, 47, 48, 49, 50, 53, 54,56, 57, 58, 59, 65, 71, 72,
        73, 74, 103, 107, 111
    Becoming a Mum, ...
        13, 14, 15, 24, 41, 42, 48, 49, 50, 53, 56, 62, 65, 66, 72, 75, 77,
        78, 81, 82, 83, 91, 93, 98, 104, 105, 107, 108, 109, 111
    Their Own Mum 13, 15, 42, 49, 50, 65, 66, 75, 77, 78, 91, 93, 109
Moving House 5, 11, 30, 52, 55, 82

Index

N

Nappy Changing 15, 61, 62, 63, 68
Natural Birth
   Vaginal Delivery 31, 37
Natural/Normal 2, 20, 25, 27, 62, 98, 100
Needles 30, 33, 41, 76
   Needle Phobic 33
Neil 3, 34, 38, 40, 57, 65, 83, 92, 100
Neonatal Intensive Care Unit
   Leicester General Hospital 34

O

Open Mind
   Keeping an Open Mind 30, 63, 65, 66, 67
Optimism 2, 48, 51, 59

P

Pain 27, 28, 29, 31, 32, 33, 35, 40, 46, 47, 55, 59
   Pain Relief 28, 29, 31, 33, 46
   Epidural 28, 29, 30, 31, 33
   Gas and Air 29, 33
   Side Effects 28, 33, 46, 47, 73, 98
   TENS Machines 32
Panic 27, 30, 42, 54, 55, 56, 108
Parenthood 4, 10, 61, 64, 65, 66, 69, 71, 86, 89, 91, 92
Patience 72, 74, 86, 89, 105
Paul 5, 61, 81, 88, 89, 105
Perfection 51, 55, 56, 64, 91, 108, 111
Periods 8, 10, 18, 28, 43, 62, 109
Pessimism 2, 48, 49, 59
Physical Aspects .. 1, 20, 23, 24, 25, 26, 31, 38, 45, 46, 50, 54, 61, 79, 80, 92, 98, 111
Play 48, 50, 61, 62, 64, 84, 88, 89, 94
Pleasure 7, 12, 60, 108
Possibility 10, 20, 27, 47, 80, 98
Pregnancy
   Planned 7, 8, 10, 11, 13, 16, 23, 24, 25, 38, 61, 64, 65, 75, 81, 108
   Pregnancy Test 1, 7, 8, 9, 10, 11, 12, 13, 15, 16, 17, 20
   Unplanned 25

121

Nine Women, Nine Months, Nine Lives

Preparing for Parenthood 1, 102
Pressure
   Peer and Family 49, 53, 56, 90, 91
Private Care 31, 89
Promises.. 64
Protective Feelings 27, 60
Proud 49, 77, 104
   Pride 36, 49

R

Rachel (See James and Charlie) ....
                5, 11, 12, 24, 26, 32, 33, 35, 39, 43, 46, 47, 48, 49, 50, 59, 60,
                61, 63, 72, 73, 74, 75, 78, 79, 84, 85, 88, 92, 95, 98, 104, 105
Reaction
   First Reaction.. 14, 15, 103
   Negative Reaction 13, 92
      Violence... 13
   Positive Reaction 13, 48
   Shock 3, 7, 8, 9, 11, 12, 16, 18, 30, 35, 39, 43, 50, 51, 57, 62, 66, 95
   Surprise......................... 28, 29, 35, 36, 38, 43, 51, 59, 78, 87, 95
   To the Pregnancy 7, 9, 11, 12, 13, 14, 15, 16, 18, 19, 21, 40, 102, 103
Reassurance 3, 34
Regret.. 56
Relationships 5, 6, 12, 13, 69, 74, 81, 85, 86, 88, 89, 90, 91, 92, 93, 94, 95, 103
   Good 12, 91, 92
Relaxation 3, 48, 55, 57, 73, 82, 83
Relief, feelings of............................ 12, 28, 29, 31, 32, 33, 36, 46
Resentment.. 51
Responsibility......................... 18, 20, 45, 61, 62, 68, 73, 81, 88, 104
Returning to Education 79, 80, 82
Rewards 49, 60
Richard 4, 17, 18, 19, 20, 21, 31, 32, 39, 42, 50, 51, 65, 66, 75, 76, 82

S

Sadie (See Paul and Alex)..
                5, 15, 16, 24, 26, 27, 35, 37, 42, 46, 48, 58, 59, 60, 61, 72,
                73, 74, 79, 81, 88, 89, 95, 98, 103, 104, 105
Sarah (See Anthony and Jack) ....
                4, 12, 13, 24, 25, 26, 33, 35, 39, 40, 41, 46, 47, 48, 51,
              52, 53, 59, 60, 67, 69, 72, 73, 74, 80, 81, 87, 88, 89, 94, 98, 104, 105

Index

Security 21
Sensitivity 27, 60, 108
Sex 56, 72
Sleeplessness
   Baby and Mother 25, 50, 53, 57, 59
Smile
   Baby's First 60, 90
Sons . . . .
       4, 5, 10, 11, 32, 33, 35, 52, 58, 60, 61, 63, 65, 68, 75, 78, 79,80, 85, 90, 98,
       108, 111, 113
Support 5, 15, 23, 37, 38, 39, 40, 41, 42, 43, 65, 73, 76, 77, 85, 91, 113
   Supportive Behaviour 37, 38, 39, 40, 42, 43, 65
Survival 3, 27, 29, 48, 76, 95, 109

T

Tanya (See Katie) . . . .
       4, 13, 15, 24, 26, 27, 30, 31, 36, 38, 42, 46, 47, 48, 57, 58, 59, 60,
       61, 72, 73, 74, 80, 81, 82, 85, 98, 104, 105
Termination of Pregnancy/Abortion 10, 13, 14, 16, 19, 20, 22
   Moral Dilemma 10, 16
Time . . . .
    2, 3, 4, 5, 6, 7, 8, 9, 10, 11, 13, 14, 15, 16, 17, 18, 19, 20, 21, 22, 23,24, 29, 32, 34,
    35, 36, 37, 38, 39, 40, 42, 43, 45, 46, 48, 49, 50, 51, 52, 53, 54, 55, 54, 55, 56,
    57, 59, 60, 61, 62, 63, 64, 65, 66, 67, 68, 73, 74, 75, 76, 77, 78, 79, 80, 81, 82,
    83, 84, 85, 87, 88, 89, 90, 91, 92, 93, 94, 96, 97, 98, 99, 100, 104, 105, 110
   Spare Time 57, 81, 82, 83, 84, 85, 90, 98, 104
Tom 4, 40, 66, 67, 80, 81, 92, 98, 102
Trauma 33

U

Ultrasound Scan 38, 39, 40
Uncertainty 31, 39
University of Leicester
   Academic Department of Psychiatry 1

V

Visitors
   When you come home 49, 50, 52, 101

W

Waters
   Breaking the waters... 28, 33, 34
   Meconium Stained Liquor 34
Will 4, 50, 60, 65, 75, 76, 78, 97
Worry 8, 12, 15, 18, 25, 28, 29, 31, 34, 42, 47, 53, 55, 62, 64, 73, 78, 93, 105

Y

Yusuf 5, 9, 28, 40, 41, 42, 54, 61, 62, 63, 87

Our Conversations

There follows eight out of the nine very frank and very honest complete conversations about the transition to motherhood for the first time. Julia requested that our full conversation was not included in the book for her own and her husband's personal reasons. Due to the fact that the transcriptions of the conversations obviously consist of spoken English, they are not grammatically correct. As a consequence they could have been a little difficult to read in places.

To limit the off-putting effect that this may have had on you the reader, the punctuation of the text has been exaggerated to try and enhance the emphases placed by the women in their speech. To clarify things further additional words have been added (sparingly) and are indicated by curved brackets. Laughter and non-verbal behaviour that convey feelings [such as shoulder shrugging and head shaking] are indicated by square brackets. Pauses for thought lasting a couple of seconds or longer… are indicated by three continuous dots. The women's words have not been altered in any other way.

Nine Women, Nine Months, Nine Lives

Emma

Emma was 31 years old when she found that she was pregnant. She had never really thought about having children. She has a long-term partner whom she lives with and considered herself to be a career woman. Whilst being shocked and unsure about the pregnancy herself, her partner just incorporated it into their life together. Their daughter Lotte was very small and had breathing problems when she was born and spent the first month of her life in the Special care baby unit at Leicester General Hospital. Nevertheless, Emma and her family have survived to tell the tale and continue to grow stronger everyday.

Thinking back to when you found out you were pregnant. Now, were you trying to get pregnant at the time?
No! [Laughs]
No, you weren't at all, were you?
No, no.
And you weren't planning on having children?
No.
Had you thought about it as a possibility? Were you dead against it?
Err, well, we weren't dead against it, just, we hadn't decided. Do you know what I mean? I don't think we'd even. We'd talked about it but we weren't, errm… It wasn't like imminent that we were going to have children.

Nine Women, Nine Months, Nine Lives

So would you say it was something you just hadn't thought about rather than something you'd decided you weren't going to do?
I think we'd both decided that we weren't going to do it, but I think we were both pleased we did! [Laughs] Do you know what I mean? [Laughs] When it came to finding out that I was actually pregnant we were both happy about it, yeah we were. [Laughs] We were both happy about it so… I think deep down we both really did want them but didn't really want to admit it I suppose, if that makes sense?
Yeah. Can you remember what went through your mind when you found out you were actually pregnant, when you saw those two lines on the test?
"How am I going to tell him?" [Laughs]
So he wasn't actually with you when you did the test?
No.
Had you said to him, I think I might be or…?
No.
So you hadn't mentioned it at all?
No.
Had he noticed? [Laughs]
No! [Laughs]
Oh God! Right, OK, So…
Well he was working away, and it's not something he would really notice.
Oh right, so he wouldn't have been around to see or notice it?
No.
So, that was your initial reaction, what did you then think afterwards? Was it the more immediate things like how am I going to tell him or was it more what am I going to do? Or what are we going to do?
It was "how am I going to tell him?" to start with, and I thought "Well, I'll get that over with"! [Laughs] Errm… I don't think we really doubted what we were going to do at all, it was "Oh fine" you know, and that was that.
How suspicious were you that you were pregnant? Had you thought "I must be pregnant"? Because obviously you did the test so you must have had an idea?
Not till I was 9 weeks pregnant.
9 weeks pregnant? That's still quite early, I mean the people who do the test 2 minutes after they were due on tend to be those who are really really planning it. Had you spent 9 weeks worrying about it or rather 6 weeks…?
No, I got to about 7 and I thought, it was only 'till I got to about then that I thought "Oh, something's not happening here"! [Laughs] And then of course I left it another week just in case I'd got my dates wrong from the month before, and then when it didn't happen again, I was like, "It's time!"
So did you want to talk to him about, "Oh God what if I am?", or did you just…?
I wasn't sure how he would react. Errm… But I thought "Well the sooner I tell him the better".

Emma

So did you have two extremes of how you thought he would react?
Yeah.
You did?
Yeah.
So you thought this could be quite a major…?
Yes, it's a major, well it is and it could have been. I think if you are planning it then it is, but if you're not…[Laughs]
I suppose in a way it's kind of like feelings that haven't been dealt with, you just don't know. Is that how, do you think you felt that way?
That's right, mmm, definitely.
I suppose if you weren't sure, then adding into the equation him not being sure, that could become, shall we say, doubly confusing?
Yes! [Laughs]
So no one was with you when you did the test?
No.
So what was his reaction when you told him? Did you tell him face-to-face?
No! On the telephone. [Laughs]
Oh you didn't?! [Laughs]
Yeah! Like I say he was working away, and I'd been to the doctor's before I even told him.
So you did a home test?
And then an appointment to see the doctor as well. And errm… It's strange really because I rang him and I said "I've got something to tell you" and he just laughed and said "Have you?" and I said "Yeah… Why?" And he said "Oh I can guess - I'll talk to you when I get home". He was coming home that night and errm… He knew! [Shrugs shoulders]
Bloody hell!
Just by my phoning him and saying "I've got something to tell you".
And the tone of your voice and the sheer panic! [Laughs]
Yeah! [Laughs] And then he rang me later in the office and he said "Are you alright?" And I said "Yeah, yeah, I'm fine" and he said "All right then, I'll see you later" which is <u>totally</u> out of character.
Really?
Mmm, to say "Are you all right?" you know, and that sort of cockiness in his voice! [Laughs] I think he had guessed before I admitted to it.
Do you think you had behaved differently when you were thinking "God I ought to do a test".
Yes.
So he'd perhaps picked up then that…?
Yeah, probably.
So how did he react then when he got back?
Oh he was fine! He said to me "So what have you got to tell me then?" and I said "It

129

doesn't really matter" because by then I thought "I can't do this"! [Laughs] And he just said "Oh, oh, all right then" and then "Well are you or not?" [Laughs] And I said "Yes" and he said "Oh, fine" and then "OK, when?" and it just went on like that.
Really? It just got accepted and incorporated?
Yeah, we just got on with it. And then of course he wanted to know everything, all the ins and outs and what I'd been doing…
Yeah of course. So had you not seen each other for quite a while then?
Errm, he was working away about 5 days a week then, including weekends, you see.
Oh right, so it was difficult.
So I hadn't seen him for about 5 days. So there you go.
The next section is your experience of pregnancy and the birth. I remember you had really bad morning sickness, didn't you?
Yeah but it didn't start until about 4 or 5 months, I was about halfway through.
Yeah, OK. What I'd like you to do is think back to before you were pregnant. How did you imagine you would feel being pregnant? Did you ever imagine?
No.
You'd never really thought about having children?
No, no I don't think I did. I saw my sister go through it exactly a year before, and she was fine, she didn't have any problems at all.
Not that you knew of?
No not that I knew of, she used to be fine really.
OK. So you hadn't really thought about it before?
No.
What about say in the early weeks, did you sort of think "If I feel like this now, it'll be a breeze or it'll be awful?"
Not really.
So you found out really when you were 9 weeks pregnant, so that's early in your pregnancy with no real symptoms to speak of. Did you find yourself wondering how you would feel later in your pregnancy? I mean did you think when you found out "My God my stomach's going to be out here…!"
I don't think it really worried me actually, no.
Did you think about how you would feel? Not just physically, did you think…?
Errm… Not really, I think I thought "Well if I do get morning sickness I'm going to have problems with work" because I do have to get up early in the mornings, and that was about it really. You know, you get the books out and think "I don't feel like that"! And then when you start reading the horror stories about birth that's when you don't even read them any more, you just put them to one-side! [Laughs]
So, you had no idea about birth or anything like that beforehand, you'd never thought about it?
No.
Well why would you?! So you didn't think about it before you were pregnant. But whilst

Emma

you were pregnant, I mean you must have wondered? You say you read a horror story - was it just one?
Yeah, just one, it was in a magazine. But I've got a lot of friends and people I work with who have had children, and you actually do hear you know birth and pregnancy horror stories, but that's about it really.
There wasn't anything that you thought "I'm really looking forward to that" or "God I hope that doesn't happen to me"!
I wasn't really looking forward to if I had to have a caesarean.
Was that a possibility?
It was towards the end. Round about December my hands started to swell up and my feet, really badly, so it was mentioned. I had an appointment at the hospital Christmas eve and one again in January but it had all gone by then so…But when it was mentioned I thought "Oohh no!"
What was it, was it because it is an operation?
Mmm yeah, I was terrified. Needles. I'm needle-phobic. [Laughs]
Really? I mean when you gave birth to Lotte you were bound to have needles or something like that near you. You didn't have to have an epidural did you?
No, no I didn't have an epidural but I was induced so, I had that thing in my hand.
The venflon?
Mmm, I looked the other way, but I was so out of it on gas and air…
You didn't really know what they were doing?
No, but I didn't look!
As long as they took the pain away you weren't bothered?
No!
So your actual experiences were they, did you think they were average? I mean you've heard other people's experiences and things, do you think there was anything about your birth that was particularly good or particularly bad?
Errm…
From your point of view, I mean I know obviously that Lotte was poorly and that was very distressing…
Errm…From my point of view everyone says you know when they give you the baby and you spend some time together, I missed all that, I didn't have any of that.
Was she rushed straight off down to Intensive Care?
Yes, yeah, so I think I missed that. I would have liked that I think, you know everyone says (how nice that is) and I have to say "No, I didn't have that". Yeah I did miss that, when people talk about that. And of course my sister had had her baby about a year before so I went to see her in hospital the next day and there were all these families sort of thing and I didn't get any of that really. So, I think I missed that bit.
Was there anything that you got unexpectedly that was good?
I met a lot of nice people, although I know that sounds strange but yeah. And I forged a very good friendship with a girl that had got a little boy on the ward. Errm… And I learnt

131

Nine Women, Nine Months, Nine Lives

a lot about myself really because if somebody had said to me "Oh you'll have to drip feed her", I'd have said "No that's not me". But I just got on with it and did as much as I could really.
Yeah, you dealt with it when it happened.
That's right, and I think I learnt quite a lot about myself really.
OK. So how did you feel when you first held your baby? With Lotte being in Intensive Care and everything, how long was it after you had had her that you actually got to hold her?
They gave me her as soon as she was born and we settled...
Do you remember it very clearly?
I don't remember much at all to be honest! I know I held her and that's all I know and that's because Neil told me. And then she started to have breathing problems again so they took her. She was 6 days old before I held her. She had wires and things coming out of her and I think I was more worried about pulling them out or making something go off than holding her close. I didn't hold her for long. Yeah it was 5 or 6 days I think it was.
And you felt pretty scared about the fact there were all these wires and things coming out of her...?
Yeah, and she was so long and so thin that I thought if I hug her tight I might break her, does that...? [Laughs]
Yeah, yeah, of course! [Laughs]
She was really really really really thin, I thought I'd better not hug too tight. But I wanted to.
Yeah, to hold her and squeeze her.
To let her know "you're all right".
Yeah, as reassurance.
Yeah that was what I was worried about. But errm... They were very good all around me. (The staff at Leicester General Hospital) So, yeah, they were very good.
So when was the first time, would you say, that you really got to hold Lotte?
Probably after she, when she was about 8 or 9 days old really. Yeah, she still had the nasal thing in but she wasn't, there weren't heart monitors, well there were but you know it was a lot easier because they would all tuck up, so yeah, she was about 8 days old.
And how did that feel?
Lovely! [Laughs]
Yeah I'll bet.
And she was awake as well, which was lovely.
She's always awake – every time I see her!
She doesn't sleep! [Laughs] Yeah, so it was really nice.
And Neil, he obviously must have held her as well. Did you talk about the fact that when you held her the first few times you felt like, you know, you didn't want to break her and things like that? Was he with you?

Emma

Neil didn't want to hold her until she was a bit older because he's quite stocky and he was even more worried, so errmm… And he doesn't like hospitals either, no he hates hospitals. I don't know why but he doesn't like the smell or anything like that. He wasn't planning on being at the birth either.
Oh that's right!
So when he saw her for the first time, because he went home to tell my mum there had been problems and whatever, he was like "Oh no!". Yeah he didn't stay very long. I don't think he handled it very well to be quite honest. But yeah, he got there in the end.
Yeah, I mean it must have been very difficult. It was horrendous for you, it was difficult for him, I mean…
He doesn't show his feelings very much.
I was going to say, did you manage to sort of acknowledge that you were feeling differently, even if you didn't sit down and say "Well tell me how you felt about this, that and the other?"
We did sit and talk, yeah we did, that weekend.
You did communicate about it.
He doesn't normally show his feelings, but he did over this, actually got emotional.
It's a shame really.
These things happen.
And she's all right now, so that's a good thing.
Yeah, yeah.
OK… In what ways was your partner involved in the pregnancy and birth of your first child? So if we concentrate on the pregnancy side of things. You said that he just sort of accepted it and asked you about things, was he curious?
He went to the (Ultrasound) Scan with me, didn't go to any of the classes because they were all like when he was working, which was difficult, but I went to a few day classes.
Did he want to?
Yeah he did, but of course he couldn't get to them. Didn't come to any of my appointments, but again it was when he was working. But he always rang me if I'd been to find out what was going on and all that sort of stuff. We went for the hospital tour together.
Oh yeah right, to see where you would have her. So was he curious about what was happening to you and the changes that were happening to you?
Yeah, because I couldn't sleep on my back at all, and I kept sleeping on my side and he said "Don't you ever sleep on your back at all?" and I said "No I can't lie there". And she was terrible, she used to lie all the way down one side, so I could only lie on my left side as well, and he would be like "Why?!" and I'd explain. So yeah he did take quite an interest.
Was he, I mean you say that he didn't want to be there at the birth, did you talk about that, did you want him there, was it a kind of a thing where…?
I did but I can't think why I did now! [Laughs] Errm… I did want him there when I first fell pregnant, then I didn't in the middle!

133

Nine Women, Nine Months, Nine Lives

Did you think your reasons changed for wanting him there?
Errm... I was scared when I first found out I was pregnant, that was why I wanted him there, and then I thought "oh no, no, I don't want him there!"
Was that when you read your horror stories? [Laughs]
Yeah! [Laughs] I thought I might want to hit him, then I thought he'd probably hit me back! [Laughter] Not that he ever has but you know... [Laughs]
No but... [Laughs]
I thought "Oh no, I can't get into a fight while I'm giving birth!" And then towards the end I thought "Oh no it might be nice if we were, you know, all there". Yeah, that's about it really, I did want him there in the end.
Were you glad he was there?
Errm... Yes and no actually. He wasn't much of a help! [Laughs] But then I wasn't expecting that anyway, I think it was just because I was a bit scared towards the end and I had been in labour for so long that I just wanted somebody there that I knew really.
How long was your labour?
27 hours from the first contraction. I think I'd still be there now if they hadn't induced me! [Laughs]
I don't think you would be! [Laughs]
I kept thinking "Oh come on, I don't want a caesarean, and they'll give me one in a minute". But no, I didn't have one. My mum had one when I was born, like mother like daughter I thought! [Laughs]
No, no not necessarily, sometimes it can be, but not always. So, he was involved in the birth, in the end. You went into labour naturally then they had to induce you to speed you up a bit more. So did Neil decide that he wanted to be involved in the birth, say a month before you were due or...?
I didn't know until the day, I didn't expect him to turn up at all.
Right and do you think it may have been because it took so long or...?
No he was there early on, it's a bit of a long story! [Laughs] He was at work in Wolverhampton and I went into labour at about half ten, and I rang him to tell him. My dad took me up the hospital and I wasn't expecting him to come across. He got to the hospital at about half eight, and they said to him "There's nothing going to happen tonight you might as well go home". So he came home and they rang him at eight o'clock the next morning to say if you want to come in, come in, and he did, so... But I wasn't expecting him to come back! [Laughs]
You were expecting him to stay out of the way?
Yeah, so he came back and stayed, only left the room once.
Do you think he came to support you? Do you think he came because he thought this is only going to happen once, the first child?
I think he came for me, yeah.
Because he thought you'd been in labour for such a while?
Well I didn't go straight onto the labour ward, because it was full. I went onto the ward

Emma

and pottered around, had a few baths. And errm... I said (to him) "I am absolutely terrified" and I think it was because I actually admitted that to him, that he thought "I'm going to come back".
And has he said anything since the birth?
No because he knows I get upset about it.
Did you kind of get the feeling that he was glad he had been there?
I think so yeah. Just the once he had to go out when it started to get a bit scary, they were taking some blood of Lotte's head with a needle or something because she was in distress and he said he couldn't handle that so...
It was understandable?
Yeah, so he went out which was obviously before she was born, but he was there when she was born.
Yeah. Are you OK? [Upset at this point] These things do work out, don't they?
Yeah, yeah.
OK, Do you think his overall reaction, thinking back to the pregnancy and the birth, do you think that was more or less than you hoped for?
More. Yes, more, a lot more.
Yeah, you sound like you...
Yes I was totally and utterly surprised that he was there, yeah! [Laughs]
You were pleased?
Oh yes, very.
And how was his behaviour different to what you expected? During the pregnancy in particular, which was obviously longer than the birth, although it might not have felt like it! [Laughter] Do you think he was more or less supportive, or maybe supportive in a different way?
A lot more supportive.
On a practical or an emotional level?
Practical, yes, very practical.
You were glad of that?
Yeah I mean he does a lot as it is but yeah he was just brilliant really. "You're not carrying that, I'll do the ironing" - he was very good.
You said that he doesn't really express his emotions very much or talk much about how he feels. Did you feel like you wanted him to or did you feel you knew where you stood and...?
Well I've known for a long time where I've stood. I mean it's just one of those things in a relationship I think. So then if he ever did say anything it was like "Oh right!" [Surprise] And then we would have quite a long conversation, but it wasn't like a continuous conversation we had every day, but you know when we needed to, we did.
So you knew what to expect from him and his responses to things and you didn't feel let down or disappointed in any way?
No not at all, no.

Nine Women, Nine Months, Nine Lives

That's good. Right the next bit is your experience of early motherhood. Yours was one hell of an experience!
Yeah, yeah it was. I wouldn't want <u>anyone</u> to go through it to be honest.
So how long was Lotte in Hospital for?
A month, she was exactly a month old.
Right. Can you think how your pregnancy may have affected early motherhood, say up until the first three months. So things like, if you had had a caesarean you'd have had an operation so you can't lift and you can't drive. Was there anything about your pregnancy at all that meant that you couldn't do things? You weren't unwell towards the end of your pregnancy?
No, no.
You said you had the threat of a caesarean?
Yeah my hands were swollen and my feet, I couldn't wear the same shoes, I had to buy new shoes! [Laughs] But no nothing like that at all.
So your pregnancy didn't really effect early motherhood. Did the birth effect early motherhood? Now this can be taken from all angles, from your experience of it or from the physicality of it, if you had to have stitches, any thing. I mean the birth for you was...
I didn't feel completely a mother until I brought her home.
Mmm, I remember you saying that before.
Because she was like, you just had to leave her and it was just like, I don't know, I don't...
Did you feel like she was yours?
Yes and no. When I was there yes and then when I was at home I thought "Well I know she's there and I know she's mine but..."
You didn't have the evidence, as it were!
No, and it was quite difficult when you were walking around, people knew but they couldn't talk to you.
They were people that knew that Lotte had been born, and they saw that you didn't have her with you, and people would stop or wouldn't stop...?
I think I noticed it more with the neighbors because I obviously, Neil told the neighbours down the road and of course it was like...
Circulated?
You know what it's like. And every morning I'd go see her, and I used to get in the car and I'd see people walking about but nobody dared ask, do you know what I mean? And then as soon as I brought her home I had a houseful, you know, that day. And the couple of days after, they let you settle in and then they were round again.
So how did you feel about that?
I could understand it.
Yes but how did you feel? I mean you can understand but...
A bit hurt.

Emma

Yeah, you can put a brave face on but...
You can only do it for so long.
So did you feel hurt when the neighbours didn't come up to you? You could understand that they were scared, they didn't want to open a can of worms as it were, ask you how she was. Did you feel hurt when they all appeared when you brought her home?
I don't know whether it's so much hurt, I think...
Disappointed?
Yeah, that's probably more, I didn't really know them that well, I knew the couple down the road, but they always waved, do you know what I mean? They always acknowledged the fact I was here and they knew there was a problem and they'd actually come and see Neil, when they knew that I wasn't here as well. Because they knew, well you get to know each other. But I was happy with their concern and that they would make an effort to find out how she was. They were here when she came home, within hours! [Laughs]
(It's) one of those things...
Yeah, it's difficult really, it's one of those things that's, there's not much really you can say about it.
No, it's happened.
OK. Had you imagined how early motherhood would be for you? I know it was very different in reality and you said you'd heard people say things like "Oo when I first held my baby" things like that. You said that for you was very brief and everything was chaos and you didn't know what was happening. Had you got a picture in your mind of what to expect?
Yes, a lot of sleepless nights, feeding, you expect people to come round, you know, you've got the happy picture basically and sharing her basically! [Laughs] So yeah I'd got a good idea of what was going to happen. But we didn't not till later...
Was it about a month/6 week's delay?
Yeah, a month.
And was the reality the way that you expected it to be? I mean it can't all have been, but...
We've had a few problems with her, she doesn't sleep! [Laughs] But she did actually sleep quite early, slept through, and now she's not doing that anymore. But I think it was more or less what I expected it to be really.
And what about Neil, do you think it's more...?
He's from a big family, six, and he's the eldest, so he'd got a good idea. I think it's a lot more demanding, no not a lot more, but a bit more demanding than I thought.
Do you mean in terms of your time or...
She's on the go all the time! My sister's little girl you see she's, when I was pregnant I used to watch her and she's just not as active as Lotte is at all.
So your niece, she could be left for a little while?
Yeah and my sister could get on with things but you can't, no way, she's constantly on the go all the time, she wants attention all the time as well. So it is a bit more demanding

Nine Women, Nine Months, Nine Lives

than I thought.
So is that the biggest thing that you would say is different from what you expected?
Errm...
I suppose the biggest in terms of having the most impact on your everyday life.
Oh my, I can't go anywhere without her now, by the time we've got in the car...!
And it's not just her, it's all her stuff too!
And the other thing is spare time as well. I don't have any anymore, not at all, not with working full-time, no. If she goes to bed early which is a total shock, then I think "Ooo!" I feel like I've won the lottery! [Laughs]
Do you know what to do with yourself? [Laughs]
No I don't!
You should be relaxing!
I tend to think "Oh I have to clean that or do that" but I never do, I just sit down and watch TV! [Pulls a guilty face]
Well that's all right, what's wrong with that? You don't have to pull faces!
It's just nice and quiet.
That's exactly what you're supposed to do with spare time, relax.
Yeah but that's different. Not having spare time.
You should put your feet up.
At the weekends we play catch up, but, you know she's worth it so...
That's the important thing. So how much would you say that it matched up? If you had to superimpose what you had imagined with what you actually have, do you think there's a fairly neat fit or do you think it's kind of...?
I think I'd got a really good idea really, I don't think I was under any kind of "It's not going to change my life" sort of syndrome. [Laughs]
Yeah but I've met a few...
Yeah, but I knew it was going to totally change.
And you seem to have tried to find out a little bit as well, like watching your sister and her daughter.
I didn't want to go totally cold in to it! [Laughs]
You wouldn't go totally cold into anything else in your life?
No, that's right, and this is very very big...
Yeah, lifetime kind of big isn't it really?
Just a bit!
Can you remember what was difficult in the early days or weeks? So let's put a time limit on this, say the first three weeks after you had her, so before you brought her home.
What was difficult?
The most difficult.
Not being able to hold her. I just didn't feel as if there was any real contact. So if there was any chance and they were like "Do you want to get her out?" I was there. I know this sounds strange but I wanted to bath her, but, she was a month old before she had

Emma

her first bath! [Laughs] But there you go. So you know, just general contact, but I knew that everybody else who had had a baby had, so I hadn't known anybody else who hadn't. Not brought them home sort of thing.
It is unusual, yeah, there must be very few people who have been through the same experience as you. I mean I haven't, in nearly four years of working, Lotte staying in hospital four weeks was the longest that any baby that I have known has had to stay in. It must have been very different indeed. I should imagine it must have been incredibly difficult. When you held her were you talking to her and things like that?
I cried the first time I held her. And then I, well, Neil used to sing to her, I used to just rock her and "la, la, la"! [Laughs] I can't sing!
No, neither can I!
So he used to sing to her.
And could you talk to her when she was actually in...?
Oh yeah, well I used to sort of put my head in the little portholes and things. She wasn't actually in that for that long, and then she went into a headbox, and she used to just pull her tubes out all the time, she was known for that. And I used to just laughingly say "you mustn't do that you know" and I'd think if anybody can hear me they'll think I'm crazy! And then the more you were there, the more you realised everybody else was doing it too! [Laughs] You weren't different!
No, no it just goes to show that your natural instincts were...
And they encouraged you to sit and hold them, so.
Yeah of course. So what would you say was the best thing? I know that these 'best things' may be very thin on the ground particularly in those first three weeks but...
Errm... Best thing ... Knowing she was going to live I think. If that makes sense! [Laughs]
It makes perfect sense.
Because to be honest I don't think they were all that sure. When I first saw her she was eight hours old and ...I kept asking to see her but they wouldn't let me see her before that and nobody could really tell me anything until the next morning. I just got "Well we don't think she's going to die but..." So when it got to two or three days and she was making much better progress than we thought...That was probably the best thing when they said to me "Oh no she'll, she'll pull through".
So that took two to three days?
Definitely not when, about the third morning, the third day.
That must have been horrendous.
Mmmm.
Were you actually staying in the hospital until...?
For a week, yeah, I wouldn't go home, and they said to me you know if you want to stay any longer you know you can. But after a week I had had enough, there's only so much hospital food you can take! [Laughs] And errm you know looking at the same four walls, and you keep seeing people coming and going and the girl I became good

139

Nine Women, Nine Months, Nine Lives

friends with she was going the day after, so...I thought I can't stick this on my own, I hadn't got any sort of support when Neil wasn't there or any of my family so I thought no this is... So I went home the day before Jennie did.
That's a pretty big best thing.
Mmm. [Smiles broadly]
In fact it's probably going to be the best 'best thing' I'll have been told. OK, and how much was Neil involved in those first few days? I mean you say he didn't want to hold her because he was worried about, I don't know pulling a tube out or just her breathing or...
The first initial two days we weren't allowed that much contact with her to be quite honest, because it was like minimum, er, minimum contact I think they call it. But after that it was just things like "Oh show me how to do that" like syringe feed and all that sort of stuff you know, and he did actually get involved then.
Was he allowed to take any time off work?
Well, he works, he doesn't work a lot of days so it was more daytime than nighttime. So with us living quite a way away I used to go in in the morning and stay 'till early evening and then I used to come home. And I used to phone before I went to bed just to see how she was so... And then I was up the next morning ready to go. So it was just like the nighttime that she was on her own.
Well she wouldn't have been on her own, all the nurses would have been there.
Well yeah, yeah.
OK. Had you talked about who would do what when you finally got her home? Had you discussed things like who was going to feed her, changing her, who was going to get up in the middle of the night, making up bottles if you ended up bottle feeding, you know...?
I think we'd decided we would try and split it. Because the original plan before anything was that I was going to go back to work about three months after I'd had her. And so we'd sort of got this plan that Neil would have her when he was at home and my mum would have her the rest of the time, it was all sorted, it was all planned. Errmm, we'd decided we were going to split the night duty! [Laughs] Half-and-half where I would do it one night or perhaps the first feed or the second feed. We'd practically decided to split it really.
So you had talked about it and got it all...?
Oh yeah and when she came home that was...
It worked? What you'd sort of expected to be doing was what you were actually doing?
Mmmm, yeah.
To a lesser or greater extent obviously.
Yeah, no shocks!
No, no, I should think you'd had about enough of those anyway!
Yeah! [Laughs]
Do you sort of update who's going to do what? Because obviously like you say at first

Emma

she was sleeping through the night then suddenly she's not, now she's teething...
Neil's changed his job since then.
Oh right, so does that make things easier? More difficult or the same?
A little bit more difficult for me. He goes, he's home Sunday, Monday, Tuesday and he's away Wednesday, Thursday, Friday, Saturday. So my mum has her Wednesday through to Friday, so I have to be organised! [Laughs] To sort of get up in the morning, feed her get her dressed and then get her to my mum so there's a bit more to it than there was before. We're getting there, it's called planning, and getting everything ready the night before! [Laughs] But I have to say I can organise what I have to do (with regards to work) so some mornings what I will do is have a late start so I haven't got to be out until about eleven so I've got plenty of time in the morning.
Yeah so it's not too bad.
It's not as if you're up at 6 o'clock every morning...
Unless of course Lotte's up at 6 and then...
Mmm and that can be quite a regular thing! [Laughter]
OK and you think that basically on the whole it worked out for the better or for the worse to date?
What, the whole thing?
Yeah.
Certainly changed my life for the better.
Yeah. So your experience of motherhood up 'till the present day. How do you think your life has changed?
Totally! [Laughs and rolls her eyes]
So your life has changed. Are you still doing the same job?
Yes but... A lot of things have changed. I don't do as big an area as I did before. I'm a lot closer to home. I don't do as many hours as before obviously because I don't drive so far away. Yeah I think actually that has probably not changed. I still do the same job.
What about contact with people like your mum and that. Do you think that is more or less than before?
A lot more.
Yeah, what with her looking after Lotte?
We are a lot more close, and I think I'm closer to my sister now because we've got something in common! [Laughs]
Were you not very close before or...?
We've never really been very very close. We've been close but you know we don't sit and talk all the time and tell secrets and stuff. But we've got a lot closer, she was very supportive when I had Lotte as my mum was as well, but ermm... I think it's brought the whole family closer.
What about Neil's family?
They actually live in Luton, so...He's been there today to see her. Oh yeah they drove up to see her while she was in intensive care, yeah I get on very well with his mum. She

141

Nine Women, Nine Months, Nine Lives

rings up quite a lot, she didn't used to before but she rings up quite a lot now. Like if I take her to the hospital or the doctors I let her know how she's getting on, things like that.
And how do you think you've changed? Your personality, you've said your whole life has changed totally.
More patient! [Laughs] I've had to be.
So, what you've learnt to be patient?
Yeah I've had to learn, I wouldn't say I was totally patient.
Do you give lessons? [Laughter]
Don't get me wrong, sometimes I could go out of the house and scream. Still do. Yeah I take more, take life a lot easier you know. I used to worry about how the house was, but now, no point worrying about it anymore because as soon as you do something about it there's somebody there who crawls around ready to wreck it anyway! So you know, people take me as they find me really, now which it wasn't before.
So, you seem to be talking about that as if it were a good thing, is that...?
Yeah, yeah I think it is. I'm a lot more relaxed about things.
So that's one of the better aspects of how you've changed. Can you think of, I mean there might not be, but can you think of something about yourself that has changed that you might feel a bit disappointed or disillusioned about yourself?
I don't think there is anything that springs to mind, not really.
OK, and do you think that is a permanent change, you being more patient, or not?
Probably not. No! [Laughter] I wouldn't like to say really, I'd hope it to be, I really really would, yeah I'd like it to be! [Laughs] I think it will be because I think you've got to have patience to be able to cope.
Yeah, so you've had to adapt really?
Yeah.
And has that been difficult do you think? Do you think you've become more patient without really trying?
Oh I've had to think about it. I've had to step back and think, if she wants feeding or changing and then she's teething so yeah. I've had to step back because I have never ever been a patient person before but, you just have to be now.
Well the next question is do you hope to go back to work but you already are so...
I already am.
And you said earlier you went back in August and its now January so that's what 5 months?
It's about six months.
Right, and did you go back to work and do full time and a bit more or have you reduced your hours since or...?
I don't do as many hours since.
Was that from the beginning, from when you went back in August?
Yeah. Yeah it was less so... And when I know Neil is at home I will book quite a long

142

Emma

day, that I know I'm going to have to be there quite a long while. And then towards the end of the week I sort of have my easier days, so I'm sort of not leaping about as much, but the travelling makes the biggest difference, that reduces a two/two and a half hour journey into an hour and ten minutes journey.
And do you think you're managing it? Do you find that you are enjoying your job and you enjoy being at home or do you find the two don't really mix...?
They do if you plan it properly. You have got to organise yourself the night before because there have been mornings when I haven't and I've paid for it! [Laughs] Definitely, yeah definitely. Yeah and you've got to, I know I'm a lot more organised than I was because I've had to be. Yeah I think the two can work quite well together. I think she's, well I know Lotte benefits from going to my mums because my mum has taught her so much. She's doing well, she doesn't not benefit from seeing my mum, because I've got a handicapped sister and my mum has to do a lot of work with my handicapped sister so it has sort of snowballed down from my niece down to Lotte, so... But we've paid for it because she comes out with words all the time! [Laughs] And she's nearly walking, mmm, climbing the stairs...
Is she climbing already?
Oh yes!
She's all right going up because she's crawling, but...?
No, I'm not even going to let her attempt...
You haven't caught her trying to tentatively shuffle down backwards or...?
Stairgate. Went up straight away. I thought "No!" Because she will, she'll just go for it, she's got no fear.
OK, and do you feel that Lotte benefits from you being at work, do you feel better for having been to work and having a break? Do you think it would drive you round the bend being at home all the time?
I wouldn't mind being at home a couple of days a week. Errm... Sort of doing three or three and a half days at work but I think she benefits from being with her Dad on Monday and Tuesday, because they're so close they really are. But then again you see, I have her every night and all day Saturday and she obviously benefits from my mum and Abigail because my mum has Abigail as well, my niece, and she's learnt, you can see how she's learning off her. I don't think she misses anything from me working.
And do you think you miss anything about Lotte when you are working?
Yeah, some days I sit and I think "Oh I wonder what she's doing?" Especially when I first went back to work, I still do now but not as badly as I did when I first went back. Yeah I was like ringing every hour to see if she was all right! [Laughter] But now you know I'll just ring once a day or if she's teething then I'll definitely ring at least once.
Do you think it's possible you could get your hours reduced or?
I'm hoping so! [Laughs]
So that's something you are looking to do?
Yeah, it's not something that's imminent, but probably by this time next year.

Nine Women, Nine Months, Nine Lives

The next question is, do you get any time to yourself? You in fact answered it a bit earlier saying that you don't get any spare time and... Without anybody around?
Yeah.
Very rare, yeah.
Do you try and make time for yourself? Have you perhaps tried to organise I don't know...?
My mum is very good, if myself or Neil want to go out, although we haven't done it very often, probably about three times, then she'll have her, but I don't like leaving her. I don't like leaving her overnight because she just doesn't go through the night so we always pick her up, she's always here! [Laughs] But no, we can make time for ourselves, I think we could actually make a bit more, because my mum is good and my sister but errmm...
Well she's getting older now so...
Yeah, I'm more confident about leaving her or whatever, she just carries on as normal, Lotte does anyway, when I leave her in the morning she will wave goodbye so...
Quite an independent young lady I would say.
Oh yes, just a bit! [Laughs]
So, in your time for yourself you say that you feel like you ought to be catching up on things like cleaning the oven and nonsense like that! But you end up watching TV and you pulled a bit of a face as if to say "Shouldn't really be doing this". Do you feel a conflict, do you feel like, I don't know, somehow guilty that you're putting your feet up and not doing something like that? Why?
Yeah because when Neil comes home he'll say things like "Oh come on lets get this done" and I'll feel guilty that I haven't done it in the week. I feel guilty for him really, that he does work in the week and then when he comes home he has to help me out. And then some days when I've come home he'll say "Oh I don't know how you cope, she's been on the go all the time". And it's then that I think "Yeah you do realise what I do!". But when he's not around and I haven't done it I think ooh he's not going to like you know, but errmm... But every now and then when he says "Oh I don't know how you cope" I think "Oh yeah". Well you know, it is difficult.
Yeah, so you feel a bit concerned about, you seem to be implying that, you think that he doesn't know what you do. That if you do have any spare time and you do put your feet up it's because you are bloody knackered not...
Yeah, yeah it is! He realises some nights it's quite late when I get home and all I do is just get Lotte, if she's, if mum's not fed her I just get her fed, bathed and bed and then I go to bed as well. Because the early part of the night she sleeps fine, and that's when I catch well grab my sleep basically and but he understands that.
Yeah, so do you think you are going to try and make more time for you just to...?
I've got to really I think.
It's not a bad thing.

Emma

No, I don't think it is.
I think you've probably got out of the habit of it.
Yeah I think I used to have...
Having the ability to do it, to make...
Yeah I used to have quite a lot of spare time, always found something to do, yeah but you've got to or else you'd crack up basically! [Laughs]
Well I think its that it doesn't do you any harm, it'll only do you harm if you feel bad about taking the time off, which is what I was a bit... concerned about.
No, no I don't feel bad about doing it at all, errmm... I just think I feel, when I pulled the face about the TV that was because it wasn't anything very exciting! [Laughs]
No but it was just brain numbing and that's what is wonderful sometimes!
Just sit in front of it and stare and think "Oh I haven't seen this in ages" [Laughter]
Oh no it doesn't do you any harm at all, it can be a good thing. Now, how do you think Neil has changed?
Errmm...
Do you think he has changed? I don't know, I'm assuming that there may be things that you've noticed.
Mmmm. He's actually a bit more loving, a bit more open with his errm... His affections yeah and he's absolutely brilliant with Lotte. Yeah he's sort of mellowed a bit, you know, if that's the right thing to say, yeah he's calmed down a lot, he was forever on the go as well, but he's just like me he just gets on with it really.
Do you think he's perhaps a bit more patient now?
Yeah, a lot more patient.
Do you think him mellowing has been a conscious effort or do you think it's just happened?
No I think it's just happened, it's just happened. I don't think he's thought about it, he's just got on with it really.
So do you think that is the biggest change the one that is most noticeable?
Mmmm I think so.
Do you think anybody else has noticed this change in him?
Yeah, my mum! [Laughs] Yeah, I think everybody thought he wouldn't get involved that much and you know just the normal things. But they're just, they're like that! [crosses fingers and holds in air] They're just so close you know, they're just inseparable, I don't get a look in really when he's at home you know!
That's the time for you to sit down and put your feet up!
It's when I come in at night and she'll go "Oh hello!" You know she'll want a hug and everything but then ten minutes later she'll be back with her dad. Yeah so I just let them get on with it really, it's good for them anyway.
Yeah that's nice, that they can be like that.
Yeah, yeah, he's adapted really well.
OK do you talk about how you have changed as individuals? Have you ever passed any

145

funny comments even like "You're getting a bit laid back in you old age!" You know?
No, not jokey no. He's started getting more homely now, he's started doing things around the house. [Rolls eyes and grimaces]
Oh no! [Laughter] What putting up shelves and things?
Gardening, yeah, he used to do a bit before but now he's saying things like when she plays out in the garden we'll have to do this and that. Bought a tool kit! [Laughs]
Does he know how to use it?
[Laughs] Put the stair gate up which I thought I'd get my dad to do, and he has actually done odd jobby bits now and then! [Laughter] But yeah more sort of homely.
Well he's got a home and a family now.
That's right. [pride in voice]
OK would you say that your relationship has changed? I mean well obviously it must of...
Yeah, for the better. We're a lot closer than we were, we were close before but you know there's that sort of like completeness really.
And do you talk about how your relationship has changed?
Not really, no.
Do you feel that you want to talk about it?
I don't think, you just, we just get on with, it's not, we know it's changed, and we've accepted it's changed but it's not...
You feel he knows it's changed as well so you don't need to say it and flag it up and say "Look isn't this great!"
Not at all. We're both aware of it.
And both pleased about it?
Yeah, we're a lot closer.
And do you try and make time for the two of you to spend time together without...?
Yeah, errm... We try. If she goes to bed early then we can grab half an hour together and then whatever. But it is so difficult because she is so....
She's into everything isn't she? From the moment she wakes up you can see her looking and thinking "What can I do next?"
Yeah and sometimes she's gone to my mums in the day and we've gone out in the day, so yeah, we do try but it is difficult with him working away. But Sundays we do spend all together.
Yeah, so is that like the family day? So you don't do oven cleaning or anything?
No, we go out or we visit or we just spend the day together playing, you know! [Laughs] Just spend the day. We do try and make time.
Just for you two?
Yeah, yeah.
So you do actually manage it. Would you say there is a fairly regular pattern that has emerged when you spend time together?
I wouldn't say it's a regular, no, errmm... We can every now and then, it just depends

Emma

on Lotte what she's like, if she's tired and we put her to bed and she sleeps then yeah but...
So you do try?
Oh yeah, we do try, yeah definitely. You need a, I know it sounds silly but you need a break, you need a break so you can be together, you catch up on things that you haven't talked about in a long while.
Yeah I mean she's only been around a year!
Yeah, but, I don't know everything about what he's doing anymore at work and he certainly doesn't know everything about my work. And yet before we knew exactly what we were doing and he knew everything about what I'd been doing and that doesn't happen any more. But we do try and catch up.
Do you feel like you want to know about things like that?
Yeah because then I don't feel like I'm neglecting Neil and everything's not just focused on Lotte, because I think you have got to spend time together.
Do you think he feels the same?
Yeah, yeah I do.
The future! We'll say your immediate future so the next 12 months. What would you say you hope to achieve in the next year? What are your hopes for the next year?
With Lotte that she gets discharged from Hospital in May [Laughs]. That's my main hope really. Errmm and just to continue being as happy as we are now really because I think we've got everything sussed really.
Just continue to build?
Yeah, for Neil to move closer to home really (with work). [Laughs] That's a hope, which he is hoping to do actually.
Yeah? Is that in the near future?
Hopefully. He wants to as well which makes a big difference.
What about you reducing your hours?
Yeah, that's going to be in about a year.
So that's something you'd hope to do within the year?
Yeah.
But realistically you think...
Yeah it might be a bit longer.
OK so do you think you'll be able to achieve it? Do you think Lotte will be discharged in May?
At the back of my mind I think so but I don't want to say yes just in case it doesn't happen. Errm... They were really pleased with her, I haven't seen them since, she's been back in November and they were very pleased with her then and on the letter I had back they put on it that they want to see her again at 18 months for a possible discharge. So I've got that in the back of my mind that it's going to happen but I don't want to sort of say it's definitely going to happen and then me getting upset because something's not quite right.

Nine Women, Nine Months, Nine Lives

So what difference will it make, do you think, if she is discharged, is that like she's been given a clean bill of health?
Yeah, yeah, basically that's what they've said to me. They're not checking her lungs or anything like that, it's developmental and at the back of my mind I keep thinking is something wrong? And until they turn round to me and say no she's fine you know she's doing what she should be doing, blah blah blah, I don't think I'll ever be a hundred percent happy, it just doesn't seem to be, it doesn't feel like it's finished. You know like, most people when they come home they think that's it really apart from health visitors and that, but I feel like I'm still attached to them somehow! [Laughs] You know, yeah, they've said to me yeah she's fine, I still feel like I am still there.
So that will make a big difference then?
Yeah.
And if that doesn't happen in May, when do you think it will happen, do you have another appointment?
No, no they usually say every three months but I only go every 6 because she did quite well, so they said they wouldn't see me in three months but in 6 months which takes me to May.
And do you think Neil will be able to actually get some work nearer?
He's got an interview [Laughs] in a couple of weeks time, make a big difference.
And what would you say you've learnt about yourself in the past year, something you weren't perhaps aware of as being present in your character or something that wasn't quite as much present before?
Errmm... Like I said before, more patient, I don't think I'd ever, I didn't think I'd ever be a mum either.
No?
No! [Laughs]
Well you seem to be doing a good job so I wouldn't worry!
Yeah, I never thought. And I didn't think I'd even have it in me.
Really?
Didn't think I was the mothering sort at all.
I suppose, now what would the phrase be, you didn't think you were cut out for it?
No I didn't, I thought I'd be like work-work-work to be honest because I've always worked ever since I was sixteen, even part-time jobs when I was going through college, or whatever, and I thought that would be it, career and nothing else, it's a big change actually. And to admit you really enjoy it! [Laughter]
Yeah you see this is thing, one or two girls have said to me it's very difficult to be pleased openly and that "I intend to take a year off for maternity leave so that I can enjoy my baby, you know, I want to be with my baby", so...
We had somebody like that at work, she was due three weeks after me, and she didn't even want to talk about the fact she was pregnant, and yet I was like telling everyone, which surprised me as well! [Laughs]

Emma

So you found out something good about yourself?
Yeah.
So what would you like to develop next year, do you think there is more unexpected things out there that you might learn about yourself?
Don't really know. Take each day as it comes, that's how I am now, you know, whereas everything before was structured. Now I structure my work but you just take it day by day, with the little one you don't always get a lot done! [Laughs]
Have you learnt anything about yourself this past year that you want to change next year?
I don't think so.
No? It could be good or bad, it could be either...
What would I like to change...Oh I'd like to loose weight! [Laughter] Errm... No I don't think I have, no.
You seem quite happy really.
Yeah, mmm, try to be.
Yeah, you've got to take the rough with the smooth.
Yeah, errrm... No, no... I'll probably think of something when you've gone!
Yes, of course! [Laughter]
No nothing that springs to mind.
OK well that's good, that is good.

Nine Women, Nine Months, Nine Lives

Tanya

Tanya was 19 years old when she found out she was pregnant. She had known the father of her child for a couple of years. She became single immediately after telling him she was pregnant. He has seen his daughter Katie once in a chance encounter in the street and had to be made to look at her. He does not contribute to either Tanya or their daughter's upkeep. She would like to return to work, perhaps re-training to a job where she can be with Katie as much as possible.

OK the first part, what I would like you to do is think back to when you were first pregnant, so when you first found out you were pregnant. Were you trying to get pregnant at the time?
No, no it was a complete and utter accident, yeah.
Can you remember what went through your mind when you found out you were pregnant?
"Oh my God, how am I going to tell my mum?"
Yeah?
Yeah, that was it.
That was the first thing you thought?
Yeah, because I was on holiday at the time, and I thought "Oh my God I'm pregnant, how am I going to tell me mum?!" [Laughs]
So, did you think about it afterwards and did how you feel change?
When, when I was pregnant? I was happy, and eventually when I did tell me mum she was OK, she was all right.

Nine Women, Nine Months, Nine Lives

You say you were on holiday, was anyone with you when you did the test?
My best friend.
And can you remember what your partner's reaction was when you told him?
Get rid of it. I don't want nothing to do with it.
So, he was like a steady boyfriend at the time? And you just basically, you thought you were pregnant, so you did the test. How many weeks were you, can you remember?
I thought I was four, but it worked out I was only three, no sorry four months sorry. I thought I was four months but it worked out when I had my first scan I was only three months, so…
So had you not mentioned it to your partner at all then?
No.
You obviously thought you were pregnant when you did the test or else you wouldn't have done it. How long had you been thinking "Oh I might be".
Well I don't know, not for, maybe a couple of weeks before I went on holiday, but I just put it down to stress because I was really stressed up at work at the time as well.
So your period was missing and you thought it was just because of worry?
Yeah, that's right, yeah.
Ok, and how did you feel about your partner's reaction?
I was really upset.
Had you known each other for a long while?
Errm… a couple of years, yeah.
Yeah? What did you think his reaction was going to be? You said your first reaction was your mum…
Yeah, and then I thought about him after, but, I don't know, I don't know what his reaction, I don't know what I was expecting from him, I didn't expect him to say what he said, but at the end of the day it's his choice in't it? I thought he was more mature than what he was, so…
Yeah, how old is he?
Twenty eight-ish.
What now, or he was then?
He's about that age, I think he is.
And how old are you (Tanya)?
I'm twenty.
You're twenty. Hmm, had he got kids from a previous relationship or…?
Not that I know of.
No, and does he still live round here?
No, he well, he lived sort of, I think Long Eaton. Last time I saw him, he said that he had moved and he weren't going to tell me his new address.
So, has he ever seen Katie or…?
He's seen her once but he didn't, I mean I had to turn the push chair round so he could see her because he weren't going to, so… I thought "Yeah you look at how beautiful she

Tanya

is!" [Laughs] "See what you are missing out on!" But he just didn't want to see her.
Did he speak to you?
Yeah, he spoke to me, he's fine with me, it's just Katie.
So he wanted you to have a termination?
Yeah.
And did you consider it?
No.
Not at all, not for a moment?
No, I don't think I'd have been able to. I mean don't get me wrong, if people, if that's what people want to do then that's up to them, but I couldn't do it myself. I just don't think I'd be able to live with myself, so, it was just, I didn't even think about it, that's the way I've been brought up, so…
And what did your mum say?
She cried a lot! [Laughs] And then she cried even more, so I cried, and then, what did she say? She said, "who is the father?" And I said, "I don't want to tell you".
Was she upset about that?
I think so at the time but, my ex-boyfriend he'd, he'd errm, oh what's the word…? He told me that if I told anybody that it was his baby he would beat me up. So I don't know where I'd have stood, if I'd have told my mum then, because he got on quite well with my mum and dad.
Oh, did they not realise…?
I think they realise now, but they still don't know till this day, but I couldn't…
No, not for sure.
But they think it's him. I don't know.
So, you don't get any support from him at all, maintenance or anything?
No, no nothing.
That must be very hard.
Oh it is. Definitely. On the benefits I get it's crap. I get the money on a Monday and nearly all of it goes on bills. It's hard, I get nappies and food for her. And then I've got like five pound left for myself. So, I mean, well me mum and dad have been helping me out as much as they can, which is really good of them, but you just have to get on with it don't you? I suppose.
Yeah, and do you think you made the right decision?
Yes, I do.
You seem very sure.
Yes, oh yes, I just don't know what my life would be without her.
OK, the next chunk, if you like, is about your experience of pregnancy, and the birth. Did you imagine how you would feel before you got pregnant? Now obviously you were very young, and you still are, but had you thought about having a baby and perhaps what that would entail physically?
Well I've always wanted babies since I was young. I've always loved kids but I didn't

153

know what it would, I mean I knew obviously that your belly got bigger and your bum got bigger and you know you just got bigger, but, I didn't really know what it entailed until I actually got pregnant.
No?
But I loved being pregnant, I absolutely loved it.
Yeah, what was the best bit?
Just feeling her kick, for the first time, that was just, that was amazing that was! And oh she was such a wriggle bum, just like she is now! [Laughs]
What did she do?
You'd sit there, (this was) when I was quite far gone because I was ginormous, and you'd see her head come out to the side or her bum, and then you'd see her arm or her legs! It was just really amazing, to know that something was alive inside you. It was just, I don't know, but I did love being pregnant.
So you had imagined how pregnancy would feel beforehand or would you say you just had a vague idea of things getting bigger?
Yeah, just, just bigger!
You hadn't really ever thought about it?
No, not really, no.
So, perhaps when you first got pregnant or first realised you were pregnant at three or four months in, then what did you think?
Ohh, errm…
Did you start imagining how it would be later on? You know like I'm this big now I wonder am I going to get much bigger?
Yeah, I seemed to grow overnight as well, and one minute I didn't have nothing and the next minute I had a big bump. Well not a big bump, but it was there you know. So that was quite strange, yeah.
So you had started to think about how it would feel later on in pregnancy. And when you think back to what your actual experiences were is there a difference?
Oh yes, definitely.
Yeah and what was the difference?
Errm, I don't know, just never imagined that it could be like it was, I suppose.
Be as good as it was?
Yeah, because obviously when you see other people who are pregnant, you see how some people get morning sickness. I mean don't get me wrong, if you get it then… I got it all day and all night, I just didn't get it in the morning I got it all the time! [Laughs] And food as well, I went off so much food, and I didn't expect that at all. I thought I'd still be able to eat what I wanted to when I wanted to but, no. The baby didn't agree with it.
OK, thinking about the birth. What did you expect would happen at the birth, had you read about it?
Yeah, read all the books, you know the ones you get from the midwife and whatever. But I was so petrified, I was just, I didn't want it to come out naturally.

Tanya

Yeah?
I just wanted them to get it out by some, by caesarean I suppose. Which is what I had to have, so I was really glad about that, when they said I had to have a caesarean, I was like "Yes!"
So, was it an emergency caesarean or were you booked for a caesarean?
No, it was emergency, because she was head down but facing the wrong way round. She was fine, but I'd been in labour 48 hours and she was finding it difficult and by this time I was tired, she was tired, so, it was classed as an emergency caesarean.
Had you thought about talking to your midwife about requesting a caesarean?
No, because I didn't realise you could do that, I just thought that you had to have a natural birth, unless there was complications. But I suppose now looking back, if I had anymore I would definitely have a caesarean. I didn't realise you could ask for one, but now I know so, that's me done! [Laughs]
So you were quite relieved when you had the caesarean?
Yeah, yeah but I was scared as well, but I was relieved.
Which bits scared you?
Everything, just everything about it, just having an operation I suppose. Because it's, it is an operation in't it?
Oh yeah, there's no two ways about that!
Yeah, I've got the scar! I don't know, just in case something went wrong or I don't know. I was quite high at the time so... [Laughs] I can't really remember very much about it, if you know what I mean, so I don't know, I didn't really feel anything, well obviously not, but like I didn't feel anything like in me brain, you know. But I do feel sorry for the anaesthetist.
Why?
I was shouting at him, I was really giving him some! [Laughs] Puked all over him as well, but, there we go...[Laughs] His hand was in the way so...[Laughs]
Oh dear, bet he was really chuffed!
I was lying there, and they had this screen here, and I couldn't feel none of me body and I says "I'm going to be sick". So he put this bowl thing here and I was like, I couldn't have moved, I could just go like that and be sick, and his hand was in the way, so I was sick and that was that! [Laughs] So I said "Oh, I'm sorry"... not! [Laughs]
I think they're quite used to it to be honest.
Yeah, he was having a good laugh and joke with me so that was good. That put my mind at ease.
Yeah, so you expected the birth to be fairly scary and you didn't think you were going to get what you want because you thought you were going to go through a natural birth, a vaginal delivery?
Yeah.
And you didn't you had an emergency caesarean, and you were quite happy, you were happier than you would have been?

Nine Women, Nine Months, Nine Lives

Yeah. [Laughs]
A lot happier, that was what you really wanted?
Yeah, that's right.
So had you read up about caesareans before hand?
No.
But yet you wanted one, or was it just that you didn't want to have a vaginal delivery?
Well, yeah, it was just that I didn't want to have a vaginal delivery. I don't know, I hadn't read up about caesareans. Actually, actually I didn't know nothing about them until the midwife or the nurse or whoever it was said to me "I think we'd best take you down for a caesarean because" blah blah blah - something about the baby and that would be more acceptable. You know she seemed to be in distress, or not necessarily in distress but… I was like "well, what does it involve?" So they told me, but it was like in one ear and out the other!
Yeah?
Because I was [Laughs] in the sky but I was like "yeah, go for it then". But I wanted just what was best for her at the end of the day, I didn't want her to be hurt or anything. I just wanted to make sure she was all right, and worry about me later! [Laughs]
Yeah, well, that's understandable. OK, and how did you feel when you first held Katie? You had a caesarean, so you wouldn't have held her straight away but…
No. I saw her once she had been brought out as it were, they cleaned her up, and then my mum held her.
So your mum was with you?
Yeah, she was holding my hand - I think! [Laughs]
She said she was?
Yeah! So she brought her to me and I saw her face and I just like stroked her on the face and said "hello darling!" And then, my dad was there as well but obviously he weren't in the operating theatre, because you're allowed only one person, so they took her to my (step) dad. And then it takes about another I think it's 45 to an hour, 45 minutes to an hour to sew me back up, and then they put me in recovery and then they brought Katie in. That was the first time I really held her and that was, and that was, oh, that was just lovely!
It was really good?
Yeah, yeah it was, I was just crying my eyes out. [Laughs]
So you remember it very clearly when you first held her?
Yeah, I was just lying there, and she was lying next to me and I was saying "hello darling, I'm your mummy". And I was just you know, gabble, gabble, gabbling away. I'll never forget that moment.
OK. So your partner was not involved in your pregnancy at all?
No.
So, going back to the decision to have Katie and he wanted you to have the termination, did you tell him that you were going to have her, or did you just listen to what he had to

Tanya

say and walk away?
I listened to what he had to say. I says "fair enough that's your decision but my decision is I'm going to have her, if you don't want nothing to do with it it's up to you". But, you know, I'm still going to leave it open, if he wants to meet up with her in the future, it's up to him. I'm not going to come inbetween that, because I know what it's like to be brought up with no dad so, I'm not going to come inbetween that.
No.
At the end of the day... But yeah, when he just told me, I said "OK that's your decision I understand that, this is my decision".
So, he was, he wasn't involved in the pregnancy at all, not even for a month?
No.
Nothing at all?
No. He must of seen me about five times while I was pregnant, but he'd just, he'd just pop in every now and, just pop in you know, just out of the blue.
What? Came round to your house?
Yeah, just pop in, you know, say he was coming in for a coffee, just passing sort of thing, so...
And would you say that his reaction, to the pregnancy, was that more or less than you had hoped for? Sounds like a silly question. It was less than you hoped for really wasn't it?
Yes. Yeah, yeah, I expected him to, be, do more than that, not say, just, you know, straight off the top of his head "get rid of it", you don't expect that from...
What did you expect?
I don't know. I just expected us to talk it through, I suppose. And, I don't know, just talk it through, not just... Aarrgghh!! [Angry] First thing he said to me was "get rid of it", and I just, I mean, that was his decision, fair enough but, I still expected him to talk it through more before he said that.
Before he reached that decision, yeah.
Yeah, that's right.
Yeah, it was a bit of an immediate reaction.
Hello?! [Sarcasm – shake of head]
So had you any expectations that you would be together as a couple, and bring Katie up with the both of you...?
When I found out I was pregnant?
Mmm.
I suppose yeah, it would have been nice.
Yeah, but was that what you expected?
I wouldn't say I expected it but, I thought it would be a possibility.
So it was something you hoped for?
Yes, yeah.
OK, the next section is your experience of early motherhood. We'll say the first three

Nine Women, Nine Months, Nine Lives

weeks, four weeks, so really early. OK, was there anything about your pregnancy that carried on into the first sort of few weeks after you had had the baby? I mean obviously you had the caesarean so stitches and things like that, I don't know if you can drive, but you wouldn't have been able to drive...
I can't anyway, but yeah I weren't allowed to drive, I think it was the first three weeks, if I remember rightly, but...
Did you have water retention or anything like that?
Yeah, oh yeah! Woo hoo! I had to stay in hospital for a week after she was born, but I didn't, I only stayed in for five days Because the day after me operation I was up on me feet and they didn't expect me to be, because obviously when you have an epidural, it numbs you and you can't walk or anything. So, well I could walk near enough straight away, the next day, so they were like "Oh my God! What are you doing?" And I had water retention in my ankles, they were absolutely ginormous they were at least three times of what they are now! I couldn't wear no slippers, I couldn't put nothing on my feet, I had to walk around with bare feet, so my ankles, yeah... And that lasted 'till I came out on the Sunday, but they had gone down slowly. But I couldn't fit my boots on, because I'd got boots with a zip up the side, couldn't fit them on, couldn't even put my foot in them! So I had to wear, my mum bought my trainers in, which would stretch at the sides, that was better. I think that was all that swelled up!
OK, and the birth, how did that affect early motherhood? Because obviously with the caesarean lifting her and things like that, did you, I mean, you were obviously able to hold her when you were sitting but...
Yeah, I was allowed to carry her and that was it, anything else no. I was allowed to carry her weight, I weren't allowed to carry nothing heavier than her weight. So for example, her car seat, I wouldn't have been able to carry that, because it's heavier, especially if she's in it! Bags, just simple things like that, if they were heavier than her I wouldn't have been allowed to carry it. And I weren't allowed to do that I think it was for the first, I can't remember how long that was for, for a while anyway, about the first six weeks. It was quite good because I had to get everyone to carry everything for me! [Laughs]
So would you say that that made life easy or difficult then after the birth? The first six weeks?
I suppose if I had been on my own with nobody to help me then it would have been hard. But because I had people around me to help me it was, it wasn't too bad, it was quite easy really, I suppose, yeah.
OK, How did you imagine early motherhood would be for you? Towards the end of your pregnancy, you say you were quite big, and I remember you saying before something about, you were really slow at walking and you kept having to tell people to slow down?
Oh yeah! That was a nightmare, I was like a snail! [Laughs] Honestly I was, like a snail!
So you must have had time for putting your feet up, did you spend time imagining what early motherhood would be like? Imagining what Katie would be like, whether she would be Katie?

Tanya

Yeah, errm, I thought she was a boy so that, I mean I had pictured a blue eyed blond haired boy, that was what I thought I was having, so when they brought out this dark haired blue eyed girl I was like that's not my baby! [Laughs] I had an argument with them! [Laughs]I had an argument with them, I said, take that baby back it's not mine! Mine's blue eyed, you know, I've got a little blue eyed boy! So, she wasn't nothing like I expected her.
So you had expected her to be something?
Yeah.
You had thought about what she would be like?
Yeah, I thought she was going to be a boy, but she weren't! [Laughs]
So did you want a boy then, or had you just sort of felt like it was a boy?
Yeah, I thought it was a boy. Just because of, I don't know, the way she was inside me. Because I was all up front, and the way she used to kick me, she used to pretend I was a blooming rugby ball, battering me she was! I just thought, I just thought all the way through, well no not all the way through, but towards the end, I just thought it was going to be a boy. Everybody had their bets on saying it was going to be a girl or a boy, so, yeah, I'd expected her to be a boy.
And would you say you were disappointed when…?
Oh no, no, as soon as I saw her I was like, I fell in love with her. I was like "oh dear there's me mouthing off to the people about 'where is my boy?'" And then they showed me her and I was like "Oh, it's my baby!" So, it was a nice surprise if nothing else.
Yeah, yeah. And does she resemble her father?
Errm, I think she's tall like him, she's quite long, because I'm not, I'm a short arse so, she must take after him!
So am I, so…[Laughs]
She must take after him for that.
What about in her face, things like that, that wouldn't upset you if she looked like him?
Oh no, no…I'm quite lucky in that way because everybody thinks she looks like me.
Yeah, I think she looks like you, but then I…
But I don't see it. Yeah, exactly, nobody knows who the father is so yeah, I suppose you do see me.
I just wondered if you know, that would be upsetting for you really?
Oh no, no.
That wouldn't bother you at all?
No, everybody's different anyway, they've got their own features and that.
And what about the actual practicalities of motherhood? You know looking after a baby, regardless of whether you thought she was a boy or a girl, whether you would love her, or whether you would grow to love her, or things like that, had you considered them?
I knew it was going to be hard, well I thought it was going to be hard, and it was. And more demanding, because obviously night feeds, things like that. I mean towards the end I didn't get much sleep anyway, and I slept all day. But I mean I couldn't do that when I

159

Nine Women, Nine Months, Nine Lives

first had her, you see I slept when she slept, like they tell you to, forget everything else, just sleep when she's sleeping. [Laughs] So I did that, I mean I still do that now, if she has a nap in the afternoon I have a sleep as well, it's just like they say. Otherwise I mean, yeah, you know, housework, so what? Forget about it, yeah, I mean you have just got to do the best for your baby haven't you? I mean if you're tired, and when I'm tired I get snappy, and I don't like being snappy with her. So I'd rather have a kip when she has a kip and then I'm all right, you know, get my energy back up sort of thing. So when she wakes up you know full of life, I'm you know, I can cope with it, just let her get on with it. I suppose it was hard for the first, well it still is hard now but, not as hard. But then you had to get up in the night, change and then feed her.
And there was only you to do it then as well?
Yeah.
I suppose it must have been doubly hard?
Yeah, yeah it was, but I suppose I got used to it, it had to be done so I had to do it. At the end of the day that's the way you've got to think about it haven't you?
Yeah. OK and do you think what you thought motherhood would be like actually matched up, with what it was?
Errm, I suppose in a way yes, but obviously there were things that I hadn't thought about, like teething for instance, but obviously you just take them as they come, don't you?
OK, and what would you say was difficult in those early days or weeks? What was the most difficult?
The night feeds, because if I don't get my sleep, I'm terrible.
And you weren't getting your sleep?
No, I mean I got used to it. But the first couple of times, it was a nightmare!
And what would you say was the best thing about those early days and weeks?
When she was asleep! [Laughs]
Now there's an honest answer! [Laughs]
But I do love you darling! [Laughs] No, when she was asleep.
What was it about when she was asleep?
The peace, just peace, oooh, you could hear yourself think! [Laughs] It was just great! [Laughs]
Now obviously your partner wasn't involved at all in the early days, now was he?
No
OK. Right the next chunk is your experience of motherhood up to the present day. So from when she was about three months old-ish up till now. How do you think your life has changed since you had Katie?
Everything revolves around her. Everything I do, revolves around her. Yeah, you know, because from first thing when I get up in the morning I've got to get her breakfast ready. I just put her first in everything I do, I get her breakfast and then her milk and then I get my cup of tea. I come and sit down and she is eating her breakfast, and then what she's not ate I feed her the last little bit, and she uses her hands, and we have a sit down and

Tanya

she has a bit of a play and I get her dressed and then I get myself dressed and then we go out. And when, if I go out, like socially at the week-ends, I make sure that she is all packed and ready because she stays at my mum's house.
Oh right yeah, that's good.
Yeah, oooh, I look forward to Saturday nights I can tell you something! I live for my Saturday nights because then I can just go out and let my hair down and just be myself. Because that's the only time that I can be myself, because that's the only time that I don't have to worry about her if she's crying, or you know, just let them look after her, and I go out which is absolutely lovely. But other than that my life just revolves around her, if people come round obviously I've got to make sure either she is in bed or she's, you know.
Were you working before, when you were pregnant?
Yeah.
But you're not now?
No, I can't. Not that I, I suppose I could go back to work eventually, but I don't want to, because I think that the first…
Yeah, weren't you going to study as well?
I wanted to go to college yeah, like a night-time course. To do maybe, just to do something with my time but, obviously with me moving out of home and getting a place of my own, I just, it's just very difficult, like I say…
OK and how do you think you have changed since you had Katie, so both good and bad aspects, temporary and permanent changes?
Errm…
Is there a facet of your personality that has suddenly come into its own or, has been a drawback?
I'm getting back to my normal self. I was a really bubbly outgoing sort of girl, always out you know. Errm… A lot of that when I was pregnant, it went. I don't know where it went but it just went! I would say hello to anybody, that was what I was like. But when I was pregnant and just after I had had her it went and I was, I weren't shy, I weren't depressed, I was just, I'd just lost it. I suppose I was too tired to be like it. But now she's getting older and having more sleep, so obviously I'm having more sleep, I'm getting back to being like that. Because when I go out I just let my hair down and I just go for it, you name it, I do it sort of thing, jut really enjoying myself. And that's what, that's what people like about me I suppose, so that's one, that's good. I knew it would come back eventually… [Laughs] It's just took its time! [Laughs]
So that was a temporary change, and something that you missed?
Yes, oh yes, I did miss that yeah.
Because you seem glad to have it back again!
Oh yeah, errm… I can't remember what the question was now?
Well, errm… How do you think you have changed?
Changed. I think I've grown up, more, quicker than what, say my age group normally

161

Nine Women, Nine Months, Nine Lives

does.
Perhaps quicker than you would have done, you think?
Yeah, yeah that's right. Obviously I've got to be more responsible, because of having my own home, paying my bills you know, they've got to be done weekly etcetera. So, got to have a good head on my shoulders to do that, haven't you? More responsible looking after her, making sure that she can't touch things that she's not supposed to, if she does, get them off her quick. So, that is a change and that is here to stay I think.
Yeah?
Obviously it's got to be hasn't it? [Laughs] Errm… I can't think of anything else
No, that's all right, that's lots. And did you hope to go back to work?
Eventually. Yeah but obviously not straight away, I mean, I still hope to go back, when she is older. I mean I could go back now and do a part time job because my dad said that he would have her in the afternoons because he works mornings. Which would be lovely but it means, but obviously I would have to earn preferably more than what I get for my benefit, so…
Exactly, otherwise…
Yeah, otherwise if I don't then I am losing out, and in the end it just wouldn't be worth it. I mean, I don't want to go back yet, give it another while, a year or so I suppose. When, I suppose I would quite like to go back when she is at playschool, something like that, even when she's at school. But you never know, because like you say, that's in that many years, I might be married I might have another kid by then, so you never know do you?
No, no that's true.
Doubtful but it is possible isn't it! [Laughs]
It's possible, anything is possible, that's right, yeah. Ok and would you say that you get anytime to yourself, for just you?
Errm…
You mentioned the Saturday nights…
Yeah, when she's in bed as well. She goes to bed, whenever she goes to bed, normally between six and eight say, depending on how much sleep she's had during the day and whether she's tired so, when she's gone to bed she wakes up maybe once, not long after she's gone to bed. Anytime after nine, that's my time, so that's quite nice as well.
And what do you tend to do with your time?
I relax. Sometimes I fall asleep down here, sometimes I have my friends round, you know. I mean I can't go out obviously because she's upstairs, apart from Saturdays when she goes to my mum's, but I just do what I want to do. I mean if I've not eaten then I'll have something to eat, things like that, watch the telly, read if there's nothing on the telly, just, do what I want to do, do what I feel like doing at the time.
Yeah, that's good. It's good that you do actually make time for yourself as well, with the Saturday nights.
Yeah, oh yeah, I couldn't live without my Saturday nights, I don't know how I would be able to cope!

Tanya

And how long have you had this Saturday night arrangement with your mum, has that always been in place?
No, she always said from the start that she would have her once a week. When I was at home I used to go out Friday nights with my (step) dad, not with my dad all the time but, I used to go out with my dad occasionally because he goes out Friday nights. But I used to go out with my friends on a Friday as well. But since I've moved in here, it, it started off once a week and then they'd be doing things on a Saturday so I wouldn't go out, and I'd miss going out. And then, I'd take it, I'd not take it out on her but I'd be, I wouldn't be myself because I hadn't been out. And then just recently it's gone back to Saturday nights, it's just like a routine now she goes to stay with grandma. Grandma picks her up about four o'clock Saturday and takes her back to her house and then she comes and picks me up too, because I go round there for Sunday lunch, on Sunday, so, it's nice, I get a lie in as well.
Yeah, you get to get some sleep.
Yeah, because I love my lie-ins! [Laughs]
Yeah, it does you good definitely. How long has it been since you moved here?
I moved in the beginning of December.
Oh right, so four months?
Yeah.
So you are quite well settled, aren't you really?
Yeah, you get into a routine of things, so yeah it is nice.
OK. Right the next part is your immediate future, so the next twelve months OK? What do you hope to achieve this year? What do you aspire to in the next twelve months?
To go on holiday! [Laughs]
Yeah? With Katie or without?
Preferably without because I would like to go abroad and I don't think it would be very nice for her taking her with me to some place very hot. Just so that I can show my body that there is some sun out there! [Laughs] I don't think I've seen the sun for about a year, no, two years! Errm, I don't know. I haven't really thought about the future to be honest, I'm one of these people who lives each day by you know, each day at a time, I suppose. My best friend, she's having a baby in September, so that's something to look forward to. I don't know, if she goes back to work then I'll be having the baby, so that would be nice. Just concentrating on Katie and, you know helping her to learn to talk and read and write, things like that, start them young and, I mean because I've got plenty of time haven't I? So, but I think the main thing is to go on holiday, definitely, have a really good holiday, a couple of weeks away, that would be lovely.
And do you think you'll be able to achieve that in the next twelve months?
Hopefully, because when I'm 21 I'll inherit some money off my grandad, so I'll use a bit of that to go away with. Hopefully if it all comes to plan, but that is what I would like to do.
Who would you like to go away with?

Nine Women, Nine Months, Nine Lives

Errm... [Laughs]
On your own, with someone else?
I don't know, no not on my own, with somebody else.
I was going to say your mum but I guess Katie would perhaps be with your mum?
Yeah, I don't know I've not thought about that one yet! [Laughs] That is one of my ambitions, to go away. I'll think of somebody nearer the time, depends, depends whose available to go I suppose, if there is anybody available to go, if not I shall just have to wait!
What would you say you have learnt about yourself this past year that you would like to develop next year?
Errm... I don't know, errm...
Can you think of the things you have learnt about yourself in the past year and whether there is any one of them you would like to develop? You've talked about things like being more mature and, you know, having more control over your life and being responsible.
I think responsible, I'd like to develop on that.
Independent? I mean you've, you've moved out from home.
Yeah, yeah I suppose I have become more independent. Yes, I'd like to develop on that as well. because obviously she's getting to the age now where she's nearly walking, so once she's walking it'll be so much easier, not having to carry her everywhere, so that would be good, taking her to places where she can walk.
So you'd like to develop your independence and help her to develop hers?
Yeah.
OK, and what have you learnt about yourself in the past year that you would like to change next year, something you've perhaps been a bit disappointed in yourself about?
Sleep! I've got to, not necessarily sleep, but if I don't get enough or if I get too much, I wake up in a groggy mood, and with her I can't, so I've got to get used to that. I mean it's still very hard because I used to sleep when I wanted to, you know what I mean, so I've got to get used to that.
What, so, realise what your optimum is and be quite firm with yourself?
Yeah, that's right. So if it means she's waking up early, go to bed early yourself, things like that.
So, flexibility then?
Yeah.
Yeah, so you'd like to become more flexible, you don't think you've been flexible enough?
Yeah, I suppose I've been quite flexible, but I need to be more flexible.
Yeah, anything else?
I don't think so, errm... Not that I can think of!
OK, that's lovely, that's it, all done and dusted!

Helen

Helen was 30 years old when she accidentally became pregnant. She and her husband Richard had been married for six months and have known each other since they were at school. She experienced a great deal of internal conflict about her decision to go ahead with the pregnancy, this continued well into the first few months of motherhood as she had never really seen herself having children. She returned to work as a flight attendant as soon as she could for her son Will's and her own benefit. This allowed her to retain her sense of self and give her best as a mother. As a consequence of her career she is away from home for half the week and therefore her husband is equally involved in their son's upbringing.

Right, OK the interview breaks down into a series of chunks. So we'll think in terms of time, and we'll start at the beginning. If you could think back to when you found out you were pregnant, OK, were you trying to get pregnant at the time?
No!
OK, I know that anyway but for the sake of the interview! [Laughs] Can you remember what went through your mind when you found out? When you did the test, when you saw those two blue lines on the...?
Anger, absolute anger, fear and frustration at having got myself into that situation.
Because wasn't it something like you were on the pill?
Yes, yeah I stopped that whilst I was on a course in Germany, and I thought "Well I'll start having a break then." So I stopped taking it not thinking that Richard might come

Nine Women, Nine Months, Nine Lives

out and visit. He came out to visit and because I had been on the pill so long I thought... And I'd really taken it very haphazardly.
Yeah I suppose it must be difficult flying and that, working out the time zones and that...?
Oh yeah, well I'm a bit dizzy anyway, I mean I'd take none for two days and then take two the next day and stuff. So I thought, I really thought "Oh I'm immune to it". Errm... And then flying as well messes about with you so I thought, well it must be OK, there's been no reason to think that it could happen. Which was so <u>so</u> stupid and I was just so livid when it happened. So errm... That was the situation. Didn't expect it. Made a silly mistake and...
Because you weren't planning on having any kids at all were you?
Well, it didn't figure in my life, I knew that at some point it would probably figure in Richard's. I'm sure it did. To be honest, I'm sure it did. And I really wanted to hold out as long as I could. It really wasn't on the agenda, it's not something that we thought "Right we'll do that in so many years". I really thought I could last out until I was almost forty, but whether that was my dream...
Well maybe, maybe not. I mean you know it's not impossible, it could have been like that. There's no reason really to say that it wouldn't have been.
Yeah it's probably just something I'd put to the back of my mind and thought "Well maybe at some stage in my life I'll want to do this" but I really don't want to start talking about it or doing anything.
So was anybody with you when you did the test?
No, no I was on my own.
Was that what you wanted to do?
Errm... Well it was during the day and Richard was at work and I just knew I had to get this test over and done with, because I knew otherwise...
Were you late?
Yeah, and errm... I felt, I'd just been to my cousin's wedding and I'd felt really ill for about a week after that.
Really?
Yeah, I was sick and oh! I was thinking "This is some hangover, one or two days is Fine but [Laughs] not a week!"
Oh my God!
Yeah, and one of my friends said to me "You know you've been sick and well you should really find out for definite". I must admit the thought had entered my head but I thought "No it can't be true, it really can't be true" and then when I did the test... It was a real effort to get out of bed in the morning to go and get the test, I mean I haven't done a pregnancy test for years, I still thought that you had to do it first thing in the morning.
Oh right!
So that shows you how long...! So I ran down to the chemist, ran back, did the test, and that explained why I was late.
So how late were you? Were you like a week or two weeks?

Helen

I'm not quite sure but I'd say it was probably about two weeks. Yeah, which is kind of major, but then I didn't really pay much attention to it because I'd just stopped taking the pill and I just thought well, my system and everything will be completely messed up.
And you'd expect there to be some kind of adjustment anyway?
Yeah exactly and plus two years prior to that what with the wedding and the travelling and errm... I'd worked as much as I could work right up until Christmas, I'd got all my hours in before Christmas. So that the day after I'd finished work we went off to Australia, and I didn't have a period that month, so it wasn't until the following month, so it, that was strange. So I just thought "Oh it's all messed up, I've been working a lot" which does sometimes happen.
Yeah exactly.
So it really didn't worry me until I was still feeling ill after this wedding.
Your 'mysterious' hangover!
Yeah, yeah, so then I knew what it was likely to be, yeah.
And what was Richard's reaction? When did you tell him? Did you tell him straightaway?
No, errm... No, I told him that day but he was very late coming home from work. And errm... It all just cascaded out, it'd been going round and round in my head that day, and oh! [Laughs] It's just that, when you know that you're all emotionally errm... So it came across from me as being the worst thing possible and, and I just blurted it out. I was just the most miserable sobbing wreck. So his reaction was pretty negative as well, but that was tinged with shock. Yeah and I, beforehand, if I'd ever imagined telling him something like that I'd thought well yeah... But as it was he wasn't as overjoyed as I thought he would be, so that was good for me, personally. But he took it really really strangely, and that wasn't...
Well yeah, I suppose I mean, did you get the impression that he was reacting to you more than reacting to the fact that you were pregnant?
I don't know, a bit of both really. I mean we'd only been married six months, and although we'd been together for so long it...
Oh yeah, because you've been together since you were at school?
Yeah, and I think all the things that we could do together, you know, get off and do some more travelling together instead of doing it separately, which we had done, and errm... That was all in the forefront of my mind. It just seemed to be at the wrong time, and also knowing how I'd always felt about having children he knew that that was a bad thing. And initially he just said to me "Just do what you think, what you want to do" and that was a hard thing for him to say, it was a hard decision to have to make.
So do you think he handed over the responsibility?
Initially, initially, as I say it was, well it was really just that day. By the next day it was like no, we've got to decide what we want to do. Then that changed over the next fortnight, I knew what I felt, that I wouldn't want to, but... And I think Richard knew that and he kept saying "It'll be OK" and then it'd be "No we can't do this, we can't have

a baby, it will change everything." To the point that at the end of that fortnight errm...
We came to a decision at the end of that, because we had to put a time limit on it, and
then we talked and he said that we would do whatever I wanted to do. And he knew what
I wanted to do, I wanted to have an abortion and that he was saying it was OK with him.
Errm... And so that was what we decided to do, made another appointment to go and
see the doctor, errm... To get it arranged basically.
To go and get the blue slip and...
Yeah, that's right and errm... Then my best friend called that night and she asked me if
we had come to a decision.
So you'd talked to her about it?
Yeah I'd talked to her as she was my best friend. And I said "Yeah" and told her what
we'd decided to do and she said "How does Richard feel about that?" And she's known
Richard for probably about the same length of time as I've known him. All our adult
lives anyway, and I said "I'll pass the 'phone over to you he's, he needs to speak to
somebody else, he's only spoken to me, nobody else has discussed it with him, nobody
else knows the situation" and I was sat on the stairs listening. Which was a strange thing,
it was quite open, and I was sat there waiting for him to come off the 'phone so I could
speak to her again. And errm... I understood that what he was saying wasn't in line with
what he had told me. So really it came across that you know he, that we would go ahead
with the abortion to please me. I, I didn't discuss it any further at that point, I just
thought maybe I need to rethink this. Because I'd spent all my time thinking "I can't do
it, there's no way I can do it" and I had never swayed in thinking that until this phone
call.
How long after you found out did you decide that you were going to have an abortion?
Straightaway.
And then how long after that was this conversation, was it a week or two weeks?
This conversation, the conversation with my friend was two weeks later and in that time
we had both gone to see our doctor. Richard's now registered with my doctor so we've
all got the same doctor. And his reaction was initially "Well you'll have to pay for it
yourself." Which, at the time was a bit of a strange thing to say.
Particularly for a GP.
It's not as if we had done this willy nilly...
It's hardly as if you used it as a form of contraception!
Yeah, quite. Well, we said that was fine and he said "And then of course there's your
age". Which kind of shook me.
How old were you?
I was 30 just under 31, yeah I was 30. And that really shook me. Because sometimes...
Because we'd always been together you just think of yourself as being 20 or whatever and
then all of a sudden it was like "Oh I'm 30!" One minute I was at school and the next
minute I'm too old to have children! And it really effected me that way and errm... I
knew that was rubbish I just thought "Thirty's not old! I know what you're saying, I

Helen

know the biological clock may be ticking but I still feel too young to do it. I don't want to do it, I don't feel responsible enough to do it."
Yeah, but if you feel too young then, well perhaps you are...?
Yeah, and then it did make me have a rethink. I'm trying to remember exactly how he worded it but he, he was implying that it wasn't always the best physical move to make for your body if you want to have children after that. And errm... Once again I kind of decided that that was something that would be...
So if you perhaps decided that you were going to in the future then...?
Which I always think of as a scare-mongering tactic. That if you have an abortion then...
Yeah, I would say that I agree with that, errm... you can have a balanced opinion. GP's don't need to have and in-your-face extreme...
Yeah, he came on quite strong, trying to dissuade me. But it did initially, the day after the doctors. Yeah, so that, that was very strange, I did the test on the Friday and we went to the doctors on the Monday, it was either the Monday or the Tuesday. Yeah because I'd already booked an appointment at the doctors, but then at the end of the conversation at the doctor he said "I think you'd better go away and make up your minds, come back in a week". So I had this time limit. "If you can't get back here in a week, get back here as soon as you can, because you need to decide either way". I'm glad we did that, and I think it was better to have the time. And then before going back was this turning point, the 'phone call from my best friend. And I didn't say anything to Richard at the time, I thought about it over night and I was going back to work the following day. And I said "I think I've changed my mind, I thought maybe this is the only way, this is for the best, but it will happen again" which is more to the point. What would I do if it happened again? I can't be picking and choosing having one abortion or more.
Yeah, it's kind of like the consistency of your decision isn't it?
Because I'm so haphazard, I always have been haphazard with the pill which is why it never scared me that I would ever be pregnant I think.
Yeah because you kind of feel safer once you've been haphazard for so long. You kind of think, well I'll be fine. I mean I'm on the pill, the times that say I've got up late, say half past ten and I think "Oh it's only three hours, I'll be all right..."
Which never phased me at all!
No, exactly.
If it was only half a day late, that was normal. Or I'd take it at four o'clock in the morning and then again at 8 o'clock at night, when I was away on trips you know. So yeah it never really bothered me. So I thought I was safe, and as much as this has frightened me, it's going to happen again, I'm sure it is, because I will just think oh I'm OK. Which is why I've not gone back onto the pill again, because it's just too stupid.
There's always going to be the possibility of it happening again
Yeah, exactly and I can't let that happen again. Because there's no way I ever want to have to make that decision again, no way. I know that I thought that this might happen

Nine Women, Nine Months, Nine Lives

again this time, so in the end I thought right just get on and do it. So will that do?! [Laughs]
Yeah, yeah! [Laughs]
And when I called Richard, err... On his mobile it was, to talk about me having changed my mind, errm... I'd actually left a note on the pillow, and he hadn't been home yet, and I told him and he said he just couldn't take it in, his reaction was just so positive "It'll be OK, I'll look after your baby, I'll do everything!" So it was <u>so</u> positive.
Really, really positive.
I knew then that what he had said to me was very different from what he was feeling. It was amazing, unreal, to think that he cared about me that much! [Laughs]
Yeah, well that's it, you know no-ones ever really certain all the time.
No, but errm, I wanted to talk to him about, not practically, day-to-day but, what would happen, how would we look after a baby? When would I go back to work? Richard's work? We talked about the realities of it all, and he just kept saying "It'll be OK". And he has been great, I mean the times that I was in a real state, that I'd been on a flight with loads of screaming children, I would come home and close the door, I just felt like I couldn't deal with it. And then he would say something like "It'll be OK yours won't be like that" [Laughter] And I was like "Oh yeah, and how do you know?!"
Oh really?! Yeah mmm.
I was like, because he is so laid back and so am I, but he was convinced "No they won't be, they won't be highly strung or anything like that" but I wasn't so sure!
Yeah, well everybody has their good days and their bad days. And so do kids, every child is different, so you know, it's true what he said, yours might not be like that! But then again... [Laughs]
So errm... Even, I think even up to the end I wasn't sure if I was doing the right thing. But errm... you can only do the best that you can, and I was trying to cope with it, thinking "I am going to have this baby - it's too late now".
Mmm, kind of dealing with it then, knowing that you were going to have to deal with it at some stage...
At some stage yeah. It was a case of really, but I've never questioned my morals like that before <u>ever.</u> I always knew exactly what I would have done. Say if I'd got pregnant at twenty, it would have been a different situation but I would always know that if the situation arose... The main thing that made me step back from it was the fact that I was married, I couldn't justify it as much as if I had been single.
Really?
Yeah, which is ridiculous but yeah, and I don't think that marriage is this big thing, I don't think you've got to be married to have children, but the fact that I was married in that situation.
Do you think marriage perhaps reflected security almost?
Mmm, yeah. Yeah maybe but I just felt that I couldn't, because I could have done it when I was single. Because Richard said at one point "If we hadn't have been married,

Helen

even if we had been living together, and you'd got pregnant, you wouldn't have told me would you?" And I wouldn't.
No, it would have been a different situation.
I mean he knew me well enough, and knew what I would have wanted to do, but errm... yeah that's the way I would have done it.
Yeah, if that's the way you feel then...
But I think it did make a lot of difference the fact that I was married, I couldn't justify what I wanted to do, other than for selfish reasons and feelings on my part.
Yeah, it is quite a big-ee.
Yeah, definitely.
OK, right we're going to move on to the next chunk, errm, this is your experience of pregnancy and the birth. Now, you obviously weren't planning on having children...
No.
So you haven't ever sat down or imagined what pregnancy would be like, or looked at your friends who were pregnant and thought "Oh God no!"
No.
Errm... when you were in your early pregnancy, did you ever look forward and think something like "I'm going to be huge soon, I'm not going to be able to bend, I'm not going to be able to work..."
No, no because I didn't, I didn't know anything about it, I didn't want to know anything about it. I just wasn't interested. I was just like, big belly, have baby, I'll deal with it when it arrives. And that was the only way I could deal with it really. I didn't want to talk to my friends, because my friends had had children, I mean my best friend has two children, but I just didn't want to ask her, I just didn't want to know. And everybody at work, because obviously everybody at work, different people all the time, and they all want to tell you their story. It's usually a nightmare and the number of times I've said to people "Look I don't want to know this, I'm not being rude but I'm not happy with my situation, don't go any further, I don't want to hear your stories, they scare me". And most of the time people did stop, so I really didn't take it much further about finding out about you know. I carried on doing what I was doing, exercised, swum, and did things you know. I just didn't let it effect me, I ate really well anyway so I didn't have to change anything, I just let it go on. So no, I never <u>ever</u> thought about the birth, really until the last month.
[Laughs] Right!
And really late on in the last month as well, I was errm, thinking that at that point I was so big that you know I was thinking "It's got to get out" and errm...
So you'd not made a birth plan or anything like that?
No, not at all. We only really knew about what was available when the contractions were happening you know.
"Give me some drugs!" [Laughs]
[Laughs] Yeah, oh yeah that was a definite. If I could have booked in for a caesarean,

171

Nine Women, Nine Months, Nine Lives

I'd have done it!
You could have! You could have requested a caesarean. I'm surprised how few people know this.
Yeah, yeah? Because I always got the impression that they didn't tell you about them as they are more costly.
I suppose they could always ask you for a contribution as well!
Although if I wanted that, it wouldn't have gone down too well with Richard.
Well, there are all sorts of pluses and negatives.
So I could have requested one?
Yeah, you can.
So no I didn't make any plans other than errm... Having some kind of drugs.
So had you asked about what you could have and what the effects of you know if you had pethidine, gas and air and...?
Yeah, but I didn't ask about specifics, I just asked whether I could take the strongest thing to make it the least painful and that's as far in depth as I went. And errm... And I, that was it really. I think the first point at which I thought about what was going to happen to me was the week before because I went down to my, to my friends in London and I'd been there about an hour and I thought I'd had a show.
Oooh, panic!
Yeah!
I'm in London, miles away, oh my giddy!
Yeah because she was pregnant as well, so what happened was, she's calm and cool and errm... Obviously didn't want to get into a panic in her situation as well, but errm... I needed to know about everything. And she had books at home so we went back to her house, because we were out strolling around all over the place and when we got back to her house I spent most of that night reading! [Laughs] And thinking Ooh! [Laughs]
Mmm, finding out...
Mmm, so it was then.
Yeah, well when you needed to read it you did, so you know, and if you found out what you needed to know then, whether it was what you wanted to know...
Yeah, exactly.
But it felt right to do it then, so you did it.
So I avoided all the nightmare stories, all the "What if what if?" stuff. I just couldn't think like that, it would have been like "Well what else is going to happen to me?!"
So you started reading then, and you found out what you needed, the drugs and...
When I needed to, in the hospital, turned out to be something minor, because I probably didn't know enough, so from that point maybe I didn't educate myself well enough. But everybody is really helpful in that situation. Initially I felt as if I was wasting people's time, but...
Yeah that's right, and it's your first baby, you couldn't know...
And I can't, I can't go on other people's experiences, it's not your experiences, it's not

Helen

the way you think, it's not the way you feel. It's not the way that you deal with everyday things, so I just asked when I got there.
Mmm, wait and see.
Late really but...
Yeah, you did the best you could do, everyone says or thinks and does...
Everyone is an individual isn't it?
Precisely. I mean you know yourself, what suits you and what does not.
Exactly!
It's like the example you gave earlier about gruesome stories, and you asked people to stop, you really didn't want to know, and you knew what you could deal with. I mean I've done a similar thing recently, about going out to Andorra. Got my PhD exams about three days after I get back, how much stuff am I taking with me? None! Because if I take it with me I'll panic, if it's not there, I won't think about it!
Yeah, just forget it, if you don't know it by now, you won't know it!
It's a perfectly normal way of dealing with it. It might seem a bit strange but...
Yeah, just feels like I am just, I don't know, escapism thinking. But then it works so...
[Laughs]
Yeah, if it worked, then fine.
The girls at you know, at work, they when they're pregnant, they ask me. And I say "Well I can't say what it was like for me, because it'll be different for you, I'm not going to tell you one thing, it might be different for you." Because I had, I had a very easy time of it, honestly. And if I said that to somebody and they did not, then they'd be like "Oh why didn't you tell me?" So I just say "If you want to know go and ask somebody else I'm not going to tell you."
How do you think your pregnancy was, in reality? Do you think it was, that there were particular parts of it that were really awful, that were a shock, and other bits that were actually better or not as...?
Errm... I think the shocking thing was not being able to do things that you could have done three weeks prior to that. You know errm... Because you are out of breath because you don't have the stamina that you had because errm... You're tired. The feeling of being exhausted when you are only eight or nine weeks pregnant, and you don't look pregnant and you know, you're not even, your heads not even round the idea, but this thing is slowing you down and making you feel a certain way. Errm... I mean luckily I wasn't very ill it was just that, other than that week, there was nothing else that was making me feel so sick or anything, I didn't have anything really of that. And being really really tired. But other than that it... Just the fact that it stopped me from doing things. And little things used to drive me up the wall errm... Walking at a certain pace, when I was working I would feel it a lot more.
Yeah because it's a physical job.
Yeah, I could feel it a lot more, after I just couldn't do a thing, you know when I'd finished work the other end. So as soon as I could it was legs up the wall when I first

Nine Women, Nine Months, Nine Lives

got in and then I would just zonk! But I needed it and it was a good time to do it so.... But yeah, the restrictions. And then later on being so big and, trying to get comfortable... And well I mean you're the same size as me, you're not used to your clothes being uncomfortable!
No, exactly!
Errm... Right down to your underwear as well! It's a huge thing, you feel like you've just got to get it sorted out. But there's not much you can do. Errm... What else? And later on that you get itchy, things that are to do with the pregnancy, the physical things that you are like "Why am I putting up with this? What can I take to put it right?" Well there isn't anything!
No, I think that's, yeah, I hear that a lot as well. That there is this, this kind of frustration really.
You're stuck with it!
Yeah, there is a lack of control.
It is a lack of control, and I, that was probably the most frustrating thing.
It's your body, suddenly, it ain't!
You can't control it, yeah exactly. What else was there? Errm... Reactions from people were quite strange, I suppose doing the job I was doing, the fact that I was still flying.
Oh yeah, because you were flying till quite late weren't you?
Yeah, and wearing a great big maternity dress, that was strange. And I suppose it was strange because people were so, open and errm... nosey. I couldn't deal with that because I'm just like, no you're not knowing any of my business don't even ask! So at work errm... to have complete strangers ask me when am I due and blah blah blah, the questions about it, that I should be really happy, I found that difficult to deal with. I should have just lied, but I couldn't get the... Do you know what I mean? It was a strange situation, I found that difficult, and errm... The fact that everybody had a story, that was pretty bad, [Laughs] I found that very difficult to deal with. Everybody had to tell me their nightmare story. My Auntie Chris would telephone me and tell me her stories and I didn't like to say no to her, she must have told me the same story six times – aarghh! [Laughs] And when she'd done telling me I would phone my mum and say "Auntie Chris has told me her story again! Oh God I've had to listen to it again!" And it's a twenty-minute story, and it's quite factual in detail, and... But she was the only one I would let go on like that, because, her memory's gone and I wouldn't upset her, and so I wouldn't upset her by saying that. So that was oh! [Laughs] And men! Men would tell me their wife's situations!
Really?
Yeah! And I found that almost obscene. Really... Odd. Really really odd.
What about the birth and everything if they were there and stuff like that?
Yeah, yeah, and I had a pilot, errm... I went in to give him his tea, and he started saying about his errm... pelvic floor exercises, his ex-wife and pelvic floor exercises [Laughs] And in the end I just had to say "Do you need anything else?" It was so embarrassing!

Helen

[Laughs]
Oh for Christ's sake! [Laughs]
Why was I forced into that situation? Telling me about his ex-wife and how she does trampolining and now she can't do it because she wets herself and, oh God! But things like, they were an encroachment into your private life. And I couldn't understand that because it was like you were public property because you were pregnant. And, one of my friends said to me "You'll also find that people will come and touch your belly" and you get so protective, complete strangers. And they do! Weird! That was just, maybe that was just the Americans. [Flies for an American Airline] Because they are very open, about the families and all that kind of stuff and, I don't know... [Laughs]
And the birth, did it match up to the horror stories you had heard?
Well I think because I had such a bad, I knew it was going to be really bad, I knew it was going to be the hardest thing that I ever did. Errm... It wasn't as bad as I thought, it was bad, but having now had a baby, the labour wasn't that long but then when does labour start? When do you count labour from? And this is what I had got into my head it was like. I counted labour from when I had real pain, which was literally, right after the drugs I was still having pain, so that to me is <u>real</u> pain.
That's pain! [Laughs] That's no nonsense pain.
Yeah, and that was really only about an hour and forty five. So that was nothing. So do people count from when they get contractions or what, because some people are in labour for like 30 hours. I couldn't, and I know they do, and I couldn't imagine that I would have that pain for all that time, maybe they do, but I don't know. And I think because I had expected it to be a long drawn out process I'd got my head ready for it. I mean I didn't ever go to any of the antenatal classes or anything like that, but I think if you do exercise you know how to breathe anyway, and that's all I could relate it to. Errm... I didn't, errm... I didn't think it was going to be any different because that's when you're pushing yourself and you think it'll be done soon and you can breathe or whatever. Errm... So no it, it really wasn't as bad as I thought it would be. And, and the impression I had [about hospitals and having a baby] was mostly from the television, of people coming and going. And, it was a bit surreal really because there was only errm... I felt like I was a fly on the wall the whole time, like it wasn't happening to me!
Was that before the drugs?! [Laughs]
[Laughs] Yeah, wait till the morning after! Errm... But there was just the errm... the midwife, yeah, the midwife. The midwife, Richard and myself. Apart from when they brought in the anaesthetist, it was just the three of us, which was so strange. I'd never really expected that so I'm glad I had no expectations, or I did, the only negative, well the only expectations that I had were negative. Because it was far better from that point of view with just the three of us. So it was quite a private, nice thing. Well it wasn't nice but you know.
It was nicer?
Yeah, you've still got to do what you've got to do at the end of the day but it was loads

Nine Women, Nine Months, Nine Lives

better the way it was done. And errm... Everybody says that at the end you want it out and you will do anything to do that, but that's for a short time when you feel like you just want it over. I don't think I realised how exhausted I was going to be, errm... Because I had felt exhausted, well not exhausted but... Doing a job on a daily or a weekly basis but you knew that if you pushed yourself too hard at each end [of the flights] then it would catch up with you. So I'd kind of thought that it's probably going to be like that. But it was much more, I was <u>ab-so-lutely</u> exhausted, because you are. I was in the room and the nurse came into the room with errm... A bottle and I thought "Oh no, I can't!"
You'd no strength to hold him and feed him?
Yeah exactly, I thought "What am I going to do? And I just, I can't do it!" Thank <u>goodness</u> they had no intentions of giving him to me. They went straight to Richard, which was lovely! [Laughs] I was just so relieved! [Laughs]
Yeah, there's all these things that you can't know until you've been there and...
Mostly I just felt relief, relief it was a boy, and relief that I don't have to do it again! [Laughs] Yeah, errm, and relief that it was over! Just the once anyway!
Yeah? Right, and how did you feel when you actually did hold him for the first time?
Like I say, I felt like a fly on the wall, and I continued to feel like that for weeks if not months. So, there was this "How can I be in this situation?" maybe total denial, maybe, I don't know actually. The whole time I felt like a fly on the wall. I knew I had, I mean I didn't know <u>what</u> to do when I was left on my own. I mean thankfully I got a room which was a Godsend because I don't know, I don't know I think it was just the time he was born there was a room free. I was <u>so</u> lucky. I realise that now. You think God that's just what you need but it's not available, so I know how fortunate I was, and errm... I think it would have frightened me being on a ward with all those babies crying and stuff. But at least I could get some rest and errm... then when I woke up he was chewing his hand and I thought "Oh maybe he's hungry" and that was the only reason that I thought I'd better do something. Still at that point I didn't know what to do, so I rang the nurse and the nurse came in and I said "I think he's hungry can you show me what to do?" And I said "I know nothing about changing nappies, so I've got to learn whilst I'm in hospital. Because I can't pretend I know everything because I don't and I haven't got enough common sense to figure it out." So yeah I just thought, God I've got to find out now. If you don't do it nobody else is going to do it" so that makes you try, and continually through, you know, through the day through the night through the weeks and months. You do what you have got to do because nobody else is there to do it and so, you just can't go through the motions.
Mmm, and how was Richard involved in the pregnancy? Was he sort of just there for you, was he interested? I know he came along to the evening class...
Oh yeah, he really didn't want to come to that. And he was the only one there. I almost had to blackmail him to come, not blackmail him but...
Yeah, I know what you mean, maybe, coerce him?
Yeah I ended up saying to him, "if you're not going to come tell me now because I can

Helen

ask my mum to come and I know my mum will come." And now he said that he felt it would be a waste of time, which is no reflection on you, but...
Oh no, but if that was his perception of it then...
Well initially when I said I was going to do it he said "You're wasting you're time – there's no point in doing it you'll be all right". You know he kept saying that the whole time, "You'll be OK". Errm... I didn't think I would be OK. And I needed to, I needed to say things I couldn't say. I would have hated to have offended his mum and dad, you know, I didn't want to upset my mum and dad. I mean they don't, they don't understand, they're from a different generation, you know. I didn't think Richard's parents would understand but they were very understanding, very. Because I wasn't even there when Richard told them I was pregnant, I didn't want to be there. I thought I'd just ruin their happiness their joy and stuff, so I just didn't want to be there. That was quite hard. He was totally supportive all the time, he was willing to give up work. Errm... He, he would have been the mother, but as it happened we managed, by sheer luck, to find him a place in a nursery. Errm... he took the place of my sister-in-laws baby, so my nephew's, in the holidays. Initially in the summer, just for two weeks. And then my sister-in-law said "Well what about the other babies going on holiday, why don't you just ask if he can slot in to everybody else's holidays?" Which we did until September, and then he, then in January a place came up so, that helped. I mean all right, it's a big expense a month, but also for what Richard could be earning working, well we just couldn't do it. So errm... But he was totally brilliant, not to work for three days or something or work week-ends to make up for the time, so yeah, he was totally supportive in that way. I don't think he could understand the way that I was thinking at the time, purely because he loves children.
So he comes from a different standpoint anyway when it comes to...?
Yeah, exactly, totally different totally. And I think once I said, I was going to have the baby, he thought well everything from this point forward is going to be OK. And it was only really the odd occasions were I just, where I was an emotional mess, that he realised it wasn't OK. And then finally when he came to the class, errm... And he saw when we were sat outside, he said "Maybe I shouldn't be here". And I said "Well it's up to you, you can either sit in the car or you can come in". And he said "Well I might as well come in now I'm here". And then when we got back out I was so grateful that he'd come, and I said "You know I really appreciate the fact that, I know you didn't want to come, but I really appreciate it". And he said "No, you needed to do this, I see that now". So that was good that he could alter his opinion so, so hugely really.
And to be willing to see your point of view?
Yeah, to accept the situation. But I mean I evaluated, it really helped me, I didn't want to... There were things I needed to sort out in my own head, which I seemed to be able to do. Because it was total strangers, errm... So it was easier. Because whenever I had tried to weigh up it had just put me in a worse state, so it helped.
And during the birth, Richard was there?

Nine Women, Nine Months, Nine Lives

Oh yes. I didn't want him to be there either, I just wanted to go away, get it done, and come back, with a baby!
So you'd talked to him about it? And you'd said to him that you didn't want him to be there, did he want to be there?
Oh yeah, yeah. And he said "Don't be ridiculous! I've got to be there, there's no way I don't want to be there. Because it might never happen again. I want to be there". I was just like, "oh for goodness sake, what difference will it make, you get a baby at the end of the day!" [Laughs] Black and white!
Yeah exactly! [Laughs]
He said "But I just want to see, I just want to experience that."
Well you're not going to experience it! [Laughs]
No, exactly. And I didn't realise how, how draining it would be on him as well.
Yeah?
Yeah, because you've got all the emotional stuff that is flying around, yeah, stamina is what it takes. But when he was there it was like just...
Was he there in the background? Was he able to, practically be able to help you?
Errm... Yeah, he was very encouraging, errm... He stayed with me, the morning after until after three, went and grabbed something to eat and then came back. Yeah, he was right on in there, as close as you could be for some of it! [Laughs] And errm... And the midwife would ask him to do stuff and he would just do it. And errm... Like at the point where it was painful, he was like "what do you need? I'll do anything", so he was there, he went through that, was very supportive. And errm... Then when errm... When the nurse came in with the milk, he was straight there because I was just...
"No, not me!"
Yeah! [Laughs] I kind of looked at him and he was just there. I didn't need to say anything he just did it [fed the baby] so.... He was brilliant. Still is.
Yeah, yeah.
So from that, I think, if he hadn't been so confident, so unfazed by it all, I think I took my confidence from the way he reacted, so he'd do stuff before I'd even think about it. And I would look and think "Oh that's how you do that, you just do that!"
What you mean when you got him home?
Yeah when we actually got home, I mean I was quite happy to stay in the hospital for about six months! [Laughs] "Oh do I have to go home and do this on my own now?"
Yeah – "Are you sure?" [Laughs] "You'd hardly notice I was here!"
Exactly, I was in no rush. Errm... I tried to stay calm, that was all I ever did. Throughout he was just full of common sense so I just learnt from him really, so that helped.
So would you say that his support during pregnancy was more or less than you had hoped for?
I'd say it was a lot more, yeah, a lot more.
And the birth?

Helen

Errm...
There may have been good bits and bad bits.
Yeah, I was going to say that knowing him I should have expected him to be as good as he was...
Mmm, but you didn't?
But I didn't, no.
It's a new situation...
I think because you are very selfish about the whole situation as well. I was anyway. I was like "Well how am I going to do, what will...?" You know. And I hadn't really given him much thought. Which is a terrible situation but I think I was so wrapped up in like...
In what you were...
Errm... Like am I really doing this? That it kind of took over everything, errm... And all the time, for the entire nine months he kept saying "It'll be OK" and all the time I'd been thinking "It won't be OK. Life is not going to be as easy as you think it will." So, and then, at the birth he just kind of, kind of held it together really.
It carried on over into the...?
Yeah, so I should have expected that he would do that but I was too wrapped up in myself really to think about, I'd say.
I mean it was, well birth is primarily your area.
Well yeah that's it. And I am quite independent anyway so I was just like well, I'll deal with it.
Mmm, I'll do it my way?
Yeah, mmm.
Right the next chunk is your experience of early motherhood. So a maximum of up to the end of the first three months. Would you say that your pregnancy effected early motherhood? Was there anything residual, perhaps water retention, the tiredness, some women still have a bit of nausea up to the end...?
Just the tiredness really, errm... And I should have taken more heed from the classes. To say "Please don't call at this time, please don't come round at this time. Give me some space". I should have been stronger in saying that. Because that was exhausting, and I was exhausted. Richard's mum was fantastic she'd turn up and say "I've brought you something to eat, just plonk it in the microwave, I've put the washing in, I've taken it out, there it is clean". My mum would come round, play with him, and then go home about half an hour later!
Yeah? Just what you need!
Yeah! [Laughs] Errm... That happened time and time again, ridiculous, awful! My dad thought it would be a good idea for my mum to come and help me in the first week but that just wore me down. And the emotional situation as well, the fact that it was just such an alien thing to have this little thing in your home, it wears you down.
And there's nothing that you can contemplate it being like.
Errm... So you've got the emotional tiredness, the physical tiredness, purely because

179

Nine Women, Nine Months, Nine Lives

of the things that need to be done.
The things that have got to be done.
Yeah, yeah. I'm sure whether you are breastfeeding or bottle feeding you would have the same exhaustion. You've just got to do it and there's no escaping it, and when there is someone who will do things for you there are still twenty things down the line that you've got to do. Errm... To eat yourself, to get some sleep, you know, but that's way down the line, because firstly you've got to look after this little baby so... Yeah so exhaustion I think was the thing, because I, I tend to... Prior to this, in my life I just pushed myself, I just pushed myself, I'd get by, I'd be OK, I would tend to think "Oh I'll sleep later on".
Yeah or catch up in the week?
Yeah, whereas with this there is no catching up. There's always a feed or something.
And did the birth effect early motherhood at all? You know stitches things like that?
Errm... Again, I think I knew it was going to be uncomfortable and sore. You just...
That was just the way it was?
I knew I was going to be pulled about, but you know, it was better to just...
So you kind of thought just get on with it, on reflection?
Yeah that bits over, it was OK.
Yeah, this I can do! [Laughs] Yeah, but if you'd done that to me today, and I felt like that...
I'd be dying but yeah.
Yeah, yeah, but at the time?
Yeah, you've got to put it into perspective, don't you, that was a short but busy time.
Yeah I'll bet it was! [Laughs]
Yeah, so...
OK how did you imagine early motherhood would be for you? Had you got a picture in your mind what Will would be like? How you would sort out the things like feeding and stuff like that?
Mmm, not really. I errm... I think I blocked it out of my mind because I just couldn't imagine what I would be doing. So everything was, each day was, was, I just ended up applying common sense to, that was how I got by.
Yeah, I remember you saying when I saw you before.
I remember Richard saying early on he was like, "well if you're hot then he must be hot."
Oh yeah!
And that, yeah, I just kept thinking that all the way along. It was just such a simple thing. You know, I need to eat every three hours because I've, I've got low blood sugar but I have, and I need to eat on a regular basis, and I thought "Well yeah, If I need that then he needs it!"
I mean he's not an alien, you know he's a human...
Exactly, <u>exactly</u>! So that was how, you know that kind of got us by. Prior to that I just hadn't given it a thought.

Helen

That's fair enough. Yeah. And how do you think it actually was?
Not an experience I'd want to repeat.
So the first few months was...
Not nice.
No, it was a shock?
Yeah, yeah, but errm... A shock but then, then you surprise yourself and think "as the weeks go by I think I can deal with this, you know, it's OK. I did that last week so I can do it this week." Errm... "And this week is better than last week, or this day is better than last week", and then all of a sudden you get a day that is just crap. And I'd think "I hate it I don't want to be in this situation, how did I, why did I decide to do this? How can I get out of it now? Right now!" [Laughs] "Can I just go?!" It's like I was desperate to get back to work, errm... And that was my saving grace. As hard faced as it sounds, and I know it does sound hard faced but, that was my saving. Because I got, all right sleeps still messed up but I got one full nights sleep a week. So I mean that was great, but it was hard for Richard because he was still here. Yeah, it was the best thing. I can't, I mean, I mean I wasn't asking anybody about anything, I didn't want to know how bad it was, that there was no escape was bad enough. For example, my friend Sam, I just couldn't, in any conversations we've had, before she decided what to do, I was like "Sam it is going to be so hard [partner walked out when she got pregnant]. It is so hard with Richard here. What is it going to be like?"
Yeah on your own. Yeah, it's unimaginable.
And that was the strongest thing I could ever say to somebody. It's harder to like be on your own, it's, it's... I don't know how young girls do it, I really don't. Without the support that you know, so it's... I mean I look at it this way, it's education without life, a life of education you know outside school, without basic things that you'll need to know. Errm... because at sixteen, eighteen, you're still a young girl.
Yeah, where are your survival skills?
Yeah, exactly, you just don't have them. I think that, I just don't know how they do it, I do believe that I wouldn't have been able to, if that had happened to me at that stage. I wouldn't have had a clue. So, yeah I think that although I had prepared myself that it was going to be bad, it was still a shock.
It was really bad?
Yeah, it was still a shock.
And what was the most difficult thing in say the first three months? The thing that really brought you up short.
Errm... The <u>constant</u> lack of sleep, and the fact that there was no let up. Errm... And because people were continually around, there was no let up when there should have been. And, and, while it frustrated me and I was trying to sort myself out and deal with it and like say "Don't come round" I also didn't want to upset anybody because I was so emotionally unbalanced at the time, I couldn't. I think that it just frustrated me so much, and the lack of sleep. Because normally as I say, when you can catch upon your sleep,

181

Nine Women, Nine Months, Nine Lives

fine. It's a different day, deal with it, but it was constant, constant, constant. Everybody kept saying he's so good, he's this, and you know, but when a baby is crying in the middle of the night...
It's crying.
I mean he didn't cry for hours on end or anything like that, he was very easy osey, and if he cried he needed something. But it was just when you're in an absolute coma sleeping because you are <u>so</u> tired, and you're woken so abruptly, to sit for half an hour forty minutes to do what you've got to do, then that's, that's hard. So yeah, probably the exhaustion with it all.
OK and what would you say was the best thing about that time?
[Pulls a face]
I know, I know, but there might be something that was not so...
Mmm, yeah.
Or perhaps the least worse thing? I don't know...
The least worse thing. Probably when they start reacting to you, and they, smile and stuff, and then that is quite nice.
Yeah?
Yeah, because before that you feel like you're just behaving like a machine. And I remember one morning, when he was about one and a half, I don't know he was maybe five weeks old, six weeks old, and I hadn't spoken to him at all, and this was by lunchtime, and this was like on a usual day. Errm... And at that point I thought "I've got to snap out of this and start talking to him like a human he's not this little thing". All right, because everything, I just did it because I knew that somebody had to do it, I was there to do it, get on with it. But that was ridiculous. I thought that was, I thought "I've been constantly doing this, just because I'm so tired". And I know that it's strange because when I'm at work and it gets to about five o'clock in the morning, I'm just like leave me alone I want to go to sleep.
Yeah, "Just go away!"
Yeah, and it's the same thing, because you are so tired. I just didn't want to ever have to do conversations, and plus they don't talk back to you, so there's no need to talk. From my point of you it was like, there was no need to talk. Errm... That was, when he, you know, when you said this or that he would smile or look at you or look for you or something, then later on when he started doing that, that was nice.
And how much was Richard involved in those early days?
Totally, he did at least as much as I did. Errm... He was still working so I would try in the night to do the feeds because at that stage I could cover, but he was there as much as I was. He was very involved as well. He never, he never just left it to me, when he'd be away, I'd say OK I'd do it, and then when I was, it was him. Life's still the same, because with me, for half a week he has to do it.
Yeah, because you're not here.
So, we always knew that it would be. But I think it, I think it was probably, errm... A

Helen

shock to me that I had to do as much as half a week! [Laughs] Do you know what I mean? [Laughs] I was like "Well he said he'd be looking after this baby, why am I doing it?" [Laughs] I was just going to go back to work! I was like "Oh God, have I got to?" But yeah, he was the most help to me, more than my mum was, he was the most help, the most understanding. The most thoughtful, yeah, I was very lucky. And again, it's only when you listen to other people you're like, "Oh my God!" Because you take it for granted... I didn't know and...
Well yeah yeah, exactly.
So errm... Like I say, I was very lucky. Just the fact that, the friend that I was with down in London, when I first thought I'd had a show, errm... And she also flies, has one baby and is on maternity leave at the minute, so because she's off, she also because she's obviously doing most things all the time, he would never think to bath their baby or he never want to be involved in bath time or... And she would ask him and he would be like, "No I don't want to do that" even though he had wanted the baby too! And I'm just like "Oh my God!" you know, and he is just one of the most lovely people so it was really shocking when I heard. And he was the one that wanted the children. You know at the time, she did want children but he, well I suppose with him being that little bit older, so he was like right, right now!
Yeah, this is a good time, let's do it!
So...
But the reality of it...?
Yeah, that kind of highlighted to me, how much he does.
It brought it home to you?
Yeah, and like a lot of fathers will do certain things but not others.
Yeah, oh yeah! God the amount of times I get, you know, I mean one girl, her partner hasn't even changed a nappy!
See, that's what he's like!
I was just horrified, and I just thought well, right, is she exaggerating or...? No she's really not. That's for real!
I mean we were at a party a few weeks ago and there were loads of guys saying that, and they all take the, this was a rugby tour party, and they all take the mickey out of Richard. But he's like... And I said to him, "Does it not ever bother you Richard, you know, you said you were going to give up work to help out?" He said "That's their problem, I've not got a problem with it". So at the party they were saying "He really does this because he wants to?" And I just said "Well what do you think, do you think his mum comes over and does it all?!"
Yeah, the magic fairy comes along and does it!
And yeah, he does go over there to eat [his mums] and stuff because he hasn't got time to cook a meal and do all the stuff. When there is two of you, one of you does it. But yeah, basically he's there, he does the same as I do if not more. This week he's doing more because I'm away for four days, so he's got him for four days.

183

Nine Women, Nine Months, Nine Lives

So he did a lot, and he still does a lot?
Yeah, yeah.
Errm... Had you talked about who would do what?
Not really, not specifics no, and errm... I think it all changed because at the time Will was born, it was just the start of spring wasn't it, March so errm... Things were just so busy for Richard. The months before hadn't really been that busy, so we hadn't really expected it, so we had to deal with what we had at the time. And at that point Richard, could, well, a couple of months after, when he was old enough to go to the nursery, he could go there and that kind of resolved the situation. Because he had work stacked up as far as you could see, so even though we had planned something, the way we wanted it initially, it just wouldn't have worked out. Or financially it would have been a bit stupid really.
To turn down the work?
Yeah, exactly. And then another work situation came up as well that was always brewing from before Will was born, and now is what Richard does. But errm... That was in the background as well, but you know, maybe later on it worked out quite well so... It's a case of well that's what we planned initially but, it's not going to come off, and I think we realised that and we worked round it. In fact before he was born, we did.
Well I suppose with his work and stuff, he must know fairly early on in advance, that he would be busy?
Yeah, oh yeah. So basically, we worked round it, and his business is going OK. And I've said it's just like well... I don't know, looking back at it now! [Laughs]
Yeah, well. Do you feel that things worked out for the best?
Errm... Having the baby, or, errm... In what way do you mean?
In terms of him working and you being at home, the way that the workload was split, and in terms of...?
Yeah it worked out to be the best situation that we could have. Errm... Had Richard gone back to work and I'd stayed at home like full-time, that would have been, madness. There was absolutely no point. And as much as you know, the people in their fifties and sixties think that that's what you should do, not all people, but a lot of people do, and a lot of people say "Oh are you going back to work? So that's you not working anymore, is it?" Well, no. Because, you know, I've worked long enough that I've worked up to a good level of salary.
Yeah exactly, and you get used to it.
Oh yeah! I have never, ever, and I'm sure you've not, been in a situation where I've ever had to say to Richard "Look, can I have this?" [Laughs] And that would needle me so much. Really, that's, that is another reason why I was desperate to get back to work, I did not like having to say, and it was no problem to Richard at all, but it...
But if that was how you felt and you felt so strongly...
Yeah, so errm... No it couldn't have worked any other way. I could not have stayed at home. I couldn't have let Richard support everything, it would have been worse. While

Helen

they're working on a garden the other guy would be off building and doing other stuff, and then they wouldn't have been paid until three months later. We couldn't survive on that, we'd have got by but that would have been it. And that's reality. I mean hopefully in time things will work out but errm... And I think, I do think, that I am better towards Will for being away.

Yes, yeah.

And I say that without a doubt. I think I would be an awful person. I don't know what kind of state I would be in if I had to be here all the time. Get away, get a break, come back, and I can deal with the situation. And Richard and I have always been used to us living like that anyway so, he's got to fit in.

OK, good. The next chunk is your experience of motherhood up to the present day. This is a big-ee, how do you think you life has changed since you had your first baby?

[Laughs] Oh hardly at all! [Sarcasm - Laughs]

Oh I didn't notice, when did that happen?!

Yeah! Errm... It's made me more errm... Responsible for my actions. Before I'd just bomb off, and come home from a trip and say "Oh I'm going down to..." All my friends live out, not all of them but the majority of the real good friends, live outside Leicester. I'd come back and say "I'm going to be here for a day and then I'm off". And that was never a problem. But I can't do that now! [Laughs] I just can't do it. So it curbs your life in every possible way. Errm... it curbs your life to the point where you have to think about whether to have a bath or a shower, you know? Down to when you eat, when you can go to bed, every possible area of your life, social life, yeah it takes a lot of juggling. You've just got to be constantly rearranging things.

What you mean you make an arrangement and then you have to change them, to be flexible?

Well, I was pretty flexible anyway but no you've got to look ahead and think "Right I can't do that I'm going to have to do this, I'd better make some arrangements for Will" on say the social things. But day-to-day, I mean like you think well "I can't get down and get some veggies or something like that until we've done this." You can't just hop out and say "Right I'm going to be there at nine thirty" because nine thirty's going to be a push it a bit. So your whole life is taken over by what you need to provide for this baby, first. I was fairly, I didn't have to provide anything for Richard before really, do you know what I mean? If I wasn't at home he would eat at his mums, or get something himself and that's fine. So, I never had those restrictions on my life before and now I feel I really heavily do. Errm... And that was hard. And I knew it would be that way which is why I didn't want any children!

Yeah, yeah.

And errm... But it is, and as I say there are ways around it but I you know, I try not to restrict the places we go to or the things we do. And just try and carry on doing stuff but there is a limit.

Yeah, well yeah.

Nine Women, Nine Months, Nine Lives

I mean it takes a lot of preparation, I mean I still do it, but it just takes a lot more thought and stuff, whereas before I was... Same for Richard really. Errm, yeah, I'd say that was the most major thing, and it just effects every single thing that you do. But I'm lucky, I've got a lot of people around me who want to help, I mean they are desperate to help out. Errm... And if I needed to use them more I could but I probably don't because I think I'd feel well I'm only at home for three or four days, I shouldn't need to take him to somebody else, but you have to do it for you own, mental well-being. Because you have to have a social, you can't cut out your social life totally.

No, well, you have to know your own limitations, you have to know your needs, and if you know they're not being met you're not being... I mean there's no point being a martyr!

There is <u>no</u> point, because you're not doing anybody any good and you only end up resenting the baby in the end, so that's no good.

I mean there's, you can't do the things you want to do at the moment because financially it's not possible. But over time, you know it'll work out eventually, and errm... As long as that is a positive situation to know that that's what's ahead of you, even if it's five years, it's there.

Yeah, errm... I mean I know it's the same for Richard, like he plays rugby and stuff, and so the nights I'm away he trains one of the nights, and makes arrangements.

Yeah, making sure everything's all right?

Yeah, exactly, and he's working a lot at the weekends now, trying to get this (new business) up and running. So he has to make arrangements there. There was a time when I was working the weekends so that he could work something out, and errm... But he's had to realign that as well, so it's not just from my point of view, he's had to do the same.

So both your lives have changed?

Totally. Yes. We should sell the baby! [Laughs]

[Laughs] Yeah but would you get a good price though?

Yeah, of course! Put him up for auction! [Laughs]

[Laughs] OK, how do you think you have changed since you've had you first baby?

Errm... I've become a lot less selfish, I was pretty calm anyway but I'm very calm now. Errm... Most things are irrelevant and petty and just don't matter. I think about what's going on, and I'm just calm. After the blast of the first few months and the fact that we managed through that, errm... And like I say I think I've become a more responsible person.

And do you think there was any sort of permanent or temporary changes that perhaps came and went, in the last year?

Errm... Yeah, errm... I can't deny it any longer – I <u>have</u> got a baby! [Laughs]

Yeah?!

Yeah, that's one of them! [Laughs] And just accepting your situation and life. You start off thinking you will do everything you want to do and everything's going to be nice. But

Helen

you can't, things slow you down, there are just some things you've just got to deal with. Errm... And I think, I think the things that have changed are, errm... Frustrations, and things because they're so... I couldn't understand because I wasn't that way so. Women with babies and children, it used to frustrate me, terrible, <u>terrible.</u> Pandering to babies you know coming up and tickling him and. I think, I'm just this way, whereas initially that used to aggravate me so much. Errm... The fact that grandparents spoil children and stuff like that. You've just got to live with it, where as you, six months ago, four months ago let's say, it was still frustrating me. But that's just a difference in personalities and ages and everything else, they have a different relationship with him. It took me a long while to realise, to not to judge people me, I mean we all judge people, but it doesn't wind me up now, not any more. Errm... That used to be a constant frustration.

Mmm, and do you think that's a good change?

Yeah, yeah. Much as I wouldn't like to admit it. [Laughter] But yeah, a good change. Bad, oh I can think of one bad change! My mind is like a sponge, but not in a good way you know, it's just like... It's frazzled really! No brain! I think it's one of those physical effects. I'll start doing one thing and then I'll swap over onto something else, I was pretty bad at that anyway but it's severe now. I wasn't here earlier when you came so...[Had arranged the visit for earlier in the day but Helen had forgotten!]

Oh no, no!

Errm... Yeah, that was a bad one. I expected a lot more (problems)! [Laughs] Yeah.

Yeah? [Laughs]

I thought it would cause problems between Richard and I, and it's not. I think if anything it's brought us closer together, than I would, I would never have imagined that that could happen. Errm...

Not with the way you were feeling?

No, no exactly. I really thought it would be a nightmare, that he'd be so adoring to the baby and I'd just be, want to walk out. But he's not, he's as strict as I am if not stricter than I am.

Mmm, OK. Now you've gone back to work and you feel like you've managed it as well?

Yeah.

It was what you wanted, and you knew it was what you wanted and it is?

Yeah.

And do you get any time for yourself? Just you, without Richard, without Will, and not at work.

When I'm at home no.

No, but when you're away, you manage to do something for yourself?

Yes, oh yeah. I, if I want to be completely on my own I can do it, errm...If I want to be with people, because it's, we've got a reasonably small base for the size of the company. So pretty much you know, at least three or four people on each trip. So if you want to be part of something then you can go out, and have a meal and all the things that

187

Nine Women, Nine Months, Nine Lives

you don't get to do as often now. Errm... Or go shopping or whatever, you know. Nice things that I took for granted before, errm... Then I can do it. But if I just want to veg' out and do nothing, not even go out of my room then I can do that. So yeah, it's nice to be able to do the little things like that, to have a shower and wash your hair, and things like take three hours to do it kind of thing. And that's lovely. So, loads of times when I'm away, but I don't find I really have very much time at all to myself when I'm at home. But that's, you know, that's life.

That's the way it is.

You've got to keep doing washing, you've got to eat properly, and there's always stuff that needs doing. I take care of him full-time when Richard's working, but Richard now, again, it's a different kind of period, and that will change.

So do you get much time to spend together, just the two of you? Like in the evening if he goes to bed early.

Errm... Yeah, we do in the evenings. At the weekends it hasn't been so good, but when we do have time together we make the most of it and we've started to go out, which is better than we used to do. But no when we're together we do stuff, I mean all three of us do stuff, like we'll go out on the bikes, or we'll go somewhere, or you know, we certainly make the most of it. But it's not as often as it should be right now, but as I say...

Has it become less often over the last year? It might sound a funny question, but it's just that you were saying about Richard's job changing, and...

Oh yeah definitely, I mean we're only talking since Christmas, it's got so like so busy really. It's busy because most of the last few months he's been working seven days a week. Errm... Still fitting in training twice a week, working a morning on the Saturday, go to rugby, come back work again on the Sunday. Errm... Because he's not earning a regular salary from that, I'm working maximum hours as well, to make up for that loss of money. And as I say we're paying for nursery full-time in advance so that, that's a big chunk. I think that was a shock to Richard because I don't think he realised how expensive that would be, and it's not any more expensive than any other nursery.

It's just what they cost.

Yeah, and he was like but that's the equivalent of our mortgage, because our mortgage is really low, so from that point of view, it's brought up all kinds of different issues but, we'll get by. It's just that right now, it's, it's tight. It's tight on time, it's tight on money, but it's a temporary thing.

Yeah, and you know it's a temporary thing.

Yeah, yeah.

Do you talk about it being a temporary thing?

Oh yeah, I mean last week, I said to him "Things can not go on like this forever more." And Richard's like well, because errm... He's taken an order for some slabs, well that's not going to kick off until Easter, but the builders merchant who he sells to he's not going to get rid of much stock before Easter.

Helen

Yeah, yeah, it's a quiet time.
So hopefully, his stock will have built up, and after Easter it'll take off. He came away with me on a trip at Christmas time, and that's why... because he knew it was going to be crazy afterwards, that he was going to have to work longer hours. Before we were fine, if I wanted to go out with the girls or whatever, and I would ask him if he would look after him, and yeah that would be fine, and we could afford to do it at that time, but right now, no. So for the next six eight months it's going to be like this. No, not for the next six or eight months, say June July. When the summer comes. It's just exhausting at the minute [Laughs] I mean I say to Richard "I can't say I'm tired, and I am, I'm shattered but I get away, I have a break, you don't. You work 24 hours everyday."
Does his mum have Will on the weekend?
Yeah, she does. And he can stay, yeah, if, when Richard goes training Will stays over at his mums. I mean initially she was coming over here, but she doesn't drive.
So it was difficult?
Yeah. So now errm... Will will stay over there at night, so there is a couple of nights a week, if I'm away then Richard has a bit of a break. And he sleeps all the way through the night, as well. Richard starts work between half past six and seven anyway so, errm... So my dad comes over and sits with Will until he takes him to nursery, and sometimes at night, because Richard's not finishing until about half five. So yeah, we get lots of help from everybody. And as much as I feel we're asking a lot from everybody around us, I mean Richard's dad works with Richard as well, for no pay, he works his back side off so, everybody around us is helping us. But I, well I always feel a bit guilty about that, and like I keep getting stuff for her [Richard's mum], like even if it's just a bottle of something, I shouldn't have done it, I'm in trouble for doing that! They say "you shouldn't worry about the situation, because it's not as difficult as it could have been".
But you still recognise that it's not making you feel good? I mean you can't kid yourself, if it's not, it's not. Otherwise how would you know when it's great?
Exactly, yeah, exactly. And I think last week was quite all right, there is some light at the end of the tunnel, because it is hard. But it's not so bad if one of you can take over at home, because it takes the load off the other one who's working.
OK, and do you think Richard has changed in the last year?
Errm... Yeah, yeah! [Laughs] When I think it's been a year, I've never heard that actually said before! Errm... I suppose he was brought up in a family where the mother did everything, and when we lived together, while I was there I'd be ski-daddling all over the place, but while I was here, I would pretty much do everything. But now he'll understand if I come in, say like I came in yesterday, he took one look at me, and I'm ga-ga because I haven't slept for thirty hours, so he...
You're not safe to cook a meal! [Laughs]
[Laughs] So he said "Right I'll take Will" he'll do stuff to make it easier for me, whereas

189

Nine Women, Nine Months, Nine Lives

before, he'd be like "Oh you'll be all right" and carry on as usual, you know, "You can't be tired!" Well I am. I think he understands a lot more. And I think he, he is so laid back anyway, that he was just happy to be a part of it. Before, as long as we could have a holiday away every year and escape for a bit, then that was good, and you know do up the house in between. But now he looks at the bigger picture of like, what's the situation going to be in five years time, ten years time, you know, even when he is retired, and he never looked at that before ever. Even as much as this work thing that was all brewing before Will was born.
Yeah, I mean it's like me at the moment. We're flying from Luton on Sunday morning at about half nine, we've got this surprise party tomorrow night for a friend's Fortieth, and I'm supposed to be going to my mum's in Berkshire! So we're going to this surprise party, leaving at about midnight, going home collecting the cat, driving there (to my mum's) and getting in at about two, and then we've got to be at the airport at Luton at about half eight! And I'm like waaah!
Oh God, and you're driving and everything – it's all down to you! [Laughs]
I know, I know, but it will be worth it when we get there! [Laughs]
Yeah it's just like when you can see a block ahead of you, and this is like the pregnancy thing! [Laughter] When the baby's just arrived and you can see the next six/eight weeks ahead of you, horrendous, where's the light at the end of the tunnel?! [Laughs] That's what I can relate it to. It's sad isn't it?! Make the best of the situation, eh?! [Laughs]
Yeah, and then you think "Oh my God what is happening to my life?" [Laughs] OK, so Richard has changed in quite a lot of ways, hasn't he?
Yeah, I think he has. The fact that he's working so much, so many hours. Errm... And Will's changed, it felt like he was doing the same things for a long time initially, and I felt like I don't want to be staying at home doing this, which I could live with at the time but now I'm away... I mean I can go away for four days and I come back and he's changed and I see that on a regular basis. There are so many things, I mean I've got no big thing about I must be the, I must see him the first time he does this, because he'll... Well, once he's done it he'll continue doing it so, that's not a problem. But I, I couldn't stand there watching over him, not all day waiting. But I can see just so many things have happened in those few days.
So your relationship must have changed, I mean you say you had half-expected things to be more strained?
Yeah, I did. I really did. I was just very negative about the whole thing. I knew it'd be a stress, I thought it'd be really bad, but errm... [Laughs] So yeah things have definitely changed. As much as I had just got married six months before finding out, I felt pretty secure anyway, but now I feel completely secure, again that might be naive but that's the way I feel. I do feel more confidant that we can do this on a larger scale.
Errm... Have you ever talked about your relationship changing? I don't mean in the sense of let's sit down and discuss this.
No, no.

Helen

Maybe in a jokey kind of way, you know like "look at us, God!"
Yeah, oh God yeah, I mean loads and loads of times, I mean errm... just in the last couple of months I've noticed, you don't realise how you are together. But at the same time you think, you know if this can bring us together it could force us apart as well. I'm not highly strung, we're quite easy unflappable people, when the baby cries yes it's annoying and exhausting, you've got to do something about it. It would never, it would very rarely, I can't say it would never, very very rarely made us snap at each other. You know saying, "well can't we do this? Can't we do that?", it does, it does happen. You know I'd be lying to say it doesn't happen. Errm... But I think, we both know that each person is doing as much as they can possibly do to put the situation right, you can't ask for more than that. I mean like a few weeks back, Will had been ill, and he'd been up the last three nights with him, on the Tuesday he'd been up and coughing most of the night. Richard hadn't had much sleep, so one night he took him round to his mum and dads just so that he could get some sleep. Errm... I came back, I missed the first bus so I got the next bus home, I got home at half past four. I went over and collected Will, didn't realise he'd been ill, Richard hadn't said because he thought with me being so far away I'd only worry so, there was no point. Richard has probably got more idea of what would be wrong with him than I have anyway, but he can always ask his mum anyway. So I didn't know he was ill when I went to collect him. So you can imagine, when I saw him you could see he hadn't been very well, and I didn't know at this stage that he had been ill. And then Richard came home, and then it all kind of came out. So it was probably about nine o'clock when I went to bed. And then when he was crying in the night Richard brought him in with us and I was like "I can't deal with this I have had no sleep, I do not want him to be in our bed." And it's a rare thing anyway, but if Richard's on his own then he will do that. But if you have had no sleep and oh I was just like "Will you just take him out of here" and the way I said it was angry "don't you <u>dare</u> bring him in here!" I was just like "Look I have got to get some sleep or I shall scream I can <u>not</u> go any more hours without sleep." And errm... Richard took him out of our room and then got up and went to work. And after he'd gone to work, he rang and I said "I'm really sorry but I was just so desperate to get some sleep" and he was fine about, we laughed about it then, but oh!
But that was the way you felt at the time?
Yeah exactly. It was just the way I said it! [Laughs]
Yeah "Don't you <u>dare</u>!" [Laughs]
I thought "Oh God no!" But yeah, it's not quite how you imagine but I think it's probably bought out the better side in both of us, so we'll cope.
Yeah, and things are constantly changing.
Yeah, exactly.
If you can adapt to it then...
And I know that we'll be faced with hard things again at different ages, but like constantly for all his life. You know even when he's thirty, he'll still be like, I know how

191

Nine Women, Nine Months, Nine Lives

I am with my mum and dad. But that will change as he grows, and we'll just have to adjust. As it was from day one, then on to week one, and month one and so on. Yes, so a major change, although a reluctant one, it is a positive one! [Laughs]
Yeah, yeah that's true.
It's no longer just black and white.
So you see the bits of grey in between, what they could have been or might be?
Yeah, yeah I do.
Do you think you kind of got yourself into a habit of doing that? Before I mean, when you were pregnant maybe?
Maybe I, I don't know, I did believe it and I still believe it [means that she was not sure about having a baby].
Yeah I remember talking to you and knowing that.
And I still get that fresh in my mind.
It's still fresh in my mind talking to you.
Yeah, and even, the first day we met, I was so, I was scared to death!
Yeah I remember you in clinic, and you were just, and your mum was there in the background.
I don't, I couldn't tell you if I've got any stronger a feeling or any less a feeling but it was still there when the baby was born. Even when he'd been here for a few weeks, I would say it'd taken until probably, if I was to put a date on it, I would say until probably about December [nine months]. It really scared me to death, I don't know what I would have done. I mean my blackest days and my blackest thoughts on it, I think I just would have walked out of here. Because I had no worries that Will wouldn't have been all right, without me. I knew that there would be people there, and some days, you can feel dreadful but I never got to that stage of thinking, but I think if it had been disastrous then that's what I would have done. So, had it not worked out… And it <u>has</u> worked out fine, we've all dealt with it.
Yeah, it's turned out OK. I mean there are a lot of girls that I see, who are having a baby and it's not working out, they're so stressed, and even when they're in the situation and it's not working, they keep going, and I'm like, "What are you going to do? It is going to happen, you <u>are</u> going to snap if you carry on."
This is why, I mean my friend, I was so surprised that she lasted out for so long, she was just…
Yeah, mmm, but when things get to be too much, and you've reached the end of your tether, you know <u>you</u> are at the end of your tether, you don't need somebody to point it out, you know it?
Yeah, yeah, but it's like, in addition to that you've got errm… The problem of what people are going to think of you. [That you are not happy being pregnant]
Yeah, yes that's a big problem.
And maybe that's why they find it hard to, to say.
Yeah, but sometimes, people are not even aware, they don't have the insight. And to

Helen

be honest, I don't think you can know until you are faced with the reality of the situation, then you can see it.
Maybe that's why they never tell you what it's going to be like. It's such a massive market, I mean the baby market is such a multi-million pound/dollar thing, because everybody wants the best for their child, so... I mean my friend Sam, absolutely realistic, but she can't pay the bills she has got coming through the door. We went shopping in Edinburgh.... And when we went out we couldn't go anywhere near shops, because she would be tempted to buy things, and she is up to her limit now anyway. And each... I felt bad, I stopped saying it in the end, because errm... I kept saying "well that can wait until you get back to work", but she was like "Oh it's all right Dad's paying for most of this out of the allowance", but like, I was like "Well what about when the baby's here and you need to get something else or just to pay for the roof over your head and the bills?" But no...
Yeah, yeah, I mean very few people actually sit down and look at their lives or spend time thinking about it.
Well, she's always been, I mean up until this time, she's been OK. And she thinks she is OK. But I still believe you can get hooked into this round of buying stuff, I mean I've no problems with buying things that are a bit big or second hand, but why not spread it out a bit? I mean I bought something for him that he wore maybe once and she was like "well look how much that cost!" and I was like "Yeah I know how much that cost, that's why I've said do this!" And she had bought this frilly dress, saying that "Oh she looks really lovely in this!" And I said "Why not wait until they have a sale on?" And I was like don't do it. She'll only fit it for a bit, it's expensive. People do, even she has been, sucked into it, this...
I mean people want to believe the best of situations, and people want an easy life, and if they are led to believe that something is going to be straight forward and happy and fulfilling, and have very little input for lots of output, you know, people think great, excellent. I mean it's like power steering for kids.
Oh yeah, totally.
I mean if you are given a choice between a car that has power steering and one that hasn't got it for the same price!
Yeah, exactly. Well, I am slightly old fashioned in that, as long as it works it doesn't have to be the newest latest thing. Some people get carried away with what they are going to wear or what they are going to put in their house or what they are driving or, it goes on and on.
So like their expectations are unrealistic?
Yeah, yeah.
What, about expectations about what babies do?
[Laughs] That was way down on the list!
Mmm, yeah, what will your baby be like?
That was way <u>way</u> down. You won't know until it is actually here, plus what people tell

Nine Women, Nine Months, Nine Lives

you is not actually the truth! Read between the lines, they're just talking for the sake of their own ego.
Exactly! When people are sad, really, people want their lives to be different, so they invent a better life for themselves, to perpetuate the myth, and you know?
Delude themselves.
Yeah delude themselves. They're not particularly going out of their way to delude anybody else.
No, I don't think so, but it's just like, people, all mothers want their children to be happy. I don't think people realise just how different it is going to be. When you are going to be stuck in the house for three months with this little thing. You can't even go out or I don't know get dressed properly or you know go out and stand and have a conversation in a pub or a party and you know, things like that. Things that don't seem essential but make a huge difference in reality.
Because I mean like I suppose, well I know that you, when you've got a baby you just have to concentrate on the baby and the baby demands your attention, you have to go with it.
Yeah, but you also, you don't have time to do anything else, and there just isn't any time left over. You are completely dictated to by your child. I mean like in conversations, with other people, you're not used to having to try and talk about stuff other than the baby!
Yeah you know "What have you been doing?" Well, what have you been doing?!
Exactly!
I mean astronauts come back from space and they...
They're molly coddled! [Laughs]
Yeah and they're put in a special room and molly coddled, and yeah "You'll be all right in a few days time, and we'll get you sorted, and get rid of the bends or whatever and then you can come back when you've adjusted"!
Yeah, exactly!
You get none of that when you've had a baby!
But I'm not listening to anyone in particular, some of the time it can feel a lot better, and some of the time it can be a lot worse. Lots of people seem to have it a lot worse, errm... But they don't seem to know that you do have a right for it to be better, saying that though.
No, but it could be. It could be made easier. It doesn't have to be as hard as it is.
Mmm, yeah.
Right the last chunk is your immediate future, so the next twelve months. What do you hope to achieve this next year?
As much as Will is concerned?
Or you, your work, your marriage...?
Right errm... I'm not saying to concentrate less on Will, but take more time for Richard and I to catch up. Where this period has taken us out of, we had just got married, this

Helen

came in the middle of everything. It still takes up everything. Errm... And I know that we have more contact with his grandparents, or our parents, and I know this will never change, it's like our relationship has changed with them. It has changed because they have this relationship with our baby, and that's it now. It's just there and that's it.
What you mean you're sort of...?
It's a totally different relationship, now, errm... But like I've grown up with Richard's family, and I'm really <u>really</u> close to Richard's mum, but I find now I can't I can't be as close or because I have this other perspective in my mind. I feel like I ought to be careful what I say sometimes because I think "Oh she wouldn't like that". Which never bothered me before, because they just accepted me as "that's just Richard's Helen". But now I feel I sometimes guard what I say, I wouldn't want them reading into things wrongly. So errm... But that's, that's something I'm a lot more sensitive to now. I would just like to get back to, maybe a little more how it was before. But yeah, I would like to pull us out some more time for us, and Will as well, but more space for us to do things together. To catch up again on our social life. We did have a little bit of a social life, it wasn't massive, it wasn't a major sort of thing...
But it was something! [Laughs]
Yeah exactly! To do those things together, to take time out and relax a bit, yeah that's my immediate thing to try and work on. Errm...As far as Will is concerned, who knows what tomorrow is going to be? Next week or whenever, I just don't know. I just, it's worked so far by just going from day-to-day so, I won't change that. I don't know what to expect. We seem to get by so. Errm... Work-wise I can only do as much as I am doing, which isn't right it's too much. And it takes quite a lot for me to say that, I'm not a workaholic or anything like that, and this is an easy job really, it's the easiest job I've ever done. But errm... I can't combine being constantly away, and having a young child it's difficult, and somehow it's just got to be done at the moment, and Richard would be the same I'm sure. We know that it's going to be...
You know that it's short term?
We know it's going to slow down soon.
Mmm, is there anything you'd like to achieve, for you?
Yeah. I don't normally set too high a like a "That will <u>never</u> happen" although saying that I always think that everything you want to do is within your sights, so in some way, if you really want to do it then you will do it. But errm... The next 12 months I don't think with the situation we are in you can expect much more than that, and that would be a big improvement really.
Yeah, yeah. OK, what have you learnt about yourself in the past year that you would like to develop next year? So something good that you feel quite proud of, that you perhaps weren't aware of before and that you want to keep going and make sure it's not lost. It may be something quite small, it doesn't have to be huge...
Errm... Perhaps, errm... It's a difficult one to answer but errm... To be realistic, you know sometimes you think "Oh yeah I'll do that and do that" and it's not always possible.

Nine Women, Nine Months, Nine Lives

So to paint them as life like, to look at them realistically and say "I can do it or I can't do it". To realise that there really are some things that I can't do. And I'm perhaps a bit more like that now, I tend to accept that there are things that I really can't do.
As much as you would like to?
Yeah, so to be more honest, be more honest and more realistic, about the use of my time and what I can do with it. And we do do that now. I think to myself "make the most of it now!" [Laughs] To be honest, to keep doing what we're doing now but make it more realistic.
Yeah, yeah, and is there anything that you have learnt about yourself in the past year that you would like to change next year? Again, big or small...
Errm... Yeah, just not get so frustrated with the situation. It's small but...
Yeah, but they are the kind of things that matter.
Yeah, I suppose it comes out, errm... In the extreme situations, like Richard says he never thought I'd be in this situation, never before thought that, it's probably the hardest thing I've had to do in my life. Full stop.
Because you didn't want children?
Yeah, yeah, because I didn't want to go ahead with this. Errm... But on the whole really it's working out OK, so yeah, yeah.
OK, well that's it. That's great! Thank you.
No, thank you. But again like when you talk about it, when you ask specific questions it makes you think about the whole situation as well. It makes you think about it. But whereas you don't have time to think about it normally. On the day-to day basis.
Mmm, people don't really talk about it. Do you look back on things that you've done and think "Well I did that OK that was all right?"
No, not really. No I probably don't, and as I say, it's only when you, when the questions are put in front of you or errm... For example maybe not seeing him for weeks. I mean which was something that happened all the time before we got married. But when you go through it together. You think "Blimey!" when you look back and compare it, that that was what it was like then and this is what it is like now. And you don't think about it, you don't notice. It's purely because someone asks you about it! [Laughs] So it's good from my point of view.
Yeah, OK, well that's brilliant – we may well be back!
[Laughs] Oh right! Maybe I'll remember you coming the next time! [Laughs]
No, it was no problem honestly, it really wasn't a problem!

Claire

Claire was 25 years old when she and her husband decided to start to try for a family. She had not even been married a month when she became pregnant! They had been planning to have lots of children but circumstances and ill health have since changed their initial feelings about parenthood after the birth of Hannah. They have their own catering company and work together, Claire returned to work as soon as she could after having an emergency caesarean section.

OK so the first chunk. If you could think back to when you found out you were pregnant. So way back when, before Hannah,?! [Laughs]
[Laughs] OK.
Were you trying to get pregnant at the time?
Sort of. Errm... Because we decided that when we got married we'd decide afterwards. So what happened was because my wedding and honeymoon were two weeks apart I messed about with my pill, so that I'd have my period in between and then I'd come off my pill afterwards and then get pregnant after the honeymoon. That was the idea! But because I'd messed about with it I actually got pregnant before I got married but I didn't realise until just after the wedding. So we were both, we were shocked, but we were both really happy, because we wanted a baby anyway so... yaay! [Laughs]
[Laughs] Yeah, you were happy?
Yeah we really wanted to have a baby anyway so, it was just a month early.

Nine Women, Nine Months, Nine Lives

Yeah, so it wasn't a problem at all?
No. Not at all.
And can you remember what went through your mind when you saw the two lines on the pregnancy test?
Well because I was, I didn't actually miss my period, I was taking, I was going to take a malaria tablet so I thought I'd just do a test first, so I hadn't actually missed my period, well I had but I hadn't realised, if you know what I mean. It was the month before my wedding, all my family were over from Cyprus and it was really hectic. So I hadn't, I didn't really realise I'd missed it, so I did this test just, I don't know why, just, you know, just did it, and there was this really feint blue line. And I thought no, maybe it's, maybe there's something wrong with it or... So I went to the family planning and they did one and they said "Oh yes we've got a blue line too". So, ooh, right!
So you had had no symptoms at all?
No, no.
What about after the test when you had seen the feint blue line, and you went to family planning, was there a large chunk of time between those two, or was it a matter of days?
Days. Errm... well I went the first, I went straight away the same day, and then I went four days later just to confirm it again because they said it was feint you see. So I went again just to make sure and errm... I was really happy. We was a bit, because we were going to Egypt, we thought "Oh should we go?" We wish we hadn't of, but you know at the time we wanted to go. But yes, happy as anything weren't we?
Was anyone with you when you did the test?
No, no.
Obviously if it was family planning...no it was just?
When I'd done the first one there was no one, and when my husband got home I said "Errm... Can you look at that for me?" And he says "Yes" and I says "Can you see a line or not?" Just to see what he'd say, and he said "Oh, a feint one" I told him about half an hour after I'd done the test, you know when he came back, so...
And do you remember what his reaction was when you told him?
Shocked! Even though he'd, we wanted a baby, he was still shocked. I think because we both thought it wouldn't happen this soon. Yeah we thought, after the wedding it would probably take about six months, that was what we were expecting, and for it to happen before... Well! because we were shocked, weren't we darling?
So, had you been on the pill for quite a long time then, was that why you...?
Yeah, yeah, because my friend, she'd been on the pill nine years and she's been having trouble for years, she has still not conceived now. So I just thought that I'd be the same, that it would probably take about six months. That's what the doctors and everyone had said to me, that it could take a while, so we weren't sort of...
Building your hopes up?
Yeah, yeah, you were a bit of a shock weren't you darling! [Laughs]
So was he shocked when, with the feint blue line, or was it when you actually told him?

Claire

No, I think we'd both realised that I was pregnant even though we went for the test. We both knew.
And did he actually say he was shocked or...?
It was the look on his face! Yeah!
Just his general sort of...?
Yeah, "Are you sure?" Kind of thing!
OK the next chunk is your experience of pregnancy and the birth.
Oh! [Laughs]
[Laughs] Now I remember, I remembered you saying about your water retention and everything, but I didn't realise that they'd got your dates wrong! [Following on from an earlier conversation we had]
Yeah, yeah, so...
OK so before you got pregnant. Now obviously you'd talked with your husband about wanting to have children, had you actually imagined what it would physically be like for you to be pregnant?
Yeah, I'd imagined it and it was completely different because I'd...
How had...?
I don't know. I'd sort of thought it'd be lovely to be sort of... Fat and pregnant and everything. And you just, you know, when you see pregnant women they just look so nice you know what I mean and I just thought it would be a wonderful experience. I wasn't looking forward to the birth, but just to be pregnant, I just thought it would be so wonderful.
Yeah?
[Laughs] But no it wasn't, it was just, I had sickness all day. Sickness for the first five and a half months so that put me off!
Five and a half months?!
Yeah, and then just as that finished I got really big, I was uncomfortable and, I just... I wished I'd enjoyed it, I wanted so much to enjoy being pregnant, but, I didn't. No. I didn't enjoy the birth either. Did we? No!
No.
No not at all. But, it still hasn't put me off wanting another one, I'd still go through it all again, because, well this is worth it.
Right, that's good, that is good. In what way did the pregnancy differ from what you had imagined? Is there any one thing that you can think of that was a complete shock?
Errm... I think, when you, when you read books and stuff they say, people say you'll have morning sickness for a few weeks and then everything goes smoothly till the end, you just get a bit big and uncomfortable. And, but I was really big, and I was really uncomfortable it just didn't seem fair. And I felt really sick as well, it was just, everything seemed to just drag on, it just kept going. I think it, it was just not very nice for me I don't think.
Well, not every pregnancy is the same.

Nine Women, Nine Months, Nine Lives

No, they say that don't they? And they say that the first pregnancy is the worst, because your body has to get used to it.
Yeah, and I mean, every baby is different and they are 50 % of the pregnancy, so...
Everyone on the round, on the chip round, tried to predict what I was having. Half of them said I was having a boy and the other half said it was a girl, so... it made me laugh! [Laughs]
Well, that was 50-50 either way wasn't it?! OK now you say that you weren't looking forward to the birth, and you have also said that you didn't enjoy it either. What did you expect would happen at the birth? Had you read about it? Talked to people about it?
Errm... I just thought, when I went in, or when I thought I was going in, I didn't want any pain control or nothing, I just wanted to see how it went, go in with an open mind. And that's what I did at first but things went wrong, but when, when, before I had her, I just thought it would be painful as the baby was coming out but I thought I could handle that, but I never got the chance, so. Because I had to have a section with her so I don't know what it would be like to give birth, in a normal birth.
So did you have any contractions at all?
Yeah! In the end I was induced. Errm... They induced me at 12 o'clock, by 3 o'clock the contractions were starting, and by half three they were every two minutes.
Jesus!
So I had to have a, what do you call it in the back?
An Epidural.
Epidural, yeah... Because I couldn't stand it because it was too much from nothing to every two minutes, and as one was ending another was coming, so it was just like fast and furious, and, a bit much really.
Yeah, so why did they induce you then, because of the water retention?
Yeah, I'd gone in in the end and said "Look, I've had enough!" And the consultant says "Oh yes, yes you've had enough" and broke me waters! Put some gel in and off we went.
So why did you end up going in and having a caesarean then?
Well I was nine centimeters dilated, this was about nine o'clock at night.
So you were nine hours in.
Yeah, I mean, it started, well they say the labour started about three o'clock, so really it should have been a quick labour. So, by nine o'clock I was about nine centimeters dilated and they said "We're going to top the epidural up, when it starts to wear off you will be fully dilated, and you can start to push". I think it must have been about half ten and she errm... When she turned on her side!
Oh no!
Just as I, I was pushing, and I thought "Oh this is easy!" And I was, and the contractions were just coming back, and I was pushing on the contractions, and I was quite enjoying that bit, and then they said "Oh nothings happening, nothings happening!" And then the doctor came back and examined me and said "Oh the baby has turned on its side, what we are going to do is leave you for a bit longer and just see if it turns back". And it

Claire

didn't, and he, when he said to me "We're going to take you down to theatre now" I went into shock. I was shaking because I thought, I knew, I knew right from the beginning I would have to have a section and I just... You know, when you just know it?
Yeah.
And he said they would use the, you know the ventouse when they try and turn the baby round? He said "Well, we can try and do that first" and they did that for quite a while and couldn't do it, and... Then I had a section in the end. That was horrible.
What the section or the ventouse, or both?
The section, when I came round the next morning, when the painkillers started wearing off, you couldn't get out of bed. You had to lie in bed and they had to bring the baby to me and then take the baby away and...
So really that was, you weren't looking forward to it, and it wasn't quite what you had expected anyway, and you say that you sort of had a feeling that you would end up going in for a caesarean anyway...
Yeah, yeah I don't know why, I just thought I might.
Had you find out about what happens in a caesarean?
Not really, I'd sort of read about it. I knew that they cut you and that it was a big cut and they, but I thought they were going to... You see I wasn't intending to have an epidural because everyone says "Oh they're horrible, they hurt and they're dangerous". So I'd gone in with the fact that I wasn't going to have one so that if I had to have a section they would have to knock me out completely you see so, but errm... As it was I had one [an epidural] and it didn't hurt I had no complications with it. I think because your contractions are so bad that you don't feel the needle going in.
No, you just... You're a little preoccupied.
It took about twenty minutes really to take effect completely. But it was wonderful then, it really was, it was like "Oh the pains gone!" It was, it's a strange pain really, it's like, I don't know, it's just horrible! [Laughs]
OK. So the birth wasn't as you thought it would be, in terms of that you did think that you were going to have her vaginally and you weren't going to have any pain relief. So do you think it lived up to your expectations? Do you think it worked out for the best in the end or not?
No, no. I wanted to have her naturally. I didn't want to have a section at all.
Why did you want to have her naturally?
Because, because... It took me ten days to get over the section, whereas if I had had her normally, OK I might have had stitches, but if I had had her normally, I might have been up and... You know when you are lying there you can see the other mothers that have had their babies, they were up and about, and I couldn't do that. For two days I couldn't get out of bed, I just, I just, I wanted to get on with it and I couldn't, it was like being held down sort of thing.
Yeah, mmm, that's not good.
No! [Laughs]

201

Nine Women, Nine Months, Nine Lives

OK and how did you feel when you first held Hannah? Obviously with having the caesarean it probably wouldn't have been straight away...
Well, when, all through my pregnancy I'd wanted a girl, and when people say to you "What do you want, a boy or a girl?" I used to say "Oh I don't mind, I don't mind" but I really wanted a girl! And the only person I told was me mum and my husband because they were the people... And he wanted a boy, though he didn't mind. When they had taken the baby out he said to me "We've taken the baby out and we're just going to..." Because they said they were just going to put the errm... The suction thing into her mouth because she'd swallowed something and I was saying "What have I had, what have I had?" And nobody would say anything, it must have only been about thirty seconds but it seemed like ages, and I thought "Oh God, there's something wrong the baby or something!" Because nobody was saying what I had had and then all of a sudden someone said "Oh you've had a girl!" and it was just "Oh thank you! Thank you!" you know, I really wanted a girl. It made it all worth it, you know the pregnancy and everything, it just made it worth it having a girl. I think everyone said "Oh you know if you had had a boy you would have felt the same anyway" and I probably would of but, I just really wanted a girl and then having a girl, you know, it was just, it was just worth it in the end.
OK.
I didn't actually hold her though, because they wrapped her up in a towel or a blanket and they took her away, and it wasn't until about half an hour after I had her that I actually held her and fed her.
And how did it feel?
I was absolutely shattered by then. But err... It was wonderful.
So what time was she born then?
She was born at twenty five past twelve.
So twelve hours?
I think it was the epidural, that makes you a bit woosy anyway but I'd just gone into shock because of having to have a section and I was shaking, I was crying, and I was all emotional, and, yeah...
So afterwards do you, you don't really recall holding Hannah for the first time?
Yeah I remember holding her because I fed her. They said to me "Do you want to feed her or do you want us to bottle feed her?" And I said "Oh no, I'll feed her" and I just fed her and then they took her off me and put her in the little crib at the side and then we both went to sleep. Later on they took us to another room. So I remember holding her and everything but I was absolutely shattered by then.
Can you remember the first time you held her when you felt all right in your self? So, maybe the next morning when you had had a bit of a rest?
I held her, well, she was a naughty baby, and she cried a lot.
I remember she used to cry a lot, yes.
It's really funny when she's...

Claire

And she snored! She snored when she came to the reunion (of the 'Preparing for Parenthood' Course)!
Oh yeah! She doesn't snore any more but yeah, I think it was up to about three/four months that she snored. When I, the second night I was there they took her away, and I didn't want them to really because you hear all these stories and everything. I wanted her by my side. Anyway they said "We'll take her away we'll let you sleep", and she cried a bit when they took her away, and I could hear her, because they were in the nursery which was the next room to where I was. Eventually they brought her back because she was keeping all the other babies awake! [Laughs]
Oh right! [Laughs] She obviously knew what she wanted!
Yeah! And then they just, if she lay in my arms with me she'd go to sleep and be all right but errm... I couldn't get up to put her back. It was just for the first couple of days really, and then as I got up and about I kind of, I got on with it and recovered pretty quickly after that. But, it was hard work, she cried for a long time.
How long do you remember she was crying for?
The first eight weeks were terrible, and then she slowly slowly got better and then I think it must have been by the time she was about nine months old that she really calmed down! [Laughs] But I mean she's brilliant now, she's such a happy little girl, she sleeps at night, she eats everything you give her, you know a brilliant eater, so, yeah. They say that don't they? If you have a very naughty baby when they grow up they calm down and they are really good.
Yeah some do... You've done your penance early! [Laughs]
She was hard work. It has taken its toll on me really.
It's bound to. I mean it couldn't not, not really.
Yeah, mmm.
In what ways was your partner involved in the pregnancy? Was he interested in the pregnancy? Curious about the baby?
Errm... He was scared! You know like if he knocked me or anything he'd go "Is the baby all right, is the baby all right?" [Laughs] Just things like that you know. I think he was very scared of my bump, very delicate around it. Other than that, I mean he came to all the scans you know, he was concerned for me and stuff like that, and, but there's not much a man can do is there? [Laughs]
No, but you know the bits he can do like listening to you and stuff like that. Just helping you to feel better.
Yeah, he tried.
Yeah, that's it. Trying is half the battle.
Yeah, yeah.
What about the birth, was he there for the birth?
Yeah, yeah, well when I first gone in, when I first went in errm... He left me for a while and went to work and then she called him in because it was all going so fast, because I was dilating so quickly, that they called him in, I think he got in about six

203

Nine Women, Nine Months, Nine Lives

o'clock. So for the first three hours I was actually by myself, and I wished he'd been there really. Because when the pain started I was on my own, and I wanted him to be there with me. So I'd, I'd sort of, you know, when you've got your own business it's really difficult, you, you've got to run it or else you're not going to get any money, so... And then he came in, my dad took over (the chip van) and errm... You know he was there for the section with me and everything, that was good. I needed him there, he was really supportive then, when I remember when they errm... First showed me her, and he held her, he was like this [mimics him being stiff and scared] because he was so scared, because he'd never held a baby before! [Laughs] And he held her like that and I looked at her little face and I could only see sort of that much [her eyes and nose] because the towel that was round her and she looked just like him!
She does look like him!
Yeah she does, she's the double of her dad!
Yes, you do don't you?!
I thought that was nice. Because you talk about that when you are pregnant, with everyone, you say "Oh I wonder what it's going to look like! What colour hair" and stuff like that and I'm just glad that it, that she looked like Tom.
And can you, when he first held her you said that he was really scared and everything. Did he relax after that?
He tried really hard. He was so scared of dropping her or what she was...
Because with you being in bed most of the time, and not quite as mobile as...
Yeah, I got out... I had her on the Thursday and I came home on the Sunday which wasn't very long really but, I came home. I couldn't really carry her about, so he used to, he sort of did everything more or less for me and then you know I taught him how to make the bottles up, I mean I didn't really know half the stuff! And I hadn't bathed her, and me personally I had never bathed a baby before, and they'd bathed her in hospital, so it was like an experience for both of us. But we got through it, didn't we Hannah? I think you, if you aren't used to babies I think you are scared anyway because they are so small and you don't want to hurt them.
So have any of your friends or family got babies or children?
My brother, but errm... I don't really get in, I see him more but, before I never really got involved with that side of it. You know they'd come round and you would have a quick cuddle and pass them back, but you know you never changed the babies nappies or... You know when babies are first born and they have those really horrible dirty nappies, well I missed all that, because I couldn't do it, Tom changed one! [Laughs] But errm... Yeah, he's learnt a lot. I mean he'd never changed a nappy before, and the first time he put one on he stood her up and it just sort of fell down!
Yeah, well, next time you do it a bit tighter!
But he did, he feeds her, and you know...
OK would you say that your partner's involvement in the pregnancy was more or less than you hoped for?

Claire

Errrm...
It might have been more in certain ways and less in others, I don't know.
I can't really remember it seems so long ago! [Laughs] Errm... I don't think he could have done any more really. I think towards the end, for the last ten weeks, because I was so big and uncomfortable, I was very emotional and he supported me that way, and I think that's the only thing he could have done for me really. Because I was so fed up with it all, I just wanted it over. And because she was late, that made it worse, it was just dragging on and on and on. And every day just dragged on and on and on. I couldn't work because I was so big. I just used to, I used to lug that settee about hoping that she'd come, and I used to really clean behind the settee, lift the Hoover up, just to.... And she never came early! [Laughs]
She came when she was good and ready! [Laughs]
I tried to keep busy by doing housework and stuff though I used to get out of breath so easily, because I was so big, I was <u>huge</u>! But yeah he was supportive in that way.
So perhaps he was more supportive than you thought he would be emotionally?
No, about what I had expected really.
And what about the birth? Was his being there for you, supporting you, was that more or less what you had hoped for?
Yeah, I think it was more than I had hoped for really.
Yeah?
Yeah, so I, I don't know I'd just, I think he was, he didn't, when I, when I said to him originally "Do you want to be at the birth?" I think he was a bit... He said "Yes" but I got the impression, I kept asking him because I got the impression, that he was very scared you know, things like that. So when he was actually at the birth, I mean it was a section so he didn't actually see anything, but he did really well there. He was really supportive, and then afterwards, when she was born, he was like, he kept... I mean well with work it was so difficult but he kept coming in and then popping out and coming back in and you know every minute that he'd got to see us both. I think it was more than I... But it was different you see, I didn't expect to have a section, I was planning on having her and then coming home. If I'd had her in the morning I was planning on coming home in the evening. If I'd had her in the evening, coming home the next morning, I wasn't planning on staying in.
Being away, yeah.
So, I mean I came home as quickly as I could really, so...
Do you think you came home too soon?
Errm...
With hindsight?
I came home on a Sunday really because I knew Tom would be there, because on Monday or whenever, I knew he would have been at work so I would have been on my own. So I came home on the Sunday because I knew he'd be there with me. And I only wanted him there I didn't want anyone else. You know like, I think it's because I'd had

205

Nine Women, Nine Months, Nine Lives

a section and I was so tired. I was breastfeeding her, I had to stop after eleven days because I was so exhausted. And friends kept coming round, and as much as you want to see them, you don't want to see them, if you know what I mean. Because you feel like you've got to make them a cup of tea, and they want a chat and I just wanted to either sleep or get on with some house work, I just didn't want to talk to people I just wanted to get on with it. But they kept coming round, and I suppose it's nice that you've got friends [Laughs] but you just errm... You know, you just don't want it if you know what I mean, I just wanted Tom but he wasn't there, so...
Mmmm, difficult.
Yeah, yeah it was. It's like that now though, I mean I work now but, I don't work Fridays but errm... Sometimes in the day, like if she's teething, she gets really ratty sometimes and I think "Oh I just need sometime by myself!" And he's always at work and you know, it's just difficult. But you get by.
Yeah, some days you get by, and some days are great.
Yeah.
OK, so you would say that his behaviour was more supportive emotionally during the birth than you had expected?
Yeah.
OK. The next chunk is your experience of early motherhood. So those first few weeks those first few months. So really up until the last time I saw you when Hannah was about two and a half months old...
So what do you want to know, how did I feel when she was a couple of months old?
Well, if you could think back to the first three months. Can you think how your pregnancy effected early motherhood, so...
I think I was very down, I didn't get postnatal depression, nothing like that I was just down because she was such a difficult baby, more than I...
What about the physical side of the pregnancy? I mean you had water retention, and that won't have disappeared overnight...
Well, it did more or less, yeah, it didn't take long. I think, I dunno, by the time I'd come home from hospital that had more or less gone. It was amazing how much weight I lost because it was all fluid, I know you lose weight because of the baby and that obviously but it was nearly all fluid. But, errm... Yeah.
So, you felt quite down then. Do you think that was carrying on from the pregnancy? Because you said that you'd been in...
Yeah, I think, the last ten weeks of it, I'd got myself in such a state, I was so fed up, and I wanted such a brilliant baby and she was such hard work, she wasn't like they tell you. She was so demanding, everyone who looked after her said that. You know they said "Oh she cried a lot, and you can't leave her and..." It just, it just wears you down, and you're trying to get over a section as well.
Mmm, yeah, so not a good combination. OK, so how would you say the birth effected early motherhood? Obviously you've said you had the caesarean, so, having stitches

Claire

and things you weren't able to lift her, you weren't mobile...
No, I did, I did though, I just got on with it, because there wasn't anyone else to. I mean like people were there off and on, but when no one is there you've got to do it. If she needs changing or she needs feeding, you know, you've just got to get on with it, so I just did it. I went back to work after six weeks so... I think that was a bit soon.
Yeah?
Yeah, I wanted to in a way, because it did me good getting away from her, you know seeing people and, but it was, it tired me out too much.
There was no happy medium? It's out there somewhere but you couldn't quite find it?
Yeah, mmm.
So you think it was too early because, going back to work that is, because you were too tired from having the caesarean and also working is hard work?
Yeah, it is.
And Hannah is hard work.
Yeah, she is.
So there was no rest really it was just a different type of, of work.
Yeah.
How did you imagine early motherhood would be for you? You've said already that Hannah wasn't what you'd expected.
No, not as I had expected!
What had you expected?
I don't know. I just thought you'd have this baby and feed it and change it and play with it and it'd be good! [Laughs] She was errm... She didn't sleep for long periods of time but, errm... She must have had a problem with sleeping because you know she'd like have half an hour and then wake up but she'd be tired. And it wasn't, and you sort of find the baby's patterns, it wasn't until she was about eight weeks old that we started realising what her signs were. It's like now, she only has to rub her eyes and I know she's tired and up she goes to bed and she's fast asleep. And it's, I mean well at that age she couldn't rub her eyes and stuff really but she sort of, she was showing signs and I was sort of picking them up and that's when, at eight weeks, it started getting easier.
Well, it takes time to get to know your baby, I mean you don't instantly have a blueprint of their personality!
That's it, it's like when we were doing the classes, everyone was saying "No-one expects you to have a perfect house, you won't have a perfect baby" and you sort of accept that. But you don't accept it! Because... I'd kept my house so clean when I was pregnant that when she came it was such a mess, and I couldn't handle the fact that the house was a mess. I had to clean it yet I had no energy or time to clean it. And she was so naughty and I used to think "Well what have I done wrong to have such a naughty baby?" [Laughs] "What am I doing wrong?" You know, that's how it makes you feel because you try and do so much. It's not because anyone expects you to, it's because you in yourself expect you to even though you know... And it's like they were saying as well

Nine Women, Nine Months, Nine Lives

that errm... If you are feeling down you should call someone. When you are feeling down, you don't want to call anyone. When you come out of it you think "I should have called someone" and you know you should of, but you just don't when you are actually in that situation.
Did you ever have a time when you were feeling down and somebody dropped in to see you or phoned you or something like that?
I was relieved.
Yeah?
Oh yeah definitely but I wouldn't have, I wouldn't have...When I was really really down I wouldn't have called anyone to say come round or anything. Because I was always like ashamed of feeling down, and I never got, well sometimes I used to sort of shout at her but I'd never, I'd never get angry angry with her. She never got me to that stage, I'd cry if anything. I'd cry with anger rather than...
You were frustrated?
Yeah, you know.
Were you angry with yourself or were you angry with her?
I think myself really because I kept thinking "I must be doing something wrong" for her to be like this. But like I say, by the time she had reached eight weeks she'd really started to calm down, she wasn't as bad. As the weeks went by she just calmed down even more until she was like she is. I think her problem was, she was too active, she wanted to be moving, once she'd started rolling around and crawling she was better, and now she can crawl and she's trying to walk she is better again. I think that was her problem, she didn't like lying still, she wanted to be, she's always wanted to be standing on her feet and I think that was half the problem, she just didn't like lying down. She was just too demanding! [Laughs]
Yes, well there's one good thing! She might be thoroughly independent by the time she's sixteen! [Laughs] OK, so you did imagine what early motherhood would be like for you and you are basically telling me that it didn't match up?
No, no.
Can you think of one bit that really leaps to mind that was the biggest frustration or shock or disappointment?
Just the fact that she cried so much, errm... I think the first night she, we'd got this big cot and we put her in our room, we put her to bed, and she cried all night. And I was up all night with her. We couldn't get to sleep she just wouldn't sleep in this cot, and the next day he went out and he bought a Moses basket. Because we'd said there's no point buying a Moses basket, it's a waste of money - they never sleep in it for long. So we got this Moses basket, it took her a while to get used to it but slowly slowly she got used to this Moses basket and she was fine. Then we put this Moses basket in the cot, hoping that she'd slowly get used to the cot as well. By the time she was ten days old she went in her own room! [Laughs] These walls are so thin so you could still hear but it made a bit of a difference, because she snored as well. If she finally went to sleep,

Claire

she snored so loud that she'd still keep us awake! [Laughs] So, we were both so exhausted because we got no sleep, but I mean she was only in her Moses basket six weeks. We took her out of it, we took her out of her Moses basket at about six weeks, and errm… we had that same problem again because she just wouldn't sleep in her cot, she just wasn't used to it. Even though we'd put it in the cot. We tried mobiles, everything, and it was just time, in a couple of weeks she'd slowly got used to it. And people say "Oh leave her she'll cry and then she'll go to sleep" but she never did! I mean how long are you supposed to leave a baby to cry? I mean now, when she's awake and she wants to get out she shakes her cot, she stands up, shakes the cot "I want to come out", so you take her out. When they are a baby they can't, you can't, they just scream and scream and scream.

Yeah, it's frustrating for them because they know what they want to do but they have no way of telling you. And even if they find a way and manage to control their limbs in such a way to do that – you don't know what the bloody hell they are on about!

Yeah! [Laughs] And then everyone used to say "Oh there must be something wrong with her, you ought to take her to a doctor" and then that gets you worried. You read all these books and they say that babies do cry for no reason.

Yeah, yeah.

You just get all these people who start interfering saying "Oh there's something wrong with her you ought to take her to a Paediatrician". And you think "Well is there something wrong with her?" You think "Is she hot is she cold? Does her nappy want changing? Is she thirsty…?" And you go through everything don't you? And there was nothing wrong with her she just cried a lot, she's just one of those babies that cried! [Laughs]

Yeah, she just grew out of it. So that was the most difficult thing in the early days. The crying.

Yeah, the lack of sleep! [Laughs]

And what was the best thing about those early days and weeks?

She was so cute. When she didn't cry, she…

She was lovely!

I can remember when she was four and a half weeks old. We had company staying over at the weekend, it was, and it was errm… Half four Sunday morning, she'd woken up for a feed, she always woke about that time for a bottle, and errm… I'd gone downstairs and got her bottle and she smiled at us both for the first time! Because we were both up, she smiled for the first time, and that was… Oh that was wonderful, her first smile, and we wrote it in her book! [Laughs]

At half past four in the morning! [Laughs]

Yeah! And after that, errm… She sort of smiled a few times a day, and by the time she was six weeks she smiled all the time, she cried a lot as well so…

But she smiled too!

Yeah, I thought it was wonderful when she smiled at us! [Laughs]

Nine Women, Nine Months, Nine Lives

OK, how much was your partner involved in the early days? It sounds like quite a lot really because of the caesarean.
Well he didn't have much choice really because he'd, we'd sort of, we came to a compromise where we just took it in turns, one got up and then the other one got up. And even now, it's very rare, but if she ever woke up in the night. Like the odd night she has a bad night and she won't sleep very well, not that she's being naughty she's just like, she loses her dummy or she loses her covers and she can't get to sleep, it's like "Oh it's your turn!" [Laughs] You know and there are no arguments about it, he'll just get up sort her out and... Like I say now she's brilliant, you know if she does wake up it's because she's lost her dummy, you just put her dummy in and she's out again.
OK, so had you talked about who would do what?
No.
In the early days?
No, no, nothing. No it just kind of came that way. I mean he, now, even now he says "Oh I don't want another baby just yet!" I mean you know she, we, me personally, I don't want another baby yet because of the way she is. And I know they say the second one probably won't be anything like it (was with the first) but until she's that little bit more independent, I couldn't, I couldn't imagine having a newborn baby at the moment. You know like some people have them so close, I couldn't imagine doing it, or being pregnant with her, even though she is really good she is still a hand full. She's a very active baby, you know she'd, I tell you what I find hard. Not long ago, it's only a couple of weeks ago, she's stopped having a morning nap. She used to watch the Teletubbies at ten o'clock, half ten she'd have a nap, and wake up about twelve then have another nap about half two/three o'clock, well she's stopped that morning nap. And she doesn't have a nap till after dinner now and I find that really difficult. In that morning nap I used to do my housework. That was a bit of a shock because she didn't have one!
You had a routine because she had one?
That's it, and then she broke it and it was like "Oh right!" Errm... You see when she's up you've got to entertain her, she does sit and play by herself but she gets so bored with the toys. So you've got to put them back and you've got to get fresh ones and then she'll sit and play again. And then she wants cuddles don't you? [Baby cuddles her mummy and says "mmmmm"] [Laughs] Oh she is such a good baby now, completely different, but as I say, it's still put Tom off wanting another just yet!
So what, did he want one quite quickly after Hannah?
Well when we'd, before I got pregnant, we were talking about having about four. And we were saying we'd have them, we did discuss whether we'd have them close together or... Because I always said I wanted them about three or four years apart anyway but I wanted about four. He wanted a big family as well and he said "Oh I don't really mind what sort of gap" but errm... It's just come about that with her being the way she is... We probably will have one when she's about three or four so you're going to get a gap but I don't know whether we'll have four!

Claire

Well, you'll just have to see. I mean you know if you don't have four, would it matter?
No, no, I don't mind now, I'm so happy I've got her and she's great.
And do you think that, you say that you didn't talk about who was going to do what or whatever, do you think it worked out for the best in the end?
Yeah, yeah.
It wasn't a problem that you hadn't talked about it?
I often find that if you try and make plans they never work, I think you just... I mean some things you do have to plan obviously, I think it was just a case of see how it went. It was like with the birth, I didn't plan the birth I just wanted to see how it went and, it was taken out of my hands anyway but, I think it's always best to go in with an open mind and that's what we did. When she was born we just sort of... Whatever happened we just took it day by day and, you know, if something wasn't working we talked. We talk really well, you know if there is a problem we discuss it.
OK, the next chunk is your experience of motherhood up to the present day. So, from the last time I saw you when she was three months old up until now when she's nearly one. How do you think your life has changed since you had Hannah?
We never go out!
You never go out?
No, well, we knew this anyway, once we'd had a baby we wouldn't be able to go out as often as we wanted to so that's never really been a problem. I mean he never, he never goes out with his mates drinking, we always go out.
Did he used to?
No, I'm just saying, he never did, and errm... So that's never been a problem, and when we do go out we go out together, so, I mean, we're quite happy. Because we work evenings, that's never a problem, so it's just the weekends. And my mums always happy to have her, so if we ever want to go out or anything. We usually just have a take away and you know. We're happy so... But like I say if we wanted to go out my mums always happy to have her, she's stayed over two nights, my mums got a cot there so...
Oh right that's good.
Yeah, so errm... That's not been a problem, going out, at all.
Is it, so, would you say you've changed?
Yes! [sounds wistful] I've aged. About 30 years!
[Laughs] You don't look like you have!
[Laughs] Well, when, up until I got pregnant I always used to look really young for my age and I personally think I've aged.
You haven't aged! [Laughs]
[Laughs] I do feel I've aged!
But you pluck the grey hairs out so it doesn't really matter now?! So you feel like you've aged?
Mmm.
You don't think you've matured?

211

Nine Women, Nine Months, Nine Lives

Probably yeah, but I just look in the mirror and think "Oh God, you old hag!" [Laughs]
So physically you feel like you've aged?
Yeah, oh yeah. I feel so worn out half the time you know just, I don't know...
So, is there a good aspect about you that has changed? Or a good aspect of your life? Do you feel closer to your partner? What do you feel?
Errm... I wouldn't have said it has brought us closer together and I wouldn't say it has, you know, drifted us apart in anyway. When she plays up that does put a strain on your relationship, but errm... No, I wouldn't have said it's changed us in anyway, not like that, not us together! [Laughs]
Yeah, right. You wanted to go back to work and you have gone back to work. Are you working as often as you did before you were expecting Hannah?
Only one night less. I used to work five nights. Well actually I used to work five nights and one dinner, and now I just work four nights so...
And who has Hannah when you are working?
My mum.
Yeah, because you're both working in the van?
Yeah, when I don't work my mum works for me.
So does she come here then? Or do you take Hannah to her?
Well, one night she'll go to my mums and then two nights she'll stay here because we're back late so she has to be here because she has to go to bed. Sometimes she doesn't go to bed until eleven, sometimes she'll go to bed at eight. I don't mind her staying up though. It's easier for me to be honest with you, if she goes to bed at eight o'clock you can guarantee she'll be awake around seven, if she goes to bed at eleven, she doesn't wake up till nine. So that fits in with me really, I don't mind that. There's no point putting a baby to bed if they're not tired.
Exactly, yeah, and if she's quite happy to be awake and she's not grizzly or grumpy the next day, then what's the problem?
Yeah, that's it.
OK. And do you get any time to yourself? Just you?
Not really, no. Very very rarely, and that's what I miss. I mean today I went up town with my mum and took her with us. But it's not really, that was nice to get out even though we were all together, it was just nice, but no not really. I mean sometimes I wish, I mean like, errm... She's good because I can put her in, she's got a walker and I can put her in that and I can have a bath and she can be in the bathroom with me, and she's not screaming or anything but... That's what I do miss. You know you could just, if I've got a job to do I can't do it when I want to do it. That's the hardest thing I think, not being able to do things when you want to do them, you have to do it when it fits round her. So that, that is difficult.
OK. And you say that you have had time for yourself, you say that you don't have it very often. What do you do in your time for yourself? Do you treat yourself?
Yeah, I do. When it was my birthday last September, my mum bought me some beauty

Claire

therapy treatments.
Oh lovely!
Yeah! So I had massages, you know stuff like that, it doesn't last very long. You know, a couple of hours and it is back to reality again, but it is nice, relaxing, yeah, just things like that. But it is very rare that I get anytime for myself. Sometimes, probably about once a month, I'll say to my mum "Can you have her for an hour or so?" And my mum will have her and I'll probably just sit and read something. Just so that I can just sit and do something, or just watch telly, or just sit and relax.
So do you, do you actually deliberately go and take her to your mums so that you can have time for yourself?
Yeah, but it's probably even less than once a month, do you know what I mean, just every now and again I think "Oh I could do with some time on my own". Or sometimes I feel like that and she goes to sleep and then I'll just do what I've got to do then, but it's usually just housework! [Laughs]
Yeah, OK. Do you think your partner has changed since you have had Hannah?
Yeah, I do, definitely. I think he's matured, really really matured.
Are you surprised about that?
No, no.
You look surprised!
No, I didn't expect it. Not that he was, not that he was immature it's just really changed him, having a baby, you know he's, he's errm… I think we both have really we're both sort of shocked, at how it's, I don't know… It's like when we go back to the beginning when you say "How did you expect it to be?" Well because it was so different I think it, it just changes you doesn't it? I mean your life isn't your own any more.
Yeah.
You've always got to think of someone else. It's like if you've got a dog, if you go on holiday, that's the only time you've got to worry about your dog. If you go away for the weekend you've got to have someone to look after it or something like that, or you can go out for the day and the dogs OK by itself. When you've got a baby, it's like when we go up North, to see Tom's parents, the car is full of stuff for her! [Laughs] I mean if you go for yourself you pack your overnight bag your toothbrush etcetera. You do it for her you've got to pack her bottles up, everything, it's just like… I remember when errm… You'll probably find this on one of your (video) tapes [of the 'Preparing for Parenthood' classes], Helen she was talking about her friend who came to stay, and she had a baby and she bought a bottle of milk and a banana with her and all this. I don't know whether you remember on the tape but that is something that has stuck in my head, because whenever I go out with her I take my bottle of milk! [Laughs] You know proper milk to put on her Weetabix! [Laughs] And a banana! And you do, you know like, she was saying that when her friend got there she'd brought this pint of milk and a banana, and she said "Well, I have milk and I have bananas here!" But you don't do it because you think they don't have it, you just do it because it's part of what your baby has. And

213

Nine Women, Nine Months, Nine Lives

it's just like you pack it as routine, like you pack nappies, you just pack it! That just stuck in my head and when she said that because I was thinking at the time "Well you don't do that, you ask them if they've got milk and banana's" but you [Laughs] You do! You just pack everything. A few toys, an extra change of clothes, and...
You take everything just in case?
Yeah, yeah. You don't imagine things like that. Until you've got a baby, you don't imagine a lot really. It was a, it was a shock.
Do you think anybody could have told you?
No. No.
Even if they had told you, you wouldn't have believed it?
Not that you wouldn't have believed them, you just couldn't imagine it, you couldn't imagine it being so hard. You know, I mean, people say "Oh if you've had one you might as well have two, because it's just as easy!" But I, if I had twins, two like her, I think I'd be grey!
[Laughs] Right!
I couldn't imagine having two like her! [Laughs] Running around, I just couldn't imagine it! [Laughs]
So you think that he has changed, you think that he's grown up a lot?
Oh yeah.
More responsibilities and things?
Yeah because it's been such a shock for him as well. Because I suppose how I, how we used to talk about it he felt exactly the same as me and then when she came out the way she did, it was just such a shock. You know, because you don't expect babies to be naughty or, you just, I don't know... You just, we just expected to have this little baby, it cries a few times you cuddle it and you know it just does as it is told. It doesn't! [Laughs]
No! [Laughs] OK, and do you talk to him about how you think he's changed? Does he ever say to you that he thinks that you've changed or...?
No not really.
Don't you ever look back and think "Cor weren't things different before we had Hannah?!"
Oh yeah, we say that, yeah we say that! I think that the only thing that we miss is the fact that we can't do things when we want to do them. That's the only really difficult thing, like sometimes you think "Oh wouldn't it be nice just to go out for a meal" but then, if you want to go out for a meal you've got to arrange cover (for the chip van). I mean most times as I say my mum will have her, but sometimes you don't want to burden people all the time so we don't go out. I mean we don't really mind, but like I say, the odd time, you just think "Oh yeah, it'd be nice if we could". I mean it's like holidays as well, you have to choose where you go on holiday because there are certain places where you can't, where you wouldn't really want to take a child. And errm... We were thinking about going to places like Alton Towers, and we thought well, we can't

Claire

really go to Alton Towers because what are we going to do with the baby? [Laughs] You know, just things like that. Once it was so simple, we could just get in a car and go, now you can't.
So your relationship has changed because of Hannah, and you feel like you can be less spontaneous?
Yeah, I think also... I've not been very well, I've got endometriosis.
Oh no.
Yeah, I've already had surgery, in January, and that's put a huge strain on the relationship as well, which doesn't help. I think that's what has really made a lot of difference to us both.
Did you have problems before?
No, not at all. Well, I must have had them when I was pregnant and not realised. And then when I'd had Hannah, errm... I was in a bit of pain, and the doctor said "Well, you've had a baby, it's expected, you..."
You'd had an operation as well...
Yeah, so I sort of put up with it and it got worse. And it got to the stage where I thought, well this isn't right, and he then referred me to a Gyneacologist and I went privately in the end because I didn't want to wait five months.
God no!
So, I went privately and they found it straight away. And errm... Then I went back on the NHS and had it done, I had laser treatment in January. I went back Wednesday just gone and they told me that if I have to have it done again I will have to wear a colostomy bag.
Oh lord!
Because of where it is, it's near my bowel you see. So it's gone from bad to worse really. From having a rough pregnancy to having a caesarean, then finding out I had this. I must admit my husband has been absolutely brilliant really.
That must have been really hard.
Yeah, I mean it's a lot better since I've had the surgery but it's just a case of, they could only take so much away and, it still hurts a bit. But not to worry, I'll just have to wait and see how things go.
Yeah.
The chances are that I might not be able to have anymore children as well.
Yeah, yeah, there is that. See how it goes...
[Laughs] But what can you do? [Looks gutted]
So when will you know like, if you've got to go back in again?
In May, I have to go back again.
And is that a check up?
Yeah, I went last Wednesday for a check up, then I've got to go in May for another check up. More or less to see what decision I've made as well. Because they said to me, "Well you can leave it and go on painkillers or..." Well, that's not really a solution "Or you can

have the operation". I mean I might not have to have the colostomy bag it's just...
That's the worst case scenario?
Yeah. Errm... and then there's two drugs I can have as well but they've both got very bad side effects and you know...
Well, they might not effect you.
I know but, it's just the thought of taking them, and the things they say may be happening, and you just think "Oh God" you know.
What kind of side effects are there?
One of them, it stops your period for six months so that you don't bleed and that stops the endometriosis growing. And then errm... It can bring like the menopause on, it can damage you bones, is it... Osteoporosis?
Yeah.
It can damage your bones, and it can make you errm... Infertile and, just things like that really. So [Laughs] so that was a bit of a shock really. Because when I went back on Wednesday I wasn't expecting him to say that to me. I was expecting him to say OK we're going to have to do it again, and it will be on such-and-such day. But he didn't and... It's been a rough year really.
Yeah.
She's worth it though.
Yeah.
Aren't you? So if we'd wanted more kids at the moment we couldn't have them, so...
I mean well, you don't... Like you say, with or without the endometriosis problems you feel that physically having Hannah like this...
It's hard work!
And having another Hannah as a baby...
Yeah, yeah that's it, it would just be...
Absolutely exhausting?
Yeah!
OK and do you try and make time for the two of you to spend time together without Hannah? You said that you've got people who can babysit and things like that.
Not really no. I mean, Saturday night, we get a take away and a video and hope that she goes to bed. But just lately she'll just sit and play but she won't bother you and you can just sit and watch the video... But no, we don't really get that much time to sort of, just the two of us, and it doesn't help with the hours that he works. You know like most couples they work during the day and then they've got the evening, we don't really have that.
OK the last chunk is your immediate future, so the next twelve months. What do you hope to achieve this year?
To feel better! [Laughs] Yeah.
Physically?
Mentally. I think I'm mentally worn down really. I think of everything, you feel like

Claire

you're just getting back on your feet and something else comes along and you get knocked down. So I think I'm, I think I'm mentally worn out. You know like I just need a holiday.
You need a break?
Yeah. I just want to be better again, and just think about, like the future, but at the moment... I mean I know it's not like cancer or anything where you know you are going to die. But you still feel that because you're ill, you still feel that you can't sort of get on with your life.
Is there ever, I mean you say that you like, that you've got pains and things like that, does that stop you from doing things?
Not, not really. It's because you don't feel well you don't want to go places.
Yeah yeah, that is difficult. [Telephone rings – it is Tom]
He says "Are you going to tell me about it later?!"
Does he think it's a conspiracy?!
I must admit when these ('Preparing for Parenthood') classes first, you know because it was like, it was like concentrated on postnatal depression, he was saying "Oh you know you shouldn't go to these classes because you'll end up getting postnatal depression!" [Laughs and rolls eyes]
Oh right! [Laughs and shakes head] OK, well you said that one of the things that you hope to achieve this year is a sort of holiday, maybe abroad. Do you want to go on holiday with Hannah, or a short break away with just Tom?
Oh no with Hannah, definitely.
Yeah?
I don't think that getting away from her personally would make me feel any better. I think it's just because of everything that has been going on and like this it's just brought me down, but... She's so much better now, it's not really her that gets me down, it's just, you know, life! [Laughs]
[Laughs] Life yeah. OK, and of the things that you hope to achieve this year, to mentally feel better, do you think you can achieve it? And if so, how?
To be honest with you I've not really, not really thought about it!
What, the future or...?
Yeah! I mean the only thing that I have really thought about is just getting better, and I've not really thought about that particularly, a lot. But no I've not really looked into the future and thought "Ooo" you know. I mean, not twelve months, I mean we have sort of said, that in a couple of years we'll think about trying for a baby, if everything's sorted out, but that's about the only thing we've ever really discussed. No, I can't say that I've looked into the future and...
And yet you seem very certain of what you want to do in the next 12 months - to feel better mentally.
Yeah, yeah, that's...
It was an instant reaction.

217

Nine Women, Nine Months, Nine Lives

Yeah that's probably the only thing because that is what is bothering me at the moment. I just want to be well. I just want it to be over and done with.
And you say that you really missed having time for yourself.
Yeah I still can't see how I'm going to get more time for myself.
Can't you make time for yourself? More often perhaps?
You get used to not having it though, don't you?
But is that a good thing?
When I think about things that make me really down, like when she's naughty, then you just, when she's crying a lot then I'll just ring my mum or something to have her, so that's like my time then, but errm... I think that's about it really.
Do you think you would feel bad about making more time for yourself?
Do I think I would feel bad?
Do you think you would feel guilty?
Yes! I think that's my problem. I do feel guilty. Yeah, I think that's it. I do feel guilty. Yeah I think that's my problem, yeah. I make myself feel guilty so, like I say I think you just accept the fact that you, that there isn't much time for yourself.
Yeah.
Because, I don't know, the day just seems... You get up, say you get up about eight, by the time you've fed her, bathed her and got yourself ready it's about ten, and then you do your housework and you cook dinner and then it's about two o'clock and then I'm getting ready for work and... And the day's just gone, so there isn't any time really.
So maybe that is something you could try and achieve this year then? Try and have time for yourself and not feel too guilty. Even if it was once every two months just an extra half a day for yourself, because it might make you feel better about a lots of things. About the endometriosis, it'd give you time to think about what you really want, time with Tom...
Yeah, I think, I think we need a bit more time together.
Because you've no need to feel guilty.
It's just difficult with work and everything.
Yeah, of course it is, yeah.
I think he'd like that as well.
Yeah? Has he ever said anything about wanting to spend more time...?
Oh he always says he wants to spend time with, he always says me and Hannah, but it's difficult for him, because of all the work he has to put in...
Yeah, but a little bit can go a long way.
Yeah, we're off in July so that's not too far away.
Yeah, I mean it's nearly Easter now, can't believe it!
Yeah, it's nearly your birthday in't it sweetpea?
Yeah, be a big girl! What have you learnt about yourself this past year that you would like to develop next year? So something good about yourself that you feel proud of.
Don't know. I'll tell you something going back a bit that I have noticed, I am more

Claire

emotional than I was, very emotional.
In a good way or a bad way?
In a bad way.
How do you mean emotional? Weepy or...?
Yeah I get upset easier than I used to. Yeah I've noticed that about myself. Errm... What was that you just asked me? See I'm very forgetful as well!
That's because you were distracted by Hannah shouting just now!
Mmm... You know when they say that when you are pregnant you are forgetful but when you've had your baby it comes back? It never did! [Laughs] I'm so forgetful! Honestly!
[Laughs] Oh no!
Like someone will tell me something or I'm supposed to do something, I have to write it down otherwise I don't remember!
Well you've got her to cater for 24 hours a day, whatever she wants, and you know then you've got yourself to wonder about as well. You know there's only so much room you've got in your head, so it's not really that surprising.
No, no. So what was the question?
The question was what have you learnt about yourself in the past year that you would like to develop next year?
Right, errm... I don't think I have.
Well the things that you've mentioned, things like you feel more mature. Do you feel more organised, less organised?
Errm... I try to organise myself, but errm... I don't always get there. I don't know, I think I'm very negative at the moment. I think I'd like to be more positive! [Laughs]
Yeah! Maybe realise your limitations?
Yeah, I'm only human! [Laughs]
Yeah. Quite. I mean, you know, if you have expectations that you can't reach, maybe you ought to lower them? Maybe?
Yeah, maybe.
If it makes you feel better...
I think sometimes I don't even realise though, that I'm like that. It's just...
You can't keep checking on yourself all the time. Like I was just saying, you've got her to think about, you've got yourself, there's Tom. And you know, life, like you said, the days go by.
Yeah they do.
And before you know it, so you have had other things to worry about as well. Your own health, I mean that's understandable that you are feeling really negative about that at the minute because it's something that you can't really control.
That's it.
It's not something you can physically see or monitor like a bruise on your arm. You can't see if it's changing, you know. But you do have a choice. Like you said with your treatment and things. If you decide that you don't want to take your medication...

219

Nine Women, Nine Months, Nine Lives

It's just whether you can put up with the, I mean they say you can take painkillers but that's not really an option for me. So...
Have you talked to anybody else who has had endometriosis?
No, I've got, they gave me a leaflet, like I say I only went Wednesday. Because originally when I found out, the consultant said to me "Oh you know we'll need to laser it away, and because of where it is we'll have to do it again". And that's what I'd sort of put into my head, and I was OK with that. I had it done once and I was waiting to have it done again. And when I went back and he turned round and said "If we do it again you'll have to have a colostomy bag, not that that would be forever, or you could have drug treatment"... It just sort of felt like a slap in the face really, because I wasn't expecting it.
It was a shock?
Yeah, yeah. But I do enjoy being a mum. I wouldn't change anything about that.
Well it's obvious that you enjoy being a mum.
Yeah, yeah. I'm dead proud of being Hannah's mum.
So maybe next year one of the things you would like to develop is still being as good as you are...
Well I can try!
Still being Hannah's mum. Still being good at it.
Yeah.
And to keep on being good at it. Because that's something to be proud of as well, not just proud of her but proud of yourself.
Yeah [A bit tearful at this point]
And soon she'll be able to tell you.
Yeah she will.
Would you say there's anything that you have learned about yourself, that you've become aware of, in the past year, that you would like to change next year? Something like you were saying earlier about perhaps not feeling guilty?
Mmm, yeah.
Making more time for yourself?
I think I've always been like that though, I've always... When you've been like it forever it's hard to change
Not straight away...
It's like, little things, like sometimes, on Friday nights for instance, my husband doesn't get back 'till about eleven o'clock and I feel guilty if I go to bed, because I think I should wait up for him. Not that he expects me to, I just think that I should be awake when he gets home. Just silly things like that. I know I shouldn't. I can tell you I shouldn't but, whether I'll go to bed or whether I'll be awake is a different thing! [Laughs]
Maybe there's a happy compromise, maybe you know, if you have a sleep early evening while he's out and then you're awake when he comes back. Is that a possibility?

Claire

Oh I do that! I just fall asleep! I've done it before, I've gone to sleep on the settee at about eight o'clock and woken up when he's come in! [Laughs]
I'm sure he'd prefer it if you felt a lot better in yourself, than if you struggle to be awake.
I mean he never says, like, there has been a few times when I have gone to bed, and he never says anything. It's just I feel guilty if I go to bed. I think I should wait up for him. It's just silly things like that. I think you put your own ideas into your head don't you?
Well, talk to him, ask him what he thinks, because you can only imagine... I mean he may be thinking "Oh God I wish she would go to bed because otherwise I feel bad about keeping her up, she's been up all day, I've been out at work, there's no point both of us being shattered".
That's it, yeah. And I feel like if he's been at work all morning... What he sort of does is he goes out about nine and he does his chips and sorts things out and comes back at lunchtime. Then he goes out, gets the van ready, and sometimes he doesn't get in until one in the morning because he's doing his fish, because it's a fish and chip business, fillets his fish... So like some days he's out all day, just comes back for a few hours and stuff like that. Say I've been cleaning, I'll sit down for five minutes have a cup of tea and watch telly, he'll always come home then! [Laughs] Always! He never says anything, but I feel guilty because I've sat down and watched telly, that's how I feel. Even though I've probably only just sat down and turned the telly on!
Well he's just come back in from work so he's stopped work too!
I know but you get, you can guarantee that just as I have sat down with my cup of tea he's come home. You know there are times where I've been doing things and I think "Oh I'll just carry on and do a tiny bit more - he should be home in a minute!" And half an hour later I think to myself I could have sat down and had a cup of tea and he wouldn't of known! [Laughs] Oh and it's so stupid – I shouldn't feel like that! I mean there's absolutely nothing from him to suggest that he thinks' that, it's just the way I am. I've always been hard working, you know, with my jobs. I've always worked really hard, and I know that, and my bosses have always praised me for things like that saying you know you work hard and things like that [baby crying]. I think she's tired because we went into town today.
Oh, did you have an exciting day?
And she only had a little bit of sleep.
Ah buying birthday presents!
Yeah!
But even though that is part of you, and you are adamant that it is, and that's fine, if it's not doing you good maybe you ought to do a little bit less of it. Not stop it completely because it is part of you and that is the way you are.
Well I try and then I think "Oh I'm lazy!" [Laughs] You try and do things, I know it's in my mind. But it's like breaking a habit and, it's like smoking, like trying to stop smoking.
What you have to try and think of every time that you do... like a lot of the girls that I

221

Nine Women, Nine Months, Nine Lives

spoke to when they were pregnant and they were still smoking, I would always say to them "Each cigarette you don't have is a good thing". Not telling them, you know "Cut down, you <u>will</u> cut down". You have to think positively, every time you sit down, put your feet up and have a cup of tea, think "This is good, this is doing me good". Because if you are sat there thinking "He's going to come home any bloody minute I know he is, I just know he is!" – are you really enjoying that cup of tea?
No! [Laughs]
No, exactly! So if you're going to have it, you might as well have it and enjoy it!
Yeah, I know, I know. I always think that. But you can't break a habit, it's so difficult.
You don't have to break the habit but you do have to alter the way you think about it because it's not going to do you any good.
No, I know, and I know for a fact that he doesn't think that.
Have you asked him?
No but I just…
Ask him and <u>remember</u> what he says.
Because he always says to me "Oh you work too hard" and stuff like that you know. But I just think, well you know, I should be doing more, I hate it if the house is ever a mess. I've become more, I think that's another thing that being pregnant has done to me, I'm like obsessed with cleaning. I'm not obsessed to the fact where I'm like everything has got to be scrubbed and absolutely spotless but I like it to be tidy. I don't mind Hannah's toys, this doesn't bother me, but like where she's put the newspapers on the floor, or the cushions aren't puffed up. And that's from being pregnant, that's what that has done to me. I never used to be, I always used to be fairly house proud, but <u>never</u> to that extent.
Do you think that was when you were at home for a long period of time?
Yeah, the last ten weeks.
So it may have become habit then, didn't it?
I didn't work for the last ten weeks because I was so big. I couldn't work, I couldn't fit behind the thing [counter]! [Laughs] I was too tired as well. And so I used to clean. And you get the house so clean that errm… When…
You maintain it being so clean?
When you can't, it's just, you know, you want to, but you can't.
So that's something that developed while you were pregnant?
Yeah.
So, it wasn't there before?
No.
So… it can <u>not</u> be there again!
Mmmm. I think all my hormones have just gone completely, and with this endometriosis as well - that's hormonal, I just think I'm just all over the place.
Yeah but you are here (in the house) a lot of the time, but also, the thing is, this is where you are most of the time.
Yeah.

Claire

And if you were in a working environment you would be keeping that tidy as well, and yourself busy. And you want to make sure that Hannah is safe and everything's clean, and that she is all right, so that's only natural...
Yeah, yeah.
But if it's getting to the point where you are doing it for the sake of doing it, that could be your time for you!
Yeah, I know. Mmmm, I've just got my own car now.
Oh that's good!
Because we, we were sharing one for a, well since I was pregnant really, and he's just bought himself a little van to help him with the business, so it's been a couple of weeks now. That's been brilliant, that's really helped, I've just started using it. Because before he used to have to give us a lift into town because it was difficult with a pram and the baby on a bus, so... He'd give us a lift and then he'd pick us up and it was always time, you know you had to rush. But today when we went up with my mum, we took the car into town and that's something I've never done before, I've never driven into town, into a car park, and so that was the first time I'd done that. I must admit I was a bit nervous beforehand, but when I was actually in the car it didn't bother me, I just got on with it and did it!
That's good.
That's another thing as well. With just having the one car, and him having it, I'd say to him "I'm losing my confidence driving!" Because, I'd probably drive once every fortnight round the corner to my mums, you know she lives locally, it's just things like that, and now I've got me own car I think "Great, I've got me freedom again!" and I'm you know starting to use that.
Yeah, that's great!
That's a positive thing! [Laughs]
Yeah, that is a positive thing. So that's something you can develop this year, your independence?
Yeah, I mean now she's getting older, I'll probably, I've enrolled her at this group, I've not started yet but, it's local.
A mother and baby group?
Yeah, I'm going to start taking her up there.
Well that'll be good, it'll be good for her, and good for you.
Yeah, yeah. And I've just made a new friend over the road as well.
Yeah?
Yeah, her little boy is three weeks younger than Hannah so that's brilliant!
Oh right, excellent!
I've only known her a few weeks, but errm... that's nice.
Yeah, that's good. OK so that's a good thing then, your independence?
Yeah.
You see, it's there if you look for it!

Nine Women, Nine Months, Nine Lives

Yeah I know.
I can understand that it is really difficult at the moment to think positively, but, it takes that bit more effort but it's worth it when you do!
Yeah, yeah, it is! You'll come back in a year's time and you'll say "What have you done?" and I won't be able to remember what I did and what I didn't do! [Laughs]
Yeah, but that's it isn't it? Everybody's life is like that I mean this time last year – God! I mean it's just completely different from where we are now. When I think about just things like my relationship with my partner, you know, and the fact that I had just bought a house and I was living in a tip, the builders were in, and I was at the end of my tether! I was thinking "Oh God!" – I was up the wall and half way across the ceiling! A year later and things are different. They could be different again this time next week!
Yeah that's it, you don't know what's round the corner!
But you have to try and, you know. You have to take care of yourself Claire.
Yeah.
You know how and what makes you feel good, even if you can't do it right there and then, if you know you can do it in the future.
Then that's something to look forward to. Do you know what I saw once on a film, it was about teenage mum's you know who were still at school having babies, and they, they made it look so easy! And like you see all these single mothers that are walking round the streets and stuff and they just make having a baby look so easy!
How do you mean?
Well, they've got these little babies in their prams and they're so good and quiet, so well behaved. It was ages before I could go shopping with her. I used to have to take her in, you know the rock-a-bye car seats, and I had to have someone else with me. I had to put her in the trolley and then have my own trolley for the shopping. And when she was a bit older I used to sit her in, you know the seats (on the trolleys) and she used to hate it, she used to scream and scream, I couldn't take her. I used to dread having to go shopping even if somebody was with me. Because she'd scream and scream, I used to have to carry her around and she used to get so heavy. And then now, she will actually sit in the, you know, in the seat bit, and she's fine now! I used to dread it, oh for months, <u>whenever</u> we went shopping.
Yeah, yeah. If you knew how many times I had heard girls say that to me! You've no idea! Everybody seems to have this idea that other people are making it look easy! There's a conspiracy going on! "How is everybody else doing this and I'm not?!"
I know, where does it come from, where did this idea of a perfect mother and everything, where did it come from? [Quite angry]
It's basic insecurity. It's just you know, everybody thinks "I must be doing something different or wrong"
Well, I had realised that to be honest with you because after I'd spoken to this girl, and it's funny and we'll start talking, and I don't know, things I've gone through, she's gone through, you just think, well it's not just me!

Claire

No, no it's not! But everybody goes through it differently. Some bits that you found easy other people will have found horrendous. You know, it's swings and roundabouts, you can do without the extra things that make you feel bad though.
Yeah, I think so.
You'll just have to see how you go and like you said take it day by day and you will be all right. OK, well, that's it!
Oh!
That's lovely, that's great, really good. Thanks ever so much, I hope it wasn't too bad?
No, it was fine, I've enjoyed it!
Good, good.

225

Nine Women, Nine Months, Nine Lives

Sarah

Sarah was 29 years old when she found out that she was pregnant. She had been living with her partner Anthony for a few months and was not planning to have children just yet. However, they were both pleased and continued with their pregnancy. Sarah has returned to work part-time as a sales assistant, not to her original job as a stable-hand, but wants to re-train so that she can spend more time with her son Jack and her partner. Having him has given her a new found strength and confidence within herself.

The first section is about when you first found out you were pregnant, so if you could think back to that time, OK? Were you trying to get pregnant at the time?
No.
No. So it was a completely unplanned pregnancy?
Yes.
Can you remember what went through your mind when you did the test? What was your initial reaction?
Errm... I was happy, errm... Yeah, I was happy.
So how many weeks did you think you were? Did you have a fairly good idea...?
Errm... I bet I was about 8 weeks. Yeah, because when I missed the second one really that, that I thought it was more likely.
And what did you think about afterwards, your initial reaction was happiness, did you then think "Oh my goodness!"?
I was shocked, mmm, a bit shocked. Well I was worried how my partner and my family

Nine Women, Nine Months, Nine Lives

would take it.
Was your partner with you when you did the test?
No, no! [Laughs]
Did he know that you thought you might be pregnant?
No![Laughter]
So you kept it a secret for all those weeks? Gosh!
Yeah, I know! [Laughs]
Were you worried?
Initially, I was a bit worried, I mean, just on his reaction really. I mean I knew he wasn't going to desert me or anything like that, he's from a biggish family, so... Yeah, it was just his reaction really.
How he would take it. Did you think "My God how am I going to tell him?"
Yes! [Laughter] Yes. He was all right, he was shocked, took him about, he got used to it and he was really happy. I didn't tell, I told him first and then I didn't tell any of the rest of the family for a while, because I wanted to be sure, between ourselves, you know, before I told anybody else.
Were you living together at the time?
Yes, yes we were, but we hadn't been living together very long.
Had you known each other long?
Yes, yeah we'd been together about 3 years but we'd only been living together about 4 months.
Oh right, so everything was new and different?
Yeah!
Yes, just ever so slightly! [Laughter] OK so no-one was with you when you did the test?
No.
No-one at all?
No, no I did a home test first and then I went to the doctors to have it confirmed, and I hadn't told anybody at the stage.
Right so you'd done a home test, then you went to the doctors and you still hadn't told anybody at that stage?
No.
How long did it take you between doing the test and then telling him?
Errm... From what when I knew positively?
Yeah.
I think it was about 10 days.
Ten days in total, so that's quite a while really. Do you think you were fretting a bit?
Errm... Yeah I think it, I was happy with it, I was happy with you know just being pregnant, but I was, I think I just wanted to get used to it.
In yourself?
Yeah.
To sort out how you felt? So perhaps you knew how you were feeling before you told

Sarah

him?
Yes, so I mean I was feeling completely positive about it sort of thing.
Then it was just a matter of telling him?
[Laughter] Yeah!
OK the next section is your experience of pregnancy and the birth. Did you imagine what pregnancy would be like before you got pregnant with Jack?
Errm... Not, yeah not, I'd thought about it but not, I'd thought about it more for the future sort of thing. Yeah errm... I didn't really know what baby's and children involve because I've got no immediate family with children, so I had no...
What about your friends?
No. I didn't really know what was going to happen or what it was going to be like.
Oh right, so do you think your, when you first found out, did you then start to wonder what it would be like?
A bit yeah, definitely at the end I was thinking how it was going to change things, and the things I could do and it would change my everyday life sort of thing.
So it would change you and what you could do?
Yes, yeah.
And do you think that was different to your actual experiences? Had what you'd imagined been fairly realistic?
Errm... Yes, I mean it did alter things a lot, I would say. I mean even while I was carrying him, it was surprising how much I had to alter things like what I was doing at work, that sort of thing, and physically feeling you know, that side of it.
Yeah, yeah very different.
Yes, I got very emotional and that sort of thing...
Did that surprise you?
Yeah it did really, yeah. For a start I didn't really realise that that was what it was, that I was like that because I was pregnant. I was emotional and we didn't put two and two together from the start.
Were you oversensitive, or upset, extra happy or...?
I'd get upset very easily, and just over dramatise things, little problems suddenly became... Giants! [Laughs] Just emotional.
So it was that side of things that surprised you more than the physical things? Your actual experiences differed, on the emotional side of things, quite a lot from what you'd expected?
Yeah.
And what did you expect would happen at the birth, did you have any idea about that? Had you found out about it?
I wasn't looking forward to it! [Laughter]
I don't think many people do to be honest!
Only from what I'd read in magazines and that sort of thing, you know sort of, did I know what to expect.

229

Nine Women, Nine Months, Nine Lives

And did it worry you, did you wonder.... ? Had you read horror stories? [Laughter]
Errm... It did worry me a bit. I think it was the pain side of it that was worrying me and whether I would cope with the pain.
With that much pain over that much time?
Yeah, yes.
And was the birth as you thought it would be, was it different from what you expected?
Labour was different from what I expected it would be.
In what way?
I don't know, it's difficult to describe, I suppose it depends how you feel at the time. I didn't react very well to the gas and air.
Did it make you feel sick?
It kept knocking me out! [Laughs]
Gosh!
I felt like I was out of control, I wasn't in charge of what was happening.
And was your partner around at all?
Yes he was with me all the time.
And how did you feel when you first held Jack?
I cried! [Laughs] Yeah I cried! Happy, very happy. But I felt, because he was an assisted delivery, I felt like I hadn't done it.
Oh right... So what, was he a forceps delivery?
Yes. I kept saying "but I didn't do it" or something like that, I felt that, yeah... I can't think of the words to put it in to, but I felt like I wasn't that I hadn't done it all myself sort of thing. Inadequate, I felt a bit inadequate, in the delivery sense because I'd had the forceps.
Oh right.
But other than that I was just emotional, emotional, yes.
And a bit relieved?
Yeah, yes! Yes I was relieved, he was in one piece.
Did you feel at all scared?
No, no I don't think so. No I don't remember feeling like that, I was just really happy seeing him.
And in what way was your partner involved in your pregnancy? He'd had more experience of children from friends and family, younger brothers and sisters. So, did he know more than you did perhaps?
I think he did, yeah. And throughout the pregnancy we tried to carry on, you know, not too much but not let it change our lives too much sort of thing. But he was definitely more experienced with babies than I was, I mean after he was born... [Shakes her head and rolls her eyes at the memory]
Were you nervous?
Oh yes, doing things, you know. I'd never changed a nappy, dressed them, bathed one, that kind of thing, so...

Sarah

Was it quite daunting?
Yes, yes, mmm. So he was a little bit more competent about things than I was sort of thing for a start and he was good, he was very good helping me.
So in the pregnancy itself did you talk about things like you feeling so emotional?
Errm...
Because I guess he must have been getting a bit fed up of getting his head bitten off?
Yes! [Laughter] He was understanding, I don't think he was prepared for how I was going to be emotionally, I mean he, or quite as emotional as I was. But as soon as we both realised it was because I was pregnant I was acting like that, and then he did, you know he accepted it, he was accepting of it. He probably got a bit fed up of me sometimes though!
Well you probably got a bit fed up of him?
Yeah! [Laughter]
So on the practical side of things, in your pregnancy, when say you couldn't lift things...
Yeah definitely towards the end. I did sometimes I did have to ask, I had to tell him, you know that like the shopping, I couldn't carry those heavy bags because it was painful or whatever. He just accepted that, and once I'd told him that I couldn't do something then he would get on and do them straightaway.
Oh that's really good. Yeah that is good. And what about the birth itself, you say that he was actually with you, was he able to support you or were you quite content just to know that he was around?
Errm... He was there and he sort of, he held my hand and, he was supportive all along. Other than that...
Did you want him there?
Yes I wanted him there and it did help knowing he was there, just a nice hand to hang on to! [Laughs]
OK. So was he curious about the changes that were happening to you, throughout your pregnancy, was he obviously interested?
Yeah, he didn't sort of errm... He didn't ask me questions much but he would listen and he was interested, you know. And I would tell him sort of thing, but he wasn't you know, he wasn't desperately curious or anything, he didn't push anything...
He was just interested and being supportive?
Yes, yes he was. When he came home, different things that had happened or how I was feeling I could you know sit down and tell him, and he was he was there for me, a sounding board.
Yeah that's it, that's what you need isn't it?
Yeah.
And do you think that was more or less than you hoped for, this sort of support in your pregnancy?
At the time I thought it was enough. Thinking back now I think I would, I would have liked things to have been a little bit different. Or again if I had another pregnancy, I'd

Nine Women, Nine Months, Nine Lives

like it to be, I'd like it to feel a bit more special, just to be treated a bit more special, I think. I think I tried to carry on too much as normal, instead of taking a step back sort of thing.
So do you think he was reacting to the way you wanted to carry on, or...?
I think he did, yeah.
Yeah, so he was taking his lead from you?
Yeah, I think so, I think I still stayed fairly independent, and he just saw that I was getting on and doing things and he just let me carry on sort of thing. He never stopped me from doing anything, and he never said "You shouldn't perhaps be doing that" you know.
Oh right.
So I think another time, I think it would have been nicer to feel a bit more special at the time, yeah.
Yeah. And the birth, the support that you had from him, do you think that was more or less than you'd hoped for?
Yes I was pleased, because he didn't know if he could be with me throughout.
Did he not want to come?
He wasn't sure, you know beforehand, he wasn't sure.
It must be difficult to know.
Yes, but errm... He was there throughout, and he was pleased he was. Once I'd gone into definite labour sort of thing he said he couldn't have left anyway, he said he couldn't have just walked out on me, so he was there.
So that was more than you hoped for then really?
Yes, oh yes I was definitely pleased that he was going to, that he was there.
Was his behaviour different from what you had expected? Was he more or less supportive emotionally or different from his usual self whilst you were pregnant, did he suddenly become more considerate or less considerate?
Errm... No.
OK. So you said that he took his lead from you, stepped back a bit, and kind of left it to you, and you felt OK when you were doing things so he thought you must be all right?
He certainly didn't change much really! [Laughs]
He didn't become more or less supportive?
No, no! [Laughs]
He stayed just the same as before?
Yeah. Errm... We, yes in everyday life he was the same, he wasn't more or less, obviously he comforted me or whatever when I was going through the emotional time. He would be you know more supportive then but then I suppose as soon as I was all right he'd go back to being you know! [Laughs] Certainly wasn't less, we never had any negative thoughts really between us, no.
Right the next chunk is your experience of early motherhood, so the first three months, if you could think in terms of that. Do you think your pregnancy effected the first three

232

Sarah

months of motherhood? How you were feeling physically or emotionally, sometimes if you had bad water retention or were particularly tired from the last stages of pregnancy that does tend to carry on through into early motherhood...
Errm... No, no there wasn't anything.
You weren't feeling particularly isolated or down?
Errm... No not towards the end no, no.
OK and likewise the birth, was there anything about the birth that carried on into early motherhood? You had forceps didn't you, I mean that must have been quite physically...
Painful!
... Different, did you, was that difficult?
Sitting down was quite difficult for a start! I had an episiotomy, stitches, so errm... It was a little bit uncomfortable [laughs at the understatement] but we settled down early, well I did personally. I think I got the baby blues.
You were a little bit down?
Yeah, I was all right whilst I was in hospital, I think it was when I came home. I felt particularly, he was very unsettled, he had bad colic, he used to be crying, and sometimes it really did get to me.
Yes. Were you managing to sleep at all at the time? He must have been colicky through the nights...
Yes sleep was disrupted a lot but I did try and catch up in the daytime. When he had a nap I had a nap as well so I was tired but I wasn't, I never got to the stage where I was absolutely exhausted.
No but it was a near thing?
Yeah! [Laughs]
And how did you imagine early motherhood would be? Towards the end of your pregnancy you must have been wondering what he would be like, what it would be like, what you and your partner would be like?
Yes we didn't, we hadn't, I hadn't talked to him about it that much but errm... It was more chaotic than I thought it was going to be! [Laughs] I wasn't quite prepared for how regularly he would want feeding and just the amount of attention that he needed really, I wasn't really prepared for all of that.
The 24-hour care?
Yeah, and if you wanted to go anywhere. Well, I particularly felt a bit stuck here with him for a start. I felt a little bit isolated with only a pushchair... I didn't, we didn't have a car for a start so that was, well an obstacle to doing things. I felt shut in.
Right, so did any of your friends live locally or?
Errm... No, none of them.
What about your family, sisters?
Well, two are in Melton, mum is twenty minutes away. She'd well, she'd come over and see us now and again, she didn't like pressure us, she didn't like just pop over.
She didn't just drop in?

233

Nine Women, Nine Months, Nine Lives

No, no! She'd come over a couple of times a week, which was nice. It was nice when people did come, I was pleased! [Laughter] Errm... Sorry I keep forgetting what the question was!
No, no you just tell me what you think and we'll carry on from there, don't worry at all! OK so how you'd imagined early motherhood, do you think it turned out to be the way you had expected?
Errm... Not, some things yes.
And some things not?
Yes, it wasn't, it would have been better if I'd been prepared for the colic. I had a job keeping him quiet and happy, so that sort of, I think that upset me a lot, I thought things would be a bit happier and a bit smoother. And errm... I was looking forward to going round and showing off my new baby and things like that, and I felt like I couldn't because he was so colicky and crying, you know you couldn't.
Not very settled?
Yeah, even when people came here he would scream the place down, and I used to look at him and think why couldn't he be a bit more smiley and gurgley and then people might come more often! [Laughter]
Yes! But, how long did it take to get the colic sorted out?
Well he got a bit better after a few months, the GP couldn't really prescribe anything for him. It didn't go until he was nearly four months old.
Gosh!
Yes, so it was a long while.
Yes, because if he had it, then in effect you had it.
Yes, yes! There just wasn't much they could do, what they did give him helped but it certainly didn't cure it at all.
So what would you say was difficult in the early days, say the first three weeks?... What did you find hard to adjust to?
A bit shut in. I was happy with him, I had no doubts about or had any bad feelings towards him, but errm I felt a bit cut off. I was glad to get out, I loved going out in the day, and once I was out I really wanted to stay out, I got a bit fed up of the same four walls sort of thing! [Laughs] Errm... but I liked looking after him. I liked bathing him and changing him and all those sort of things, I mean they didn't get me down at all.
No. And just getting to know him?
Yeah, yes that was nice.
So how much would you say your partner was involved in the early days?
Quite a lot, I mean I was grateful sort of when he came home from work! He used to leave early and then be back when it was dark. I was definitely pleased to see him! [Laughs] At night time he was brilliant, he would take him straight away because I was tired and getting grouchy by that time of night.
Did he manage to take any time off to be with you, when, just after you came home?
Errm... Not really, no, not really. Because I had him , I think he did have a couple of

Sarah

days off. Luckily I came out of hospital on the Thursday and he was at work on the Friday and then he was at home all weekend which was quite nice yeah... And on Friday nights he would be the one to get up. It was his idea that I should have one night were I could get some sleep which was great, because you know, he hadn't got to get up the next day and go to work so...
So you said that you didn't really know all that much about having children and what was involved, had you actually talked about who would do what...?
No.
So you hadn't talked about things like changing, the night feeds, bathing?
No, no I'd sort of jokingly said you're going to have to show me because I don't know much. But no, we hadn't sat down and seriously talked about the night feeds and stuff like that. I think I just wanted to feel, I wanted to know that, well that I had the responsibility, I wanted him to be there for him to help me and for him to back me up, I wanted him to know that that was how I was feeling really.
And do you think your partner was thinking the same thing?
Probably! [Laughs]
Yeah?
Yeah.
Well if the two coincided then that's fine but if the two don't quite match up on a practical level then...
He was definitely willing to muck in and help. I don't think he, he never thought of taking over he never really criticised me you know "No don't do it like that, this is how you do it", you know nothing like that, he was never keen on changing nappies but then... [Laughs]
No, no I don't think I would be if I had a choice! [Laughs]. So do you feel that that worked out really? That you'd sort of get on and he'd be there if you needed him, in case you needed him to help you do things was that enough for you?
Yes, yes because he was, yes.
Was that better than you'd expected or perhaps in some way not as good as you'd expected?
Errm... It would have been better I think if he hadn't gone straight to work so that we would have had a little bit more time together at home, but he had to go in. But I didn't I would have liked him to have been there and I didn't resent it, it's just, well it had to be done. Especially when he was crying and I couldn't shut him up!
Yeah, that makes you feel awful! [Laughs] So do you think things worked out for the better or for the worst?
For the better really, because it was his idea that I should have a night off.
Yeah that is a good idea.
Yeah it was his idea, and he didn't have to go to work the next day, I could just crash out and not have to do a thing, it was a great!
Right, the next chunk, this is your experience of motherhood up to the present day. How

235

Nine Women, Nine Months, Nine Lives

do you think your life has changed since you have had Jack?
Completely! [Laughter]
You were working before you had Jack, and last time I saw you, you were working part-time. Are you...?
I still am working part-time. I'm a lot happier, I'm a lot more confident now I've got Jack than I used to be. Because in every day life I used to be quite shy. I'm a lot more confident now, yes definitely. I'm more contented now I suppose because I know more now about the future with (having) Jack. Whereas before it was always work, not knowing where would I be going and things like that. I'm a lot more contented now. I don't worry about things like that anymore.
So did you used to worry about the future?
Yes, yeah I think so. I saw it as unknown yeah definitely. I'd be wary about work, because I haven't got a lot of qualifications, my job was a manual job so I knew I couldn't do that forever so I think I'm more... Plus I did want to settle down eventually and be a mother, find out if I could do it.
Is it possible? [Laughter]
I worry more financially now. Errm... The house is mortgaged, we can pay that every month but there's not a lot left.
And you're only working part-time as well?
Yeah so things are tighter at the moment, a lot tighter now. But errm... We're happy and that's what counts.
Yeah. OK and how do you think you have changed in the last 12 months? You mentioned confidence...
Yeah, there's that.
Is there something you have become aware of that wasn't there before?
I did used to be, well I think I used to be fairly self-centered, you know just looking after yourself, but not anymore.
I don't think you have much choice really! [Laughter]
I think I have changed for the better, yeah.
Yeah. And do you get any time for yourself?
Not a lot, no!
But the time that you do have for yourself, is it a regular thing?
No, no, although it is nice just to get away from him occasionally. I can't say as I always look forward to it but when I'm actually out I do enjoy it. But I need to know that he's all right whilst I'm not there, he'll have him or my mum so...
Yeah I suppose it does defeat the object of the exercise if you are spending your time for your self wondering if he is all right! [Laughter] OK so what do you tend to do in your time for yourself, do you sort of just relax or do something...?
I take the dog out.
For a nice walk?
Yeah, go across the fields, and play with him and I can be a bit more active when I

Sarah

haven't got the pushchair. When he was smaller I could carry him in a sling, I could still get out and about but I wasn't quite as free. It's just knowing that I haven't got that responsibility for that short time but it's not a regular thing.
So you don't get much time just for you?
Not without him, no. Very occasionally. My partner will take him out at the weekends! But... [Laughter]
That's a good use of his spare time, yeah! And how do you think your partner has changed? Do you think he has?
He tried not to let it.
Really?
Yeah, I think so. Especially with other people. When he is at home he loves Jack to bits and will sit and play with him, yeah, but when other people are around he tends to be a bit more reserved! [Laughs] He still goes out with his friends, plays football on a Saturday, because I wouldn't stop him. [Laughs] No, and he knows that I wouldn't stop him from going football training with his mates or whatever, you know he likes to keep it, I suppose it's just his way of, you know of keeping that side as it was.
So he's not changed as a person?
Not from the way he was.
So have you changed as a couple? Your relationship, has it developed into something...?
Well it's a lot steadier. Errm... I mean we don't, well we used to have silly little arguments, things like that, but we don't so much now. I think we're more on a level, certainly, with things.
So, what do you mean by you're more on a level?
We used to have a lot more differences of opinion or you know I'd want to do something and he'd want to do something else. Just wanting different things whereas now we're much more compatible.
Do you agree with each other more or do you just agree to disagree?
Errm... A bit of both really! We certainly do agree more, but instead of getting into an argument we tend to just walk away now, when we can see that we're definitely going to have a row we just don't. We certainly don't argue as much.
And do you talk about how you have changed as a couple?
Errm, generally in a jokey sort of way! [Laughter] I don't think we're that aware, we haven't sat down and thought about how we've changed, I think we're both aware that we have changed.
Do you think he has noticed that you have changed?
Yeah, yes. I mean he, I think he didn't think he'd be a father.
Really?
I don't know why!
Oh well that's good. Do you try and make time to spend together without Jack?
We don't really, no. I think perhaps we should do. I think that we should spend more time together, not that I don't want Jack with us, but...

237

Nine Women, Nine Months, Nine Lives

No of course not.
Just for us to be together on our own. I work in the evenings and it sometimes feels like we barely spend any time together, we don't sit down and talk like we should. He leaves for work at six in the morning whilst I'm asleep, and then when he comes home I go off to work and when I get back in again he's asleep so... I feel that we should spend more time together.
So you feel that he doesn't think it is as necessary?
Yeah I think he thinks we're just going along just fine.
Do you think he maybe feels that you can't see where you can make room in your lives for doing that? Making time to do it, I mean it's all very well in theory but do you think he's on a practical level thinking this won't be...?
Yeah, I think he thinks it might be more trouble than it is worth! [Laughs]
Do you think he might, and this is me playing the devils advocate, that he thinks this will mean him having to give up some of the time that he does his own thing, to spend with you?
Errm... maybe, he might see it like that.
Because if you are so busy in the week, the weekends are the only real...
Yeah, the weekends are quite important to him, but I'd like us to spend you know time together. And errm... I do get a little bit annoyed sometimes even, when I want the three of us to go out together, even just if I want to take the dog for a walk, or to go down the shops, he'd rather go in the garage! [Laughs] That does annoy me because I think we don't do much as a family we don't go out much as a family, things like that.
And you feel it would be nice?
Yes, I think it would be nice, and I think that we would all enjoy that time together.
Mmmm.
It'll probably be better, you know, when he's toddling about a bit more.
Yeah when he's a bit older it might perhaps be easier for you two to be together, and maybe in the evenings...
Yeah.
OK. The last bit is your immediate future, so the next 12 months. What do you hope to achieve in the next year?
Errm...
What are your hopes?
Difficult! I hadn't thought about this before! [Laughs] I haven't exactly got any major goals.
I don't mean anything in particular that is major, not career goals things like that, you know, sort of, maybe to spend more time together as a couple?
Definitely, yeah. To spend more time together, all together as a family, yeah, that time is quite important to me. Errm... Yeah just time together really. Maybe him spending less time in the garage and football and things. I know that's his right, and I don't maybe want to change him, he enjoys doing that and I'm quite happy for that to carry on, but

Sarah

a bit more spare time for us really. Maybe, I don't know, I might be able to find a different job, and we could spend more time together, so I'm not just disappearing in the evenings. I hope I can achieve these things!
Do you think you can achieve them this year?
Hopefully, yes, I mean we're quite settled we're not planning any drastic changes. We're still going to be here. Errm... I'm quite happy with the way things are going in general, it's only little things that you know... The overall pictures not bad, we're quite comfortable, we're quite happy.
Yeah, yeah it seems to be, you just want to tweak it a bit.
Yeah! [Laughs]
What would you say you had learnt about yourself in the past year that you would like to keep going, or keep up next year?
Definitely me being more positive, and, and just keep being a good mum! [Laughs] Being someone you know with responsibilities, I quite like that, I quite like having the responsibility, being a mother.
Have you been to any mother and baby groups, or anything like that?
No.
I'm sure there are some, either at your health center or local village Halls. And they are quite nice to go to in the mornings because there are people there you can chat to, you know, get a bit of human contact.
Yeah? [Laughs] Yeah I think we ought to be doing a bit more, mixing with other children a bit more. Well there is another girl near here who's had a baby recently and she comes round, Jack is quite happy to play with him but he won't play at all with older children, he's not sure of them, he'll sit and watch them, he won't interact with them yet. So I think I ought perhaps to start looking at the side of getting him involved, and I'd be making some effort towards getting out and meeting people too.
Yeah, because there are some local groups or meetings.
I wish I'd started and maybe gone to them earlier...
Well there are a lot of girls who don't go early, some join later, some only go for a while. It's not going to be the same people turning up every week, you won't be completely new and stand out. Quite a lot of the time it's just a matter of dropping in, your local library might have some information about it, or the doctors?
Yeah, yeah I think I have seen some posters about a playgroup.
You could always get involved as a helper, they always need helpers, and you do get paid sometimes.
Oh, do you?
You see that's an option, and it would be during the day, he gets contact, you get to do something you enjoy, he's with you so you don't need to pay for childcare, I don't think you would be paid much, but it could be something...
The idea appeals, definitely!
Most people who have had their first baby feel a bit lonely now and again.

239

Nine Women, Nine Months, Nine Lives

Yeah, yeah, I might give that a go.
Yeah, why not? The last question, what have you learnt about yourself in the past year that you would like to change next year?
Errm…
Is there anything that you would like to, I don't know, not necessarily something you feel really bad about, but perhaps something you could improve?
Errm… Perhaps be a bit more organised! [Laughs] And to think more about my future, plan ahead you know…
Do you not think of your future then?
I tend to think about his future quite a lot, what he's going to be doing, where he'll go to school, silly things like that.
That's not silly! Why is that silly?
He's hardly a year old! [Laughs]
I know but look how quickly it's gone!
I would like to get it planned.
Well, it is too early to do anything about it, but, at least you are thinking.
Yeah, I think so. And I would like to go back to work, financially I would.
Yeah it must be tight.
Because things are quite tight, we haven't got any money for extras you know, and, well, I mean we don't let it take over, but it's important, there's not a lot of spare about. He comes first! [Laughs] And I think we've not bought anything for ourselves really, and it would be nice not to struggle. So from that side it would be nice.
Yeah.
You know when he's a bit older, I'll perhaps get out and do a bit more. But at the minute, my mum will have him now and then but she wouldn't want him like regular like every morning nine till twelve, sort of, she wouldn't want him. So we will have to wait until he goes to a nursery, which I'm not sure about, at the minute, I don't think I could give him up and go full time!
Have you thought about retraining and stuff? Because you know you are entitled to various sort of benefits, he can go into a free crèche at the college, there might be something there that you might quite like in the daytime?
Yeah, there may be.
He'll be looked after and you can do something different.
I've thought about it vaguely but I've not looked into anything, or probably not even thought about it seriously but, I have vaguely had that idea go through my mind.
Yeah, well that might be what suits you.
Some people do go back to work straight away but I don't want to be apart from him.
Yeah, it depends how you feel. If you want to spend time with him then who's to say that is wrong or right? But if it starts to be that you feel as if you want to be able to go out more and perhaps have some free time to yourself and know that he is OK. For him to be able to get sociable with other children in the crèche or playgroup or mother and baby

240

Sarah

group, then it can't do any harm to find out...
Yeah it's good to know you've got options.
Yeah, yeah, I mean I'm sure there are more things than I know about, there is always lots of information, the problem is that you will have to ask for it, and you don't always have the time or the inclination, so...
Yeah, yeah.
Well that's lovely, I hope that wasn't too bad?
No that was just fine, not a problem at all!

Nine Women, Nine Months, Nine Lives

Ameena

Ameena was 22 years old when she became pregnant after being married for two years. Her marriage was arranged through her family. She continued with her career after marrying and indeed after having her daughter Ayesha. Although they had been trying for a child since marrying, she was glad it had taken two years to conceive as this enabled her and her husband to get to know and grow to love each other. At the time of the interview she was experiencing a conflict within herself about the balance in her life between work and home.

If you could think back to when you found out. Were you trying to get pregnant at the time?
Gosh, it seems like ages ago! It's nearly two years ago!
Yeah, time flies...
We were just starting to talk about it. We'd been married for two years and, we weren't desperate for children, we wanted to spend some time together get used to each other, then we planned to have children. On the day that I found out I was pregnant I had just got back from work, and errm…I think I was two weeks pregnant. I was two weeks late, and… Oh, I don't usually like to say things like this because, because I'm sure people think "What a ninny!"
No, no, go on.
I, I somehow, felt pregnant. I don't know whether other women get that or not, but I just had that feeling. Not that I was expecting to get pregnant or feel pregnant but, after a while I thought I'd better do a test, but then I decided "No, let's leave it a week". I didn't tell my husband at first, I was acting a bit peculiar and he asked me if I was all right. It was funny because it must have been the first time I'd said "No, I'm not!"

Nine Women, Nine Months, Nine Lives

[Laughs] I reckon he thought I'd got backache or a headache from work! [Laughs] So I sat down and said "Look I think I might be pregnant"... Well! [Laughs] And then because he manages a pharmacy, he went back to work and got a test. Rushed back home, I wee-ed in the pot, and he looked and said it was positive and he was like "Oh wow!" Really happy! [Laughs] And then he had to 'phone everybody, he was thrilled!
That's nice.
Yeah, so, it did come as a little bit of a shock, but it was a nice shock.
So, why didn't you want to do the test? You said that you felt pregnant...
Yeah, I think it's, it's the unknown. I mean you hear about it don't you, "Gosh my life has changed". I just thought "Oh my God" because I was really into my job and we had plans, like redecorating the house and that, but then you just think "Uh-oh" and then time just stops there you know. Errm... Have I answered the question?
[Laughs] Yeah, yeah, you've answered the question! You've answered a couple more actually!
[Laughs] Oops, sorry!
So can you remember what actually went through your mind when Yusuf told you? Quite often the girls I have spoken to do the test themselves, see the two blue lines, but you obviously didn't look at it.
No, no.
What do you think your reaction was? What was the first thing that went through your mind?
I was really happy, more than anything because I'd always thought I would never have children.
Why?!
Well because... [Whispered] We never used anything from when we were married and it just never happened, so... [Normal voice] I did want children but had gradually come to think that if this was the way it was going to be... If I'd pinned my hopes on it and then never been able to have any, that would have been devastating so... And his side of the family's a bit, well the generation would have stopped there with him because his sister can't have babies, his other sister's got a girl, she's nine years old now but she's split from her husband, she's divorced so you know, for him to, well...
So what was his reaction?
Oh! He was, he was jumping around, he was so happy. He loves children, and he's good with them. He had his doubts whether he would be able to cope, but he's really good with Ayesha. I think we both couldn't wait to tell my mum! [Laughs] She always used to go "When are you going to have children?" So he 'phoned her up and said "She's pregnant!" [Laughs]
Yeah? OK, the next part is your experience of pregnancy and the birth. Had you imagined how pregnancy would feel before you got pregnant? Had you wondered how it would actually feel to be pregnant?
I always loved children, but to think you will have children of your own one-day is a bit

Ameena

"Oooooo"... [Scared face] You know you play with other peoples kids and then you hand them straight back at the end of the day, but with your's you can't, they're like there all the time, 24 hours a day! [Laughs]
So had you imagined how you would feel, you may not have done?
No, no, I don't think I had thought about it.
When you were still in the early stages of pregnancy, say at about 6 weeks, did you then start wondering what pregnancy would be like?
The only thing I was worried about was the pain [Laughs] the labour pain! Not one... I mean I was happy because you know you don't get your periods when you are pregnant! [Laughs] I never really stopped to think about it.
You didn't find yourself thinking "Well I'm OK at the moment, but maybe when I get more heavily pregnant...?"
To be honest, no, no I don't think so. The only thing that worried me was the clothes, I couldn't get into any of my clothes! [Laughs] You know, after about 7 months, yeah 7 months, I just found myself wearing the same old jeans the same old top, day in, day out.
So you didn't go out and buy anything else apart from those clothes?
I did initially, but towards the end, I mean I just started with larger clothes anyway when I bought some earlier on. You know when you're about three or four months pregnant, you think "Oh these will last" but I didn't realise how big I was going to get at 12 weeks. And I didn't want to waste any more money, because I did spend quite a bit initially, so I'd got a small wardrobe by the end!
Yeah, yeah! So your actual experiences. Would you say they were very different from the little bits you had thought about?
The main difficulty I had was that I couldn't asleep. I'm not, I didn't know whether it was to do with, whether it was because I was uncomfortable or whether it was just... because towards the end I was getting really stressed out. By seven months I was just getting really <u>really</u> stressed out. I kept thinking "I bet I have to be induced everybody else has been induced" and I was induced, so maybe I should have not got...![Laughs] But errm... I couldn't sleep, and I suffered a lot of leg cramps, they were really bad, horrible.
Right, what did you expect would happen at the birth? You've already mentioned that you had some concerns about the pain side of things. Had you read up about the birth?
I didn't think about it before I attended the workshops [Preparing for Parenthood and Parentcraft] and errm... It did show the actual birth and pain control, water birth, basically how to manage the pain in your back and, but, you don't really know what to expect until you have been through it. So, I think when I was about nine months yeah, I started worrying about the pain. Throughout I had but after nine months it got worse. And I thought "Oh no, how will I manage?"
So when it got closer?
Yeah, closer. But towards the end, because she was late as well, I couldn't care less

about the pain, I thought I just want to, to have the baby, get it over and done with! So I wasn't really too much bothered about the pain in the end. And it's really strange to say that because my mum had said to me "You'll be all right" but they were all thinking "She's not going to be able to do it". They said "I'll bet she'll have to have an epidural" but [Laughs] luckily I didn't... I'm quite crap so! [Laughs] I mean the minute we got into the delivery suite, Yusuf was like "Quick, quick, where's the nurse? Who do we talk to for an epidural?" And I was like "Yusuf, hang on a minute!" [Indignant] And he just looked surprised. I think he felt sorry for me more than anything! I think he thought "Oh she has to go through all that pain!" he just wanted me to have the epidural. I didn't, I wanted to do it, I wanted to prove it to him! [Laughs]
What do you mean prove it to him?
That I can do it without the pain, the painkillers.
So was the pain really bad then?
The pain was bad, but, to be honest, I don't remember it now. But I know at the time it was bad.
Errm... And you said earlier that you expected the birth to be really bad, was it as bad as you imagined it would be?
Somebody once told me that labour pain is ten times worse than period pain, and I had really bad period pains. I <u>always</u> suffered with period pains, always, for eight or nine days every month. Thinking back now I don't think, I think it's, it's... You can cope with it, you can do things, breathing exercises helped. No, no I think it wasn't as bad as I had imagined. Having said that I, the only... It's not really a regret as it wasn't, but I didn't want to be induced. Other than that...
So were you a couple of weeks over then?
I was 14 days over so they had no choice but to induce me. That was my greatest fear.
Why were you so frightened? Did you know someone who had been induced before?
Yeah, my friend was induced. She said although she was induced she, the contractions weren't coming, so... I thought "God!" I wanted it all naturally, but the consultant said "You'll have to be induced" and I thought "Oh no". I remember I thought it was through the arm but... I didn't know they were going to do it down there! [Laughs] Oh gosh, that was so painful, that was more painful than giving birth itself! [Laughs]
Did they have to break the waters?
Yeah, yeah, errm... It took, I went into labour at about 10.30 in the morning, and I think it was 8.45pm by the time they'd actually manage to break my waters, I just couldn't, I couldn't cope with that stick! [Laughs] Oh God, it was so painful. That was the worst bit, the most appalling, the doctors and the midwives saying things like "You've got to have this baby today, if you don't then there will be problems." [Said in a stern and strict voice] So in the end they had to find the doctor to come and do it. I felt such an idiot!
Why?
Oh God! I think there were about six of them and one by one they came in and tried it

Ameena

but I couldn't let them do it. I thought "Oh no, it's so embarrassing, they are going to think I'm a right baby!"
Why?! Because you were scared?
Yeah. Because it's not a big thing. But it's not nice having you waters broken.
Yeah... How did you feel when you first held Ayesha? Did you hold her straight away?
I think Yusuf held her first, yeah, and then she came to me.
So, you had a straightforward vaginal delivery?
Yes, a straightforward delivery. I think it was five minutes, yeah after about five minutes I held her. But after the long labour, and with being induced, she was quite a heavy baby, I just could not carry her, I was so tired! [Laughs]
So how long were you in labour for?
The actual labour was only six and a half-hours but all the hanging around before they broke the waters...
Yeah, so she was born in the early hours of the morning?
Yeah, yeah she was.
So when you actually held her for the first time, that you can remember, how did you feel?
Wonderful! It was such a relief to have her out, but other than that I just felt so tired. And I always wanted, secretly I always wanted a girl. And I know in the Asian community it's always "Boys, boys, boys, boys, boys and I hate girls", you know, but gosh! I was so thrilled. I can't, I can't express myself I was so happy, <u>so</u> relieved! [Laughs]
So it was an intense high then really?
Yeah, yeah it was, definitely. But yeah, he held her first, and he was just, because she looked so much like him he was just... [puffs herself up with pride and laughs] Very chuffed, <u>very</u> chuffed "My girl!"
OK, and in what ways was Yusuf involved in the pregnancy? Did he help out round the house, listen to you, take an interest in how you were feeling?
Yes, he was quite, I think... He works long hours as well which was quite difficult, because he couldn't give me the attention, or the amount of attention that I'd have liked, but yes he was very supportive throughout the pregnancy. I've no complaints about that because before I became pregnant, he never used to lift a finger in the house, my mum used to get very upset about it. Because I used to do everything all he had to do was go to work, come back and that was his day, but he had to change. Especially when I was four or five months and you could see it. He must have thought "Oh gosh, Ameena really is pregnant!" When it was visible he was really supportive. I mean I used to have these, I used to have all these mad cravings and he used to run around getting them for me! [Laughs]
The birth, he was there throughout, was that what you had discussed beforehand?
Yeah.
That was what you expected to happen, what you both wanted? And was he quite

247

Nine Women, Nine Months, Nine Lives

supportive? Was he able to help you or did you kind of feel he was an extra?
Errm... Mixed feelings really, I mean I was really thrilled that he was there throughout. He had to hang around all day, take a day off work on the Friday and get something sorted out for the Saturday. He was there from 10 on the Friday until three in the morning on the Saturday. Before we actually went in to the hospital we had a good walk round the block, a good half-hour, and then we went to the hospital and he went to pray. He never normally goes on a Friday but that day he decided he had better get in front of God! [Laughs] So, he went to Friday prayers, and that was the only break he took away from the hospital, he came straight back and was there until maybe five or six on the Saturday morning. He was very good in there but I think he was very worried, I think he was more worried about anything and everything. I mean when they broke my waters, when they did break my waters, there was a gush of water and then quite a bit of blood. He stood there, and he just froze Sandra, he was like "Oh my God she's bleeding so much, I... Oh!" And he started panicking, and I thought "What?!" [Laughs] And I said "You can hardly see anything! What are you looking at?!" And then the doctor started laughing, and she goes "Oh love, this is nothing! You've got a lot to see still!" [Laughs] And literally, he was so worried, he started panicking, but he'd been fine until the moment before, until we actually got in there and got going with the labour and the delivery. He was really worried! He ran off to see the nurse or midwife to say "I want my wife to have an epidural!" Luckily, I shouldn't really say this but, they were short staffed and to have an epidural you need to be under constant supervision, so when the... I forget the name of the doctor who sets the epidural up, is it the anaethetist? When they walked in he said "I'm afraid we can't" Yusuf's face just dropped and mine lit up! "Oh wonderful!" I thought "Oh I'm so pleased!" I mean you do hear a lot of horror stories about the epidural don't you? I mean, even then I wanted everything natural, to be induced was bad enough, but I was like "If you think I'm going to have an epidural you've got another thing coming!" So I was really pleased, and I'm glad I didn't because, well, you <u>can</u> do it! [Laughs] It's not as bad as they make it out to be! I mean I'd do it again! The pain is really bad Sandra but, at the end of it you have well, I'm sorry... [Getting a bit emotional] I'm sorry.
No I hear this kind of thing nearly everyday, and I hear a mixture of...
You don't get bored about it?
No, no! Because everybody is different, everybody's perception of... Everyone's starting point is different, you know? Some people manage pain, some people don't manage pain, some people are worried about not doing it naturally, some people say "I wanted as much drugs as possible" and you know, the way things work out is different again, so you get all of the different combinations of experiences.
I can't manage pain.
No?
Even if it's a headache, the whole world will hear about it! I used to have really bad period pains – I would take time off school, take time off work, and I'd just sit there on

Ameena

the couch with my hot water bottle and loads of cuddly blankets and soft toys and just weep with pain. I just couldn't manage it. But, the labour pains, such a powerful pain, but it was, it was an enjoyable pain. I don't know whether it's psychological, that you can see that at the end of all this that... I mean it's going to be over soon, and at the end of it you get a lovely baby.
So you felt like you were working towards something? Something that was worthwhile?
Yeah, yes, yes, exactly! You're working towards something. I quite enjoyed the pain [sounds surprised] it sounds a bit daft but...
Would you say that you actually enjoyed the pain itself, or what the pain was leading you towards?
I actually enjoyed the pain. It sounds really stupid but, I, I saw it as a challenge. People always say it's bad. Mum used to say "Don't worry about it, but yeah, it's really bad". Until I had actually experienced the pain I was terrified, but I did, I liked it! You must think I'm mad! [Laughs] Yeah, yeah I enjoyed it!
Yeah, well that is unusual I must say, but if that's how you feel then... [Laughs]
Following on from that - I can take pain now! [Laughs]
Really?
Yeah, I stay away from paracetamol and all of that.
Have your periods been as painful or not?
No! It's really better, I don't get, I mean that's not to say that I don't get pains at all because I do, but it's not as bad as it used to be. And I suffer with back pains everyday, and I stay away from paracetamol and that so...
OK, So would you say that your partners support in pregnancy was more or less than you had hoped for?
A bit more, a tiny bit more.
In what ways, emotionally more? Or practically more?
Practically a lot more, and emotionally more. He was brilliant.
And during the birth, would you say that his support for you, emotionally and practically, was that more or less than you had hoped for?
Thinking about emotional support during the birth?
He may not have been able to give you any emotional support or practical support during the birth...?
He was quite comforting but... My mum was there doing that. I didn't want my mum there, he thought it would be a good idea in case I wasn't able to cope. He was worried that "Gosh what if he..." He was worried that he would faint and he thought "God I can't cope!" He was more worried about himself, not being supportive towards me so, my mum was there. She was the main one, if she hadn't been there I wouldn't have been able to do it. He was very comforting very supportive, he was doing the things she was doing as well, and if I didn't decide to have him there next time I would definitely take my mum! [Laughs] And I'd say to Yusuf "Don't worry about it, you don't have to be there, don't worry about it, go to work and I'll let you know when it arrives!"

249

Nine Women, Nine Months, Nine Lives

Yeah?! [Laughs]
But my mum, she was brilliant. You know it's funny, I thought it would be the other way around. I thought he would be rubbing my back and saying "Don't worry darling everything is going to be OK", he was just, well he was just not up for that!
Well, at least you did have a contingency plan, just in case. At least he'd planned for if he couldn't be there. And practically, do you think he was more or less supportive at the birth?
Practically he was... What do you mean though?
Well, things like rubbing your back, helping you with the breathing...
OK, well, he was there, but because my mum was just basically taking over, in a nice way, she was a great comfort, doing all of these things she gave me a lot of confidence and support. I don't think Yusuf felt the need to do all those things, but emotionally he was great.
OK, errm... Right the next chunk is your experience of early motherhood. So the first few days, weeks, the first few months. So, that's what I would like you to think back to. How did your pregnancy effect early motherhood? Perhaps the fact that you were overdue, you had water retention, and must have been tired, did that carry on over into those first few months?
After the birth, the back pains did carry on, the water retention that was fine that went quickly. But the nurse, who was a student I think, did my stitches and I didn't know to... I was washing my stitches in warm water, you should use cold water. Because I did this quite often, I was making it sore and oh God! That was the worst bit, those stitches, I couldn't walk. I had internal and external stitches because she tore me and the actual tear went the other way. The actual stitching wasn't too bad but after that, oh God! I was in agony, and what I did was silly... I couldn't bring myself to go to the loo, you know, and then I couldn't go so, oh it was just so painful! I'll never forget that! [Laughs]
So was that one of your fears then, that the stitches would perhaps come out?
Oh yes, that was my greatest fear of all. That I would go to the loo, and the stitches would come out and I would have to go through it all over again!
So did you go to the doctor's and get something for constipation or did it just sort itself out?
No, my midwife, she said just eat, she actually advised me to drink a lot, a lot, a lot of orange juice, which I did. I went through gallons and gallons and gallons of it! And she said "Let me tell you girl when the urge is there, you will, you will go, because nobody will be able to stop you!"[Laughs] But when the urge was there I just panicked! And you know when you tense yourself up, you then don't want to go. That went on for a good four days, four or five days, and they say the sooner you can go the better...
Yes, yes.
And breastfeeding as well, you lose a lot of water. And the, you get much more constipated so, so that was a horrible experience! [Laughs] But when I did go it was

Ameena

such a relief. But I think that was the worst bit, definitely.
So yeah, the next question was how did the birth effect early motherhood, you've already mentioned the stitches, was there anything else that you can think of from the birth that carried over into the first few weeks?
I think mainly it was the stitches.
The stitches, right. Errm... During your pregnancy did you imagine how motherhood would be for you? Did you imagine what your life would be like, how Ayesha would be?
Hmmm, I don't know...
I mean even if it was just tiny little, something very small.
Yeah, I mean every week-end we used to go shopping, looking for things for the baby, every week-end, week in week out, clothes, nappies, furniture!... I can't really remember! So when I was pregnant, did I ever imagine being a mum?
Yes.
Hmmm, I can't say that I did. I suppose I did...
Did you imagine, well do you think there is a difference between the things that you had imagined, and the things that have been a shock or a surprise? Because that would imply that you had an idea of it, even though you may not have sat down and consciously thought about it.
I don't, I mean I don't think, I probably did but I can't remember whether I had thought how I would feel. Ayesha used to give us lots of sleepless nights, she used to cry and cry and cry a lot, and then she got into a pattern whereby she would sleep for two and a half hours at a time and during those two and a half hours I used to be trying to do everything, and oh!
Oh yes, I remember now, when I saw you before...
I remember being so exhausted. I suppose when you are , you are pregnant, everything is hunky-dory, everything is flowery and happy, the sun is shining, you picture a scene where the grass is green. And then you have them and she has eczema and asthma and then it is a totally different story.
So would you say the first three months have been different from what you'd expected?
Yeah, I was really tired. I mean I remember being, I mean I'm always tired now, always needing to sleep, can't sleep but want to sleep. The house was always a tip...
Oh good Lord!
Yeah but the things like that, But (a) I don't have the energy, (b) I don't have the time and, I didn't, she's ever so ever so demanding during the day, and at night. That's one of the reasons why I've decided to go back to work full-time, so that I can get even more of a break from her! [Laughs] because I'm like, she's not up, physically up most of the night, but she is awake, you can hear her being awake and well her back is quite sore [she has bad baby eczema] so she's not comfortable. I went to see the doctor and he suggested I took her to see a specialist and she was to have some medication. It helped, but I can't afford to keep going back and forward to it. And then some nights you think "Ooohhhh!" and you just get so fed up. And Yusuf can't feed her so I'm there

Nine Women, Nine Months, Nine Lives

doing it. It just gets so much that you just want to dump her in the cot. And when she falls off to, when she does finally fall to sleep, you put her in the cot, and then in the next minute or minute or two, you think "Oh maybe she'll be all right". But then she's up again because she doesn't want to be in the cot. I sometimes think, you know how you just want to change something?
But if you're really tired, you know, maybe working...
I know working, it's hard being at home, with me working, she's a lot closer to my mum than she is with me [her mum looks after Ayesha when Ameena is at work]. When I get back from work, she'll go running up to my mum. She won't, sometimes she will go running up to my mum like, she's so clingy with my mum that it's, I think it's a danger and... Oh I don't know I just think that's dangerous. I don't think she's bonded to me...
Well she looks perfectly settled with you, she looks bonded to me [baby is actually cuddling mum at the time]
Yeah, I know, but, well... She needs her bottom changing!
Oh I see, it's a type of cupboard love! [Laughs – baby goes to have her nappy changed] OK, errm... Oh yeah, we were talking about imagined motherhood, and whether it actually matched up to what you had sort of thought, and you hadn't really thought intensely what it would be about. You hadn't got many expectations, but there were one or two things that were a shock or a surprise. Like every two and a half-hours her waking up and not being able to sleep, and feeling so tired.
Yeah and another was the eczema. I mean you hear about dry skin, these days a lot of babies are suffering with that condition, but when Ayesha actually had that, I thought "But how? But why? Is it because I, is it something that I've done wrong or..." I don't know you just... I sort of went through a guilt trip. because I know initially that her skin was dry when she was born, but that was because she was late, she was overdue, and it was improving and it became very nice and soft. And after three months following the injection, I did, I did see her skin getting quite dry but, I carried on giving her a bath everyday, using baby powder, I used baby powder. I keep thinking in my mind that it was the baby powder that made her worse because of the talcum powder. I thought well maybe that if I'd just stopped using that...?
Well maybe, but you don't know. You won't know. How is her skin now?
A lot better.
She looks a lot better.
A lot better, I don't know if you remember, but when she was about six months old, it was just...
Oh yeah, I remember, because I'd popped round hadn't I? I'd come to drop something off....?
Yeah so when she was six months old it was really bad.
Yeah, and you'd been going down to London, once a week. Was it once a week?
Yeah, for the Chinese medicine. And I had a car accident, because of going to London, and it cost me so much. It was such a headache and a hassle. But I'm glad we did go

Ameena

to Africa because she was...
Oh of course you went on holiday there and her skin improved!
The sun and seawater did a lot. I did hear someone once say that if you stay up to I think it was three months it would probably cure it, it would just disappear. But oh I would love to! Financially... Oh you just can't. I mean we were there three weeks and it did her a hell of a lot of good, she was sleeping through the night as well, I couldn't believe it! [Laughs] And then when you come back it's three hours!
Yeah, but when you were there she was probably busy during the day, more active.
Yeah and the sun as well.
Yeah the sun does make you more sleepy.
And Yusuf's got a lot of family over there and she was just from here to there to here to there!
OK so what would you say was the most difficult thing in say the first four weeks? What can you remember that came as a real shock about motherhood?
Breastfeeding! [Laughs] I don't know, from day one when I became, when I knew I was pregnant, you're always asked by people, you know, am I going to breastfeed or am I not? Am I going to do this or am I not? So you just, what was I saying? Oh yeah, I did want to I was very positive about it and then gosh! It was so painful and she just wouldn't latch on, and my sister had no problems, her baby was six weeks older than Ayesha, she said no just, no pain at all it's just an enjoyable experience. Every time she would cry for a feed, I would cry because I would think "Oh no not again". But then I didn't want to bottle feed her, obviously because of, and especially when I heard that she's got eczema as well, it would probably be better for her immune system. So I thought no, I'm going to pursue it. I'm really glad I did. The doctors also gave me a pat on the back, and still are, because obviously it's helping her a lot with her immune system. And especially with the fact that she can't, well we suspect that she can't tolerate dairy products, so she... Well she's missing out already on cheese and milk and custard and yogurts, at least this way she is making up for it. But I put her on Soya milk, she doesn't like it, so she'll have three ounces a day mixed with a rusk for breakfast and that's it. And that's it. But three ounces a day for a growing baby is not enough. I mean I am so glad that I am still feeding her.
Yeah, yeah, but like you say, you're putting it on the rusk and that, you know you have to be a bit more imaginative. If she can't taste the flavour, I think you're doing really well, to see if you can try and get the milk in some how. I mean have you tried whipping it up into a mouse or something like that? Like with a Multipractic, adding some I don't know some pureed banana or something like that?
Errm...
You know, if you take something that she really likes and mix it with the Soya milk...
You mean make the Soya milk less or more...?
Yeah put some bananas in it and liquidise it.
OK, yeah, And I can put other things in too!

253

Nine Women, Nine Months, Nine Lives

Even if you end up watering it down a bit, at least you know, it's getting into her system. You know, when you're going to work you don't stop and think about it! [Laughs]
No, of course you don't.
But I'm glad you've mentioned that, I'll do that, see what happens.
Yeah, you can try it, I mean she may spit it straight back at you but...! [Laughs]
But she likes bananas so that might work.
Yeah see what she does, she may not like it, she might.
She likes Soya yogurts.
Does she?
Yeah, obviously it's really sweet and...
Well maybe just add a little sugar to it, you know warm it up, add some sugar, cool it down and then...
But you know how sugar is not very good for teething babies?
Yes, yeah. Well that's why I thought of fruit really. You could get some fructose stuff as well, but it depends whether she likes it or not. But if you know she likes something, and you can actually combine it with that, and she will eat it then, give it a whirl...
Because I always think she is missing out on the dairy and cow stuff.
Yeah, for now. She may get more tolerant of it as she gets older.
Yeah, I suspect she will, because I've just recently started giving her, cheesy stuff, and she's taken to it.
Well she might like the flavour, yeah.
Do you think she's quite tiny for a one-year-old?
Tiny?!
Yeah tiny?
No, she's dinky, petite, she's not, she's, height wise she is about average I'd say. She's not, you see some babies that are very big build, and you see some babies that are very dinky.
You see that's what I always imagined.
No, I mean everybody's different. Well look at all of us [me Ameena and her sister-in-law] all three of us are all differently built, aren't we? So you know...
Yeah, yeah, I always think and Yusuf does as well. We sit there saying "Oh God isn't she small?"
She's not small, no!
[Laughs] We always think that!
I mean when you go to the doctors, you're bound to see other 12 month olds, like if you go to mother an baby or mother and toddler or something, the amount of variation is the same as it is with anybody else at any age. And she's perfectly happy, she's healthy...
I think it's because you always imagine babies are going to be all cuddly and chubby! [Laughs]
She is cuddly! Yeah, but you do have to remember that babies can be overweight as well, you know that's one thing you should always... I mean people don't really think that babies can be overweight but they can be, and to be overweight at such a young age puts

254

Ameena

such a strain on their frame as well, particularly when she's starting to walk about. It would take her a lot longer to become that mobile if she was carrying extra weight, and it doesn't do their bones any good, they're still relatively soft at this age.
A bit of positive thinking, yeah.
Yeah, so, yeah she's all right, she's fine!
It's little things like that that you sit there thinking about and worrying about.
But you know if you ever do get worried about that then talk to your health visitor, or go to your GP. They will be quite happy to give you an honest answer. If they think that there is something wrong they would be more likely to tell you than to wait for you to ask.
Yeah, that's true.
OK, and what was the best thing in those first four weeks, the first month?
The best thing was after all that pain was "Oh I've got such a lovely baby to hold and cuddle and pamper and dress up" you know with her being a girl, I've got all these frilly frilly things. Just holding her, it's just so peaceful, such a pleasure. Because you think, I've been through nine months of carrying and the birth and the initial teething problems up to three months, the stitches and the pain, when you've got your child you think "Wow!" When you look in their eyes, you think "Oh she's got my eyes, oh she's got daddy's hair and oh" it's such a pleasure, <u>such</u> a pleasure.
And how much was Yusuf involved in the early days, those first few weeks? You say that you went in on the Friday to be induced, and you had her early morning on the Saturday. You said that Yusuf was off at the weekend, was he back at work straightaway on the Monday? because you went to stay at your mum's didn't you?
Yeah, I did go and stay at my mum's. He was very, obviously, you know, first time proud dad and he wants to be with her as much as I do, so he actually moved in with them as well! Because I think that the two nights that he spent here and he couldn't sleep, tossing and turning, missing Ayesha, so he moved in as well for two weeks. I think he took about four days off in total. But then the nature of the work he's in, he couldn't take more. But he used to look forward to the weekends, and the bank holidays, it'd be "Ooh time to play with Ayesha!" [Laughs] Yeah.
OK, and so was he involved in sort of like, errm... Changing her and things like that, night feeds?
No, he always saw that as a mother's role! [Laughs]
Right. So had you talked about who would do what?
Yes, no we hadn't talked as in the sense, I mean I always used to tell him "Look, whether it's a boy or a girl you have to get involved in nappy changing, giving the baby baths, pushing the push chair". Simple things like that, if she needs feeding you know, but he never has! [Laughs] He never has got involved in any of that! Only recently he has started, when, when I'm giving her a bath he'll join in and splash water at her and bring her toys. But, I think he's only ever had to change a nappy once when I had to go out, and I left her with him and she... I think it, no she didn't pooh otherwise he would

255

Nine Women, Nine Months, Nine Lives

have had to do it, it was something he tried, he thought "Right let me give it a go!" But ever since he's never changed a nappy. In the whole year only once! [Laughs]
Yeah, so he hasn't really done anything practical?
Yes, yeah.
So you had talked about it, and you had basically said that you would need him to help. So things like feeding, like at night, had you talked about that as being something you'd need him to help you with?
Yes, I mean he'll stay awake , like if she's up and at week-ends he'll say "Oh it's OK, you rest I'll take her downstairs and play with her."
OK so, that obviously didn't work out. You've ended up doing the majority, the lions share of the work, errm... Would you say that was something you had discussed and said "Look it's easier for me to do it" or did it just happen?
It just happened.
Do you think it was a kind of natural division of labour that it worked out like that?
Yeah.
Do you think that was primarily because you were at home or, perhaps you feel more able to do it and Yusuf doesn't?
Errm... A bit of both really because I spend, I mean I took unpaid leave so I was off work for about 10 months, so I didn't feel I could turn round to him and say "Right Yusuf, the next nappy change is yours". I just got on with it really.
And was that OK? Or did you start to resent it towards the end?
No, it wasn't a problem.
So you didn't feel let down? That's all I'm really saying, that you discussed it would be one way, and it was actually different...
Yeah. So I mean we did discuss it and that was before Ayesha was born, he used to say "Oh don't worry we'll share everything out and I'm going to be a Dad as well" and I think at that stage, at that point in time they look forward to it. They think "Oh wow!" you know, and then when the little one does arrive, it's such a shock to their system. It is quite tiring, it is a huge responsibility, and then working full-time 9 to 7. I mean, I mean personally, I don't mind changing her feeding her and giving her a bath, so... It doesn't really bother me if he doesn't change a nappy or...
So he sees her in the evenings then when he gets home from work?
Oh yeah, she's the first thing he'll look for when he gets in! He'll open the door "Ayesha?!" [Laughs] It's not me any more! [Laughs] Not "Oh where's my lovely wife?!" [Laughs]
No, it's "Oh where's my lovely daughter?!" Now! [Laughs]
Yeah, he always says "Oh she's going to be daddy's girl" and then I always say "She's going to be...?"
OK so would you say that on the whole that worked out for the better or for the worse? On reflection...?
For the better.

Ameena

Yeah, for the better. Because if you enjoy doing those kind of things, and you're quite happy to do them...
I'm quite happy, but I do still nag him, you know put him through that guilt trip saying "Well you never did change her nappy!"
Well you know, it wouldn't really do him any harm to do things like that because you know... If you weren't around for any period of time, I mean God forbid of you were ill or something like that, your mum might not necessarily be able to be there for Ayesha.
Yeah, but I think that he does understand that if that were the case then he would have to pull his socks up and get on.
So he'd be capable of doing it?
Oh yeah definitely.
But at the moment it's just not the way that you work?
Yeah, he just thinks "Oh Ameena is there, if I don't do it she's going to. The baby's not going to be left there". He does recognise his responsibilities, but he... [Laughs]
OK, the next chunk is your experience of motherhood, up until the present day. OK? So... very nearly a certain young lady's first birthday. How do you think your life has changed since you have had Ayesha?
A lot, a considerable, considerably, too much! [Laughs] Sometimes I think "What?!" you just turn around and think "What?!" Yeah it's changed a lot, especially now that I've started working again, I mean, physically I'm there but mentally I'm still with Ayesha. Errm...
Is it very recent that you've been back at work?
Yeah, about two and a half months. Errm... I enjoy being at work but as I say my mind is always with her. Is she OK? I wonder if she's had anything to eat and...
She stays with your mum?
Yeah, she stays with my mum. And my mums brilliant, she runs around after her, I mean when she's exercising this one is giggling, they, they just get on like a house on fire. So in that respect, that's not the reason why I worry. But if I did have to leave her with a child minder I would never have gone back to work. But because mum's there and she's babysitting for me, she's happy with that arrangement, this one's happy so no qualms about that. But, it's like, well, am I losing out? Errm... When I'm 60 years old, old and grey sitting there on my rocking chair, will I be...?
Looking after your granddaughter?!
Yeah, hopefully! [Laughs] Will I be sitting there thinking "What did I miss out on and I shouldn't have gone back to work and why did I go back?" Will I be sitting there regretting... so that's that's my only...
So that's something that you think about?
I mean I still do, I have decided to go, mainly because I have to go back. Not financially, not because my husband is telling me to, but partly because I do want to go back full time.
So are you back part-time at the moment?

Nine Women, Nine Months, Nine Lives

Yes, I'm back part-time.
Is it afternoons?
I was doing five mornings, but recently I've changed my hours to three full days. I don't know whether to increase it by one extra day or just go back for the full week. But then, I do want to, but then, part of me is saying I'm already leaving her for two days and I feel as if I'm missing out so what's going to happen when I only have week-ends with her? Especially with the fact I was explaining earlier that I feel that she's bonding with my, well that she loves my mum more than she loves me, and obviously that's not the case, but, it's a dilemma.
Mmm, a bit of a quandary really. What do you think you'll do?
I think I'll end up going back full time.
Is that what you want? You don't look like that's what you want...
No, 75 per cent of me wants to and...
Why do you want to? Do you think it would be good for you or errm... It's something that you...?
It would be easier for me because working part-time it's very demanding, the role is very demanding, and it's very difficult to... You start a piece of work, you've got to leave it for four days and then go back to it on Monday morning when there are that many more messages and you...
Did you feel like you are doing the same amount of work that you used to do but in less time?
I'm doing the same amount of work, yeah, that's my main problem.
And your time is now more precious?
Yeah, more precious, a lot more precious.
So maybe you went back an extra day, say four days that might be a balance between having more time to do the work in, less time away from the work, more time with Ayesha and it would be quality time you think?
Yeah, that's exactly what Yusuf said to me yesterday. because we only just discussed this yesterday and my manager wants to know by Monday what my decision is.
Perhaps it would be better if you start yourself off lower and work your way up? Is that a possibility, I don't know if your employer would be that understanding?
I haven't put it across to them but I will certainly suggest it, I mean he keeps saying "Just stick to part time" but he doesn't understand there's a lot of pressure at the moment, and mentally I can't cope part-time, to be honest, because of the work load. And I'm doing, as you said, a full weeks work in three days, and it just gets too much. I mean today when I woke up I thought "Tut! I could have been sat in the office I could have got that done, I could have got this done. I've had to leave it for four days and go back to it on Monday, oh!" [Laughs] But that's what we've discussed whether I can work the Thursday and then have the Friday off, if my boss says "Yes!" then that will be brilliant. Errm... I'm not doing it for the money, well partly yeah because then Ayesha can have a nice life and I can buy her all the things that I want to. But I want to continue working,

Ameena

I don't want to lose my skills and my confidence.
It's the social side too?
Yeah, I want to get on with the rest of my life, with my life rather! [Laughs]
Well, yeah, yeah, I know what you mean!
And then you think, all right OK, let's have another baby! [Laughs] And you go back again. It's not easy.
OK? So your life has changed considerably?
Yes.
OK, and how do you think you have changed since you have had Ayesha? That can be good and bad changes, permanent and temporary.
I like that question! I think I've changed a lot. I mean we were just saying yesterday. Errm... I was saying to Yusuf's sister yesterday that, that gosh yeah I used to buy this and that for myself and walk down to the shops and say "Oh I like those trousers" and I'd pick them up and pay for them but I can't do that anymore. Not that, it's not that I haven't got the money, it's that I won't do that anymore, it's like "Lets go into Mothercare and get Ayesha a nice dress" instead! So in that respect I've changed, so it's altered my responsibilities. I think she's frustrated as well because she wants to be at my mums. In the morning when she gets up, she'll be like "Nanny nanny nanny!"
So she has quite a routine there as well?
Yeah, so I mean it's a sudden change for her and I don't think she enjoys being here.
It's a little disruptive perhaps, maybe, yeah.
Because my brothers are always in and out, [at her mum's] my brothers friends are always coming in and out and mum and dad are always out and...
So it's quite a social kind of thing as well.
Yeah, and it's so quiet here when she's like this, so...
OK right, so getting back to how you think you've changed, since you've had Ayesha.
I've become more responsible, I think I've matured that little bit more.
Do you think those are permanent changes?
I think so, yeah. Initially, straight after the birth I lost a lot of confidence, but I'm beginning to rebuild on that, regain confidence. I mean I used to sit there and cry, but now I get in the car and go. So that was a temporary change, I feel better now I'm building on that again. Errm... I've changed in the sense that I worry a lot more now. I get really stressed out.
Really? In general or specific?
In general, but I worry more because Yusuf's not, not keeping very well. He's been having a lot of back pain and the pains been travelling to the front, and he's recently had a full medical which has indicated that he's got a high liver enzyme. And of course then he starts thinking "My liver's going to pack in!" [Laughs] And err... I worry a lot about that, I worry about Ayesha, I worry a lot these days. Sometimes I just sit there worrying over nothing, but I worry. [Laughs] So I have become a big worrier, and that's become a big worry in itself! [Laughs] I get really stressed out, I never used to.

Nine Women, Nine Months, Nine Lives

You have a short fuse do you think?
Yeah, I think that's partly due to, because I'm always tired, I'm always feeling lethargic, I just want to sleep, but I can't sleep. Even when my mum says "Right I'll have Ayesha for three or four hours – you go to sleep." I go "Right, brilliant, brilliant idea" and then I go up and get into bed and I can't sleep! I think because I am so used to being awake now, especially when she was suffering with her eczema, I couldn't sleep, didn't sleep and I could cope with it. But I think it's bottled up, bottled up, and it's at that stage now where even if I do want to sleep, I'm really desperately tired, I can't, and that ends up in frustration losing my temper, eating chocolates, having a binge! [Laughs] That, that's changed, I'm always, I'm always looking at the time.
Yeah?
Just yesterday I was thinking about it. Get into work, only just got there, I'm just so conscious of the time now, I think it's so that I can get back home, I'm thinking "I've got to do this, I've got to do that, what time is it, gosh!" There are just so many things to do.
So there is this pressure with time, that you haven't got enough of it?
Yeah, I have not got enough time. I wish I could, I wish I could, clock, I wish I could stretch the clock! [Laughs] Not enough time to do all the things that I want to do.
Mmm, so what would you include in 'all the things' that you want to do?
I don't have time for myself anymore. I don't, I like going out, I like seeing friends, specially my friends who, and it's soo long... I haven't seen Claire, she's always ringing me, she's always knocking on the door, and she's stopped doing that because, I, I don't...
You don't reciprocate, you don't feel like you've got the time?
No! I haven't got the time. You know people say things like "Maybe you have got the time but you're abusing it, you're miss managing the time", but, I know, sometimes I think "Yeah all right OK, if I do five minutes less of this, I can have five minutes more to do this" but I know that I haven't got the time. And I, that's a worry because I've only got one! And I'm already stressed out! [Laughs] And Yusuf wants to have more babies, one more, and I'm thinking "Gosh! If I can't cope with everything with one I don't know how I'm going to do it with another one!" So, that's been a change.
I mean, have you talked to Yusuf about this? About you feeling you don't have enough time to do everything?
Yeah I have, and he always says "Look, get yourself a cleaner, get somebody who will come in and do the ironing" just, just to... Not yesterday but the day before, I was saying that "Look I need to let them know whether I'm going to go back full-time, staying part time, what my hours..." And he kept saying "If you want to go back full-time" because I kept saying " I want to go back, I want to go back" without explaining to him why. And he said "All right then, do go back, but, I don't want you to get stressed out with the housework, with the cooking, with the this with the that, you know. because we can always get a take away three or four times a week, that's not a

260

Ameena

problem, get somebody in to do your ironing for you, employ a cleaner, because you can't do everything by yourself". So he's very supportive in that respect, but I want to do everything. Why should I have to employ a cleaner to clean my home? Why can't I do it?

Would you rather worry and do the cleaning? Or would you rather let somebody else do it and have time to spend on yourself?

Option (a). That is me... That's something that I need to change.

If you have a cleaner in once a week, you know that you are going to end up doing the cleaning again at some point in that week don't you? So you could actually manage to have the best of both worlds. Whereby you have somebody who comes in and does the nitty gritty, you know get everything spotless, and then you can do a quick sweep round in the week. And you still feel like you are taking care of your family, and you'll still feel like you are doing the best for Ayesha and, having an input into the home, you know, whilst you are at work. Because if you go back to work another two days a week, or even just another one day a week, that's a big chunk of time that you've already moved. You know, and you say you haven't got enough time now?

Even now when I'm only working three days a week, but I still...

Three days is a lot Ameena, it's not "only"

Yeah.

It is a lot.

You see I always put myself down, why should I say I'm only a part-timer, or I only work three days a week?

You are a full-time mother, and you work part-time, that's a ten-day week!

Yeah, sometimes it's, it's, yeah... I don't know, maybe I need to change my way of thinking a little bit. Well even now, working three days a week, and I've got two extra days, I've got the weekend. But I'm still like mopping the floor at eleven o'clock at night and I'm still dashing clothes into the washing machine at nine o'clock in the evening, so...

Yeah, but why?

Do you see what I mean? [Laughs] Yeah and then when I'm working, well hopefully when I do go back full time, I'll probably be sat here hoovering at three in the morning! [Laughs]

Well that's not going to do you any good, it's not going to do you and Yusuf any good, and it won't do Ayesha any good.

Yeah, yeah, I need to change.

Well it's not so much that you need to change. You need to sit down and think about what things are important to you, and kind of rank them for what is the most important thing for now. It's like you say, when you are 60 and you look back, would you rather look back and think I had a clean and tidy house and went to work full-time and I saw my daughter on the week-ends and she ran towards her nanny and not towards me. Or would you rather say, I worked part time and thought stuff the house and the cleaning,

261

Nine Women, Nine Months, Nine Lives

we had take-aways, we had a good life, we enjoyed the weekends because we spent time together as a family. You know, you've got to look at the extremes of the situation, yeah, you won't get to one or other of the extremes but you've got to work out where the in between is that will work best for you. And if you try one thing and it doesn't work, try another, try it slightly differently. It's like what I was saying about, it doesn't have to be all or nothing with work, it doesn't have to be, 50 per cent of the time or a hundred per cent. You know, you can get the 75 per cent, you can do the four days, if your employers are willing then obviously you know, they will get the best of you. Because you then feel more able mentally to concentrate on your job because you know that in the three days that you are away from work, you won't be thinking "If I were there now I could be doing this or I if I was there I could have done that". And that way you won't be resenting either not being at work and being at home, or not being at home and being at work. But I mean it won't, it won't solve itself. And you are thinking about it, which is a good thing.
Yeah.
So the best thing you can do is sit down and think about it. For yourself. You'll know what feels right, you'll know what you want to do, and that's, if that's what you want it can't be that bad.
I need to, there's a lot that I need to sort out.
It's just a matter of re-evaluating. And if you shift things round, you know, like I say, if it doesn't work maybe go back to what worked before. Change one bit not all of it, try going back to work four days a week and getting someone in to do the ironing.
Yeah.
If you like doing the cleaning, and you feel like that's what you want to do, do it. You don't have to have a cleaner. But if you're not particularly fond of ironing then Christ! Get it sent out.
[Laughs] I think I'm not getting my priorities right.
I don't think you know what your priorities are...
Well, yeah.
You've only been back at work two and a half months, you know, everything is still new. It's new for you and it's new for Ayesha, so... So you've changed in the past year, and you are going to continue to change.
I'm changing now! [Laughs]
Yeah, of course!
I think sometimes you have to change, sometimes you don't want to but you have to.
So would you say that in this last year there has been some changes that you haven't felt you wanted to or didn't expect you would have to make? Do you think there has been any that would fall into that kind of category?
Errm... Probably, there must be something, I just can't think of it.
Yeah, probably, I mean I know that in my own life there has been, you know, I couldn't tell you exactly what but there's, but you know you always go through life having to make

262

Ameena

certain compromises. When they are sacrifices, then that's a little bit more difficult to deal with because you may feel a little more reluctant about what is involved, but if there's a compromise, then that's life, that's the way it goes.
I think it's going to be a continual thing. I mean as kids grow up, things change, demanding. because these days it's not easy to bring them up, like the way we were brought up.
Yeah exactly, from one generation to the next it's very different. OK, so you've gone back to work, would you say that you've managed it? Would you say that you feel happy about being back at work? No matter how much time that you spend at work or not spend at work or that you see that that situation is going to change in the near future, do you think you've managed it?
I think I've managed it. I think I've managed it well. It, it's difficult when you've spent what nearly ten months at home, just me and her and the four walls! [Laughs] And my mum and her four walls! [Laughs] To suddenly go back to people, it's a big shock.
Yeah?
Yeah, it's a hell of a shock. You put up that façade, you put that façade on, don't you? You put a bit of make up on and power dress! [Laughs] And you turn up at nine o'clock on the dot. And now it's nine thirty! [Laughs] Errm... Yeah, it was a shock going back to work, but I think I've managed it well. I enjoy it, but I mean obviously there are days and sometimes you think "Oh a jobs a job" but you get on with it.
Yeah, everybody feels like that sometimes.
But yeah, I'm glad I'm back at work. Especially with her not letting me sleep at night, and Yusuf's always praising me, saying "You are brilliant, you are a good mum, you are a good wife, so you are good at work too, because you look forward to it everyday". I mean he goes "I don't know how you do it, if I wasn't sleeping well at night, all the nappies, and the washing and the house and the paperwork, and..."
You are still at work. You come home and you are still at work.
Yeah, exactly. But I'm glad, I'm really glad that Yusuf understands that, that he recognises the amount that I'm doing in the day. I think that's a bonus and I think that's what makes me feel proud of myself, I can say "Yeah, I'm a working mum!". But I won't say it's easy! [Laughs]
No, no. Do you think as Ayesha gets older, if you're going to go back four days a week, if Yusuf wasn't particularly keen on things like night feeds, I mean you'll stop breast feeding at some point in the future, and she's going to get a lot easier to cope with in terms of that she doesn't need physically so much, like nappies bathing things like that. Do you think Yusuf maybe could take his turn at putting her to bed maybe two nights a week? because then you're not working and then coming home and continuing to work?
Yeah, [sounds dubious] yeah.
I mean if you just came home and put your feet up for two hours and let him get on with it. Because you know he may find that he really enjoys that, you know.
I think if it came to the crunch, like now he knows the arrangement. Ameena works

263

Nine Women, Nine Months, Nine Lives

three days a week, she comes back she does a lot, dinners always on the table, the house is always clean, errm... Ayesha's always happy, and I've got nothing to complain about. He understands all that, he recognises that. But I think he has, the thought must have crossed his mind thinking "Gosh she's already doing a lot but she's got the two days and then she's got the week-end. She's sort of like catching up in the sense that she's got the time to rest, catch up on the rest, and catch up on the sleep. She can put her feet up on the Friday..."
Do you?
Not really.
There you go!
But he obviously thinks that you know "she's not working Thursday, Friday and you've got Saturday and Sunday. She you know, she's a lady of leisure!" [Laughs] But, I forgot what I was going to say.
Well maybe, you going back to work full-time or four days a week, maybe now is the time to sit down and say "Look, this part of my life is changing, I only have 24 hours in every day, I am tired now and I know my limitations". And if you haven't told him what your limitations are, like you say, you assume he must have thought that on Friday's you put your feet up, but you've just said to me, no you don't get time. So unless you tell him he can't know. So maybe now is a good time to sit down, whilst you are not actually at the point where you are at screaming pitch, when you are working four days a week and you are resenting the fact that you are coming home and playing catch up for three days. You know, not that hopefully a situation like that would ever arise, but you can't do any harm to sit down and talk about it in a calm way. And now she is that little bit older you know, she's going to need you physically less, for a start if you're not breast feeding she doesn't need you for that, so...
I mean I am hoping that things will get better, and errm... I've tried on many occasions to stop breastfeeding and it's not easy.
No of course it's not. But you know when the time comes, you will, I'm not saying that you should be doing it now, but it will happen, and that will be a natural thing whereby, there is more room in Ayesha's life for her father to come in and to do things like feeding her and that.
That's what, my friends have said to me. I'm sure that when I do stop, but then he works longer hours, and he can always argue that I come home from work physically, but home is working as well. But then his argument would be that when you get back at five, you don't need to do anything else, the time is yours!
Well let him try it!
Yeah, but...
And then see whether he still thinks you don't need to do anything else!
But then who's going to get the food ready?
Well you can work it out so that you get mum and dad's tea ready, and he does Ayesha. Or you do Ayesha when you get home from work, give her her tea, and then when he

Ameena

comes in at seven, quarter past half past whatever, then he gives, he then takes over from you. Baths her, puts her to bed, reads her a story, and you know, then you get a chance then. Even if it's just an hour, to sit down phone up a friend, sit in front of the telly, and glaze over – I mean wouldn't that be a wonderful?!
Yeah [Laughs] Sounds nice!
You'd be amazed, you really would be, that hour could be so precious, and he, you can never appreciate what somebody else does unless you've actually done it.
Yeah, true.
You know you can't, explain that to him, don't explain all the nitty gritty bits or he might not want to do it! [Laughter] But you know, give him, have the courage of your convictions, give it a go. And you know, he might actually realise that he has been missing out on something, wouldn't that be dreadful? And at least you'd found out early enough to do something, so, if you look at it from all ways...
So I wouldn't be doing nothing?
No, no, it's just you know I mean obviously if you...
So like sharing her care.
Exactly, yeah. I mean I only hope that when I have children that I can sit down and talk to somebody. Because when you are in the throws of doing something, I mean it's like me with work, in the throws of actually working it's very rare that I sit down, and, sit down and think " Oh I could've done that, and that would have been so much better than this! And if only I'd known about this wouldn't it have made my life easier!" and you know talking to somebody else about it, it just spurs you on.
Yeah, yeah.
Give it a whirl, see what happens! The worst thing that can happen is that you end up where you are now, and you are already here, and you are already thinking "Well I could do this or that" so...
Yeah.
You say that you don't really get much time for yourself?
Not really, not as much as I would like to.
What do you do in your time for yourself? Go swimming, something like that?
Even when I do go swimming I have to take her! [Laughs] It was only last Tuesday that we went swimming after a very long time of not, I mean Yusuf takes her on Sundays but I can't go with them because of my dress code, so he takes her to the local pool but on Tuesdays it's women only so. But yeah I would like to maybe even go one day by myself. Even like Yusuf and me don't get time for ourselves. We used to go to the movies a lot but we don't get time now. My mum is there and I know I can always knock on her door. But then I, I sit down and think I'm not with her when I'm working so it's not fair for me to say "Oh mum can you have Ayesha whilst me and Yusuf go and watch a movie?" And I know she's not going to turn around and say no but it's... I feel guilty! [Laughs]
Do you know if there is a reason to feel guilty?
Only because my mum might think, "Well look at her, she goes to work, she is leaving

265

Nine Women, Nine Months, Nine Lives

Ayesha here, and now she wants to go to the movies." [Laughs] So it's, you sometimes think…
Yeah, you wonder about that, I can understand that you want to take that into consideration, but, if you spoke to your mum about it…?
Yeah.
You said she might think that you are leaving her there and you are going off to do this that and the other, you don't know that that is what she thinks. And if you sit down and explain to her that it would make the world of difference to you to be able to go swimming on a Tuesday, and, or you want to go out with Yusuf one evening and it may not be a regular thing but would she mind if you gave it a whirl? Errm… I mean if Ayesha is there in the daytime, you know, you could think about leaving her there over night, it might make you mums life a bit easier rather than you coming and dropping her of and then coming back and collecting her. because if she has her in the days when you are at work, you know then maybe your mum would like to be involved in things like bathtime and bedtime.
We have talked about that. My mum is always saying "Well why don't you leave her here, I'll see if I can train her into sleeping through the night." Because when I did speak to the health visitor he did say that all you need to do is train her for four nights out of five and then she'll, four nights and then she'll sleep in her own cot in her own room. I mean that would be difficult for me, as a mother, but my mums often said, that because, I'm not, I don't think I'm breastfeeding because I want to breastfeed, I think I'm breastfeeding because it's easier for me to keep her shut, to keep her quiet. It's not often that she does cry, and when she does cry in the middle of the night, put her to the breast and she's quiet…
Have you tried her with a dummy?
I've tried her with a dummy, I've tried a water bottle, I've tried Soya milk, but nothing seems to be working. But, it's what she wants, I fear, that fear is that because she doesn't feed during the day, unless if she's really cranky then I'll feed her, but well, it's very difficult.
You'll have to see how it goes.
Yeah, mmm.
Errm… And how do you think your partner has changed? Do you think he has changed?
He's become more supportive, more co-operative, listens to me more, we have a lot more to talk about now. We used to talk about work, you know how your day was, anything exciting that was happening at work and that's it. But now we have a lot more to share, a lot more to talk about, because I always used to think, he's so quiet, <u>so</u> quiet. Now he makes the effort to initiate conversations with me now.
Right, that's good.
Yeah, so he's changed a lot.
Do you think that's a positive change?
Definitely.

Ameena

And how would you say your relationship has changed?
Quite a lot. Errm... He's very comforting, like I still, you know like I had the baby blues and a bit of depression, I sometimes still feel very low. I've nothing to feel low about but I'll just feel every now and again like "Oh I could just cry" and he is there, his shoulder is always there. He says "Oh come here" and he'll give me a hug, he's very supportive now.
Mmm, that's good. So do you talk about how you have changed as individuals? Does he ever say you know...?
No, no.
Do you think that you need to?
Yeah, I think that's one thing that we are both failing to do. Errm... I'd like to say to him more "Yusuf you're so special, you're so nice" but I can't! [Laughs] Errm... No we never talk about positive changes to each other, about each other. I'd like to sometimes. I think I'll tell him he's special tonight.
He'll probably look at you like you're mad! [Laughter]
Yeah!
He'll probably think what has she broken? Has she crashed the car?! [Laughs]
Yeah [Laughs]
Yeah give it a go, I mean if it's something you think might make a difference, then yeah...
Especially when you've gone through an arranged or introductory marriage, you think "Oh God, is it going to work?" and...
Mmm, it must be very difficult.
I mean they say that you grow to like each other, you grow to love each other. But you always have that thought at the back of your mind, when you do know him after about four years time, that you are going to get fed up of him or bored of him. You develop that relationship, that understanding, a lot through respect and caring for each other. Yeah I think more than anything it's, it's the caring.
And do you try and make time for yourselves as a couple? I mean for instance with Ayesha if she does fall asleep in the evening?
Yes, yes we do, initially it was... Yeah, yeah we do.
And do you manage it quite often?
Yeah, now, now, errm... When she was depending heavily on breastfeeding it was very difficult because she was, every, about every half an hour every hour she was so demanding that, but now with that change, it's a lot better.
So it's a lot easier now?
Yeah, it's a lot easier now.
And do you sort of, what kind of things do you do? Are you at home most of the time when it's like that? Like get a video out something like that?
Yeah oh yeah, always! [Laughs] Yeah and it's always, what is it... Action?
An action movie?
An action movie, and he knows I hate that! [Laughs] But as long as he enjoys it.

Nine Women, Nine Months, Nine Lives

You'll have to get a slushy one out then!
Yeah, I'll get him to get me a slushy one , yeah a lovey dovey one! [Laughs] And then he'll be nodding off!
Oh well can't be all bad! [Laughs] OK the next and final chunk is your immediate future. So the next 12 months, so the next year. What do you hope to achieve in the next year?
Is that in terms of personal achievements, or Ayesha?
Personal, Ayesha, it includes everything and anything. Any area of your life that you are trying to work towards or would like to work towards?
Gosh! I could go on about that!
OK, then, do!
I've got so many hopes and dreams! Can I start off with career?
Yes, of course you can.
I'm not, I'm not a career woman, but I'd like to either have my own business or start thinking about setting up my own business, or if that failed then change my job. because this one is really stressful! [Laughs] Errm… That's the career side. Errm… 12 months, I'd like to conceive again, I think, only because Yusuf wants to! [Laughs] He doesn't have to go through the process! [Laughs] But no…
Do you think you'd be thinking about having another baby towards the beginning of this next year?
No I think in about six month's time.
Yeah so you'll have a gap in between, at least a couple of years.
Yes, initially we were thinking when she is about three or four years old, but then I don't want to leave such a huge gap. I mean we're not getting any younger!
Well, you're not getting any older are you really?!
Yusuf is! No I'm only joking! [Laughs] And she'll need company, so we want to have one more baby, strictly one more! [Laughs]
Yeah, no more!
No way! For Ayesha, I want to spend more quality time, quality time with her, errm… I mean she's developing and after a year it's like, I want to spend more time with her. I want to go through picture books, maybe it's too early, but I want to start introducing number work to her, I want to do all then things. Maybe I am pushing her [Laughs] pushing her a bit too fast but I want to spend more time with her. I don't get enough time with her. Errm… I want to move house, but that's not something that will happen in the next twelve months time.
No, but it's something you are thinking about.
Yeah, that's it really.
Mmm, yeah.
Can't be too greedy!
No, but there's a lot of things we can hope for. I mean you know there is no harm in hope. And do you think you will be able to achieve those aims? Do you think that they

Ameena

are realistically going to happen in the next twelve months?
I always do like to set myself realistic aims and goals. Errm... But, there's nothing wrong in dreaming! [Laughs] I do hope to achieve them with a bit of positive thinking and support from family, from friends, from my husband. I hope to achieve them. Well especially the job and the business front. I don't know what more to say about it.
No, no that's fine. As long as you feel that you can achieve it. It's not as if you feel it's something that is out there and you can't get hold of it.
No, no.
It's something that you feel you can do, then that's good.
Yeah.
And what would you say you have learnt about yourself in the past year that you would like to develop next year? So something about yourself that you feel particularly proud of, or particularly pleased about that you think you want to keep and you want to make a permanent change.
Errm... Sorry can I go back a step?
Yeah, of course you can.
As you were saying that I just thought of something else! [Laughs] That I want to achieve in the next twelve months. I want to lose weight! [Laughs]
Oh right! [Laughs]
I want to lose weight, I really do. I won't will I eating all those chocolates and chips? No, no I want to lose weight. Sorry, going back to the question...
No, no, that's all right. So what would you say that you have learnt about yourself in this past year, something good, something you feel is good, that you would like to develop next year? Perhaps, maybe not, sort of like, make it better but at least keep it there?
I'm not really sure to be honest.
Something that you feel is an achievement that you feel you have done in the past year that you would like to, things like gaining your confidence going back to work, regaining your independence and your peace of mind, becoming more patient errm...
I wouldn't, I don't...
Realising you limitations?
Yeah, yeah, getting my priorities, well knowing my priorities and then getting them right.
Yeah well trying to do something about them, not getting them right, because it won't ever feel like "Oh, done that done that", you'll never get that feeling!
Mmm, there must be something, it's just that I can't get to it right now! [Laughs]
OK, well lets think about the opposite then. What have you learnt about yourself in the past year that you would like to change next year? Something that you have discovered about yourself that you've thought "Oh my God! That's awful, I really must do something about that, I must become patient, or I must" you know...
As I was saying earlier about being so stressed out, I would like to, actually go on a

269

Nine Women, Nine Months, Nine Lives

stress management course. Yeah, I want to be less stressed, I don't want to worry as much as I do, even though Yusuf is always saying "You worry too much." And I mean it's like the little things, like we were in the pool the other day and errm... I mean I've lost my swimming skills somehow, I mean I used to swim when I was at school, at school, and then I stopped swimming, and I can't swim anymore. My mum was with Ayesha and errm... Pritty (Yusuf's sister) was trying to teach me how to swim again. Errm... All I was worried about was "No, no, no watch that lady, you're going to bump into her!" and she goes "For once in your life just turn around and think this pool is yours!" [Laughs] So yeah, I want to stop worrying, I worry too much, about others, about. So I'd like to change that?
I think that's the key to it really, you seem to be particularly concerned about what others do, what others think, and how they perceive you, and what will they think, and...
I'd love to change that!
Well you can try and change a little bit at a time.
I mean it's not going to happen overnight.
Oh no, no.
I am the world's greatest worrier! [Laughs] But the sad thing is I don't ever sit there worrying for myself, about myself. I worry for this one or that. I mean yesterday we had an incident, somebody in the community committed suicide. And I sat there and I was crying and I was sitting and I kept ringing my brother and I let the whole world know "God she's so worried". I was worried about his wife and his three little children, and I'm sitting there thinking "Well how come it's not affecting anybody else as much as it is affecting me? Why am I the one sitting here worrying?" And my brother gave me a good kick up my bum and said "Look woman, sort yourself out, sort your life out and then worry about others!" So, I want to...
Start thinking about yourself?
Yeah, I want to start thinking about myself, which I always fail to do. I always fail to think about myself.
No, I don't think that's true – and it's on the tape! Because you've started to think about what you want, you have! [Laughter] You have – I've got it! I'm going to type it out and I'm going to send you a copy!
Oh thank you! [Laughs]
You have! Well think about it, you've started to think about part-time isn't suiting you, not three days. So you've started to think full-time, four days?
But then am, I being selfish? I'm not being selfish am I? because I think well why am I going back full-time, is it because I can't cope with the pressures of work so I'm going back without realising that that extra day I won't get to spend with my daughter. So it's partly, do you see what I mean? Whenever I stop to think about myself I always think "Uh-oh I'm being selfish".
I think, no you're not being selfish you just haven't necessarily considered Ayesha up until that point in time. And just because you realise you that haven't, it doesn't mean

Ameena

therefore you are selfish because you've realised "Oh hang on a minute, if I'm there then it means I'm not with her, and how will that make me feel? How will that make her feel? How will we handle that?" So you know, you're not...
Well, if I think positively, it sounds so silly, but if I think positively, I mean I could comfort myself by thinking that the extra amount I'll be earning I can spend it all on her! [Laughs] So, it's me compromising with myself within, isn't it?
Compensating I would have thought would be a better word.
Yeah. I'm a mixed up case! [Laughs]
No you're not, because you are aware of your limitations, and you are aware of the things that matter to you and your just not sure how to go about making it slot together. You know because it's slotting at the moment but you don't feel as if it's balanced. So you just need to tweak it a little bit, and you'll spend the rest of your life tweaking it one way, tweaking another bit another way, and tweaking something else yet another way. That's, that's what life is about. You know you are aware of what you want and there's nothing wrong with standing up and saying "look, this is driving me crackers being at work three times a week. I'm working full time I'm getting paid for three days. I'm away from Ayesha, I'm not enjoying the time that I'm away from Ayesha because I'm thinking about her and when I'm with her I'm thinking about work! And that makes me feel guilty!" So you know, you've got to try and, you won't get rid of those guilty feelings but you'll at least have a sensation of having done something. So there's <u>loads</u> of thing, loads of things, that you can change, make better or you can stop. I think you don't necessarily worry, you consider, you spend a lot of your time considering other people. Errm... And being concerned about their welfare, which is only natural because they are the people closest to you and you love them dearly. But you have to have a little bit of self-preservation in there. OK. So one of the things that you want to change next year would be starting to develop, start implementing what you think and how you feel?
Yep, I agree.
So what would you say would be a good thing that you have learnt about yourself that you would like to develop next year? Going back to the previous question, would you say that comes under the same thing?
Recognising that I exist! [Laughs] Errm... Gosh, that's a difficult one to answer. I think it more or less ties in with the second one.
Yeah, because they are sort of direct opposites really. Do you think you will be able to, to start and sit down and think about what you want?
Yeah.
Have you thought about what the consequences might be if you don't?
I'll be hurting myself, I'll be, well it's it's valuing yourself isn't it? It's almost that I always put others first, I should learn to put myself first.
If you feel that is what you want and you feel that that is what will make you happy, then that's a good place to start.
Yes, yeah I think I'll stick by that.

Nine Women, Nine Months, Nine Lives

See how you go, see what happens. It'll be all right.
Yeah [Doesn't sound convinced]
You know you don't have to be scared of change. I mean if you think about it you've coped very well with like the last two years. They've been, if you think about it, it's been change. Throughout your pregnancy every month was different, and it was visibly different because you got bigger and then you had scans and things like that as you got closer to the birth. It's the same thing now, every month is different. And Ayesha gets bigger not your tummy. So, you'll have to see how you go.
Mmmm...
OK, well that's it. I hope that wasn't too dreadful?
No, no, it was quite good and I'll take that really positively, because it makes you step back a little bit and think because obviously all that we've talked about is real life, isn't it?
Yes.
Day in day out.
And they are things you don't get time to think about in real life!
Yeah, yeah <u>exactly</u>.
Because everything is going by as well. When you spend every minute talking and thinking about the next minute, it's very difficult to sit back and take time to think about yourself.
Yeah and I always think it's nice because you see Ayesha growing up and I always feel that the next day the following day I want to sit back and think, to think back basically.
So you find yourself looking forward a lot?
Yes, almost always all the time. But it's nice once in a while to sit back and think "Oh Yeah! I was pregnant once!" [Laughs] And the problems I had...
Yeah, and you don't have those anymore.
Yeah, I don't have them anymore, I've moved on!
Yeah, because of the things that you did. Because it was in your control to do something about them and you did.
Yeah, it's really nice to. I think this is the first time, well it is the first time I've ever sat down, obviously she is a year old, and I've never, never ever <u>ever</u> thought about when I was pregnant! How was I feeling and what was I wearing and [Laughs] and how did I cope with the pain and? You just look forward don't you? Which is a good thing, but sometimes it's nice just to look back. I mean it's all memory now isn't it? It's all history! So it's nice to go back and also talk about it [baby joining in] and she agrees! [Laughs]
Yeah! OK, that's lovely.

Rachel

Rachel was 27 years old when she found out she was pregnant for the first time. Her partner was in the process of moving from London to Leicester to be with her and they decided that they would probably have started a family together in the future and so went ahead with their pregnancy. However, Rachel continued to feel unsure about having a baby right up until the day of the birth. She wanted to return to her job as soon as possible after having her son Charlie to continue building her career. When she had her son she left returning to work as late as she could and continues to feel a conflict between motherhood, which she unexpectedly found she loved, and her career.

If you could think back to when you were first pregnant, when you did the pregnancy test. OK, were you trying to get pregnant at the time?
No. No, no!
Absolutely not?
Definitely not, he was a complete accident! [Laughs]
So can you remember what went through your mind when you found out you were pregnant? When you saw those two blue lines...
I couldn't believe how quickly the pregnancy test changed. I'd only moved here in the March, and I'd only just started my job, so I thought "Oh my God what do I do?" And then we also had an OFSTED visit at the school, and I was like, a bit preoccupied with that, and I thought "Oh I'm going to let down the Head". Those kind of emotions really.

Nine Women, Nine Months, Nine Lives

And then James was at school as well for a parents evening, and I thought, "Oh God I can't tell him yet, not when there's all of these parents".
So James is a teacher as well?
Yes.
Right.
So, no he wasn't planned, it was a bit of a shock horror to begin with!
I bet.
Because James hadn't moved up here yet either, so it was like "Oh my God have we done the right thing?!"
Yeah.
Weren't you, you were a bit of a shock! [Talking to baby]
OK, was anyone with you when you did the test?
No.
You did it on your own?
Yes, yes I did.
How many weeks were you when you did the test?
Five weeks.
So you had an idea that you were pregnant?
Yes.
And had you talked to James about the fact that you thought you might be before you did the test?
Yeah, the day before, I'd spoken to my friend as well and she said go and do the test so... I thought I should really, so, so I did it.
OK, can you remember what James's reaction was when you actually told him that you were pregnant, did you say it face-to-face, on the telephone?
No, I told him face-to-face, we'd just got in and made a cup of tea and I said "I'm pregnant." [Laughs] Because I hadn't told you that I was going to do a pregnancy test had I?
Husband: No, no I think you'd just said you thought you might be.
No, I hadn't told him I was going to do the test that day. And he just gave me a big hug really and then errm... We went out for a meal that night to try and get things in perspective really.
To try and sort things out?
We decided that we were in a good relationship, and the fact that we hadn't lived together yet didn't matter.
Yeah?
So once we'd recovered - that was that! [Laughs]
Yeah it was a bit of a shock I expect...
A bit of a shock! because I'd found out the day before that my brother and his girlfriend had had their baby.
That's right I remember you telling me that you'd gone round to see them a few times.

Rachel

Yeah, yeah.
And you'd witnessed it all first hand throughout?
Yeah, yeah that's right. I wasn't looking forward to pregnancy because Jane was sick throughout hers.
Had you had any symptoms then up to five weeks?
I'd had tender breasts that was all. I think that was how I knew really, they were a bit, sore.
Yeah so you had an idea that something wasn't quite right.
You were more keen for the baby than I was weren't you? [Talking to Husband]
Husband: I'd got to thirty and thought well...
Now or never?!
Yes! [Laughs]
The thing was that you'd got the job already and you were planning to actually move up here anyway. [Talking to Husband]
So you weren't living together at the time?
No, because he'd got the job ready to come up.
So you were planning to live together?
Yeah.
It all sort of came to a head at once then?
Yeah, a bit sooner than we expected though!
Right, the next part is your experience of pregnancy and the birth. OK. Before you were pregnant had you imagined how you would feel when you were pregnant?
Errrm...
Had you thought about having children?
I think I just thought "Oh I'll be like my mum" she was sick through out her first pregnancy and I just sort of expected that really.
So that was before you were pregnant?
Yeah.
So when you found out you were pregnant did you start thinking more deeply about it?
It amazed me how hungry or tired... Yeah when you were hungry or tired, how sick you felt. Where usually when you felt sick you wouldn't want to eat anything, but being pregnant you seemed to need to eat when you felt like that. And I couldn't believe how tired I was in the beginning, and I thought I'd just fallen asleep for ten minutes, but it'd be an hour and a half or two hours! [Laughs] And I'd think "Oh God where has the time gone?!" The tiredness really, I don't think I expected it quite so early on, and the changes in your body so early on, I just thought it came later. Everything came quite early on for me.
So the physical side of the pregnancy came a lot sooner than you thought?
Yeah, and the actual link with your doctor.
The what with your doctor?
The link, that you had much more contact.

Nine Women, Nine Months, Nine Lives

Right, so you established quite a good relationship with them?
Yeah I mean I saw them initially and the midwife as well. I just thought that, you know, it was such a big thing in your life that you would see them in the beginning and more towards the end. Again that was a strange thing, even though I didn't want to be pregnant, although I was, I didn't want to go because I couldn't cope with it. But when you go past your miscarriage probability and you know you're going past the dates when you could have a termination I think that was really difficult to come to terms with. Which I think, when you go past your probability stage for miscarriage or termination...
So you think that once, so when would you describe your dates for miscarriage?
Up to three and a half months, it was when I'd gone past 14 weeks that I then thought "Right, I'm going to carry this baby now". I focused my mind to that, that I was going to have a baby. We had talked about terminating it but obviously... But we did consider it what with the way we were, and I didn't know how the hell we would get on.
No, that's right.
You know with the added pressure that goes with having a baby? I don't think I'd have had the baby if he hadn't been so sure, we didn't really want to terminate the baby, but then we weren't sure if we, so that was a bit of a...
Yeah, yeah.
And then a bit later in the pregnancy, about seven weeks before I was due, I had a bleed and they thought it was coming from the placenta. I'd just finished work the Friday before, and they were considering keeping me in until the end of the pregnancy. The thought of staying in hospital for seven weeks, oh my God I couldn't face that!
Oh no!
And then the thought of having an elective caesarean, I was like "Oh my God!"
So you hadn't expected any of those things?
No, no. I think as well, in the beginning when you get stomach pains or your back hurts it doesn't say in any of the books what these are. Sometimes you think to yourself "Well am I going to lose the baby?" because these things feel more like period pains and you think "God, am I losing the baby?" You're just not sure what is happening to your body really. So... And your emotions! I don't think I've cried as much, ever been so tearful about things!
So were you quite sensitive then?
Yeah I was, too much really.
And that was different from what you expected then?
Yeah, I don't think I expected that, and I put on weight really quickly as well, I'd put on loads by the time I was eight weeks, I felt really bloated, I found that really hard to come to terms with so early. Especially as we were supposed to be going away and I was trying on clothes and I was thinking "I've outgrown my wardrobe – I have no clothes that fit me!"
Oh no, how awful! OK and the birth. Had you thought about the birth before hand, whilst you were pregnant?

Rachel

Whilst I was pregnant, well we went to some NCT classes...
Oh yes, of course you did, didn't you?
And they were really useful, pain relief, caesareans, and things like that. So they were quite useful. I mean I had some trial contractions, and they were always in the night, I didn't want to wake up James and they kind of died after two or three hours, they went.
So what you had them sort of like mini-contractions if you like?
Yeah.
So just for a couple of hours?
Well they were fairly regular, about every fifteen minutes and then they sort of went. Everybody's labour is slightly different, I'd talked to other women about having their babies, and they told me about their contractions and that. Oh yes, and my waters didn't break so they had to be broken.
So that was, was that a surprise then?
Yeah, although mum said when hers had, they hadn't gushed they'd sort of trickled, so it was not like kind of a complete surprise then. And my sister-in-law she'd had her pregnancy, she'd gone over her due-date so they broke her waters.
So she was induced?
She was induced.
What about the pain side of things, was that as you had expected? Did you feel like you were quite well prepared? With regards to pain relief preparation, the birthplan...
Yeah, I mean I had a TENS machine which I think kept me at home for quite a long time really. I'd been in labour about nine hours by the time I'd gone in, I think that just kept me at home longer than if I'd, not that it actually stops the pain it's just I think that, psychologically, you feel as if you are almost doing something with your body.
So that was good then, being at home?
Yeah, James was quite agitated to get going, but I didn't want to get sent back home, told "You're not in labour!" So errm... I had had a show as well, the day before, so I mean people I'd talked to that was different too. I mean I had gone over my due-date.
Oh right.
Although I was... I really did not want to be induced.
No, I can understand that.
And errm... Anyway that was the day that the consultant had said "If you haven't had baby by then..." So I would have had to be induced. So it was quite a relief really!
[Laughs]
Yeah, I bet you were!
It was like, a mixed emotion. You know like, "Can I get through this?" And sort of kind of being excited and looking forward to it, I felt quite a lot of things all at once...
Yeah, well, you never feel only one thing about any event in your life, so it's no surprise really...
I think because we were apprehensive when it started. I remember when, because I had a ventouse, and errm... He was thrown on my stomach when I wasn't quite expecting it

Nine Women, Nine Months, Nine Lives

and then whisked away straight away. I thought that was a really horrible way to be introduced to your baby. He was just slapped on and then gone straight away, you know, that was my only sort of negative part of it really. But the staff were really great, really helpful. I didn't get on with the gas and air, I didn't like that at all.
No, did it make you feel sick, or make you woosy?
No, I just felt like I was really drunk, and my mouth was really numb, and I didn't feel like I could make important decisions do you know what I mean, I was like...
I suppose also if you felt like you couldn't feel your mouth you wouldn't have been able to speak, you wouldn't have been able to tell them what you wanted or didn't want?
Yeah, that's right. I felt like it was better not having as strong a painkiller, but I had an epidural, even though, with that I did wonder about the side effects, but...
Did you have any side effects?
No, I didn't have any. Although I did expect the epidural to make me have a weird sensation, I still could bear down but I wasn't able to push when I was fully dilated, that went on for two hours and I was really tired. When I had the sensation of wanting to push but not being able to push that was weird.
That must have been hard.
Yeah, it was really tiring as well for two hours.
Yeah to keep trying.
Yeah and then they said "Oh you can have a ventouse" I was like phew! [Laughs]
[Laughs] Had you not thought to ask if there was anything?
Errm...
Because you sound like you knew quite a lot, you'd read quite a lot, you knew about side effects for the epidural...
I don't think I particularly wanted... If I could I was going to do it naturally really, and I didn't think I'd be overly long in labour put errm... I did start to push and then they said well, and then they did actually break his waters when I was dilated because they thought that might help, with being dilated and they said that that should do it. And they noticed that he was in quite a lot of distress, because of the waters, you know, they didn't really give me much of an option did they? [Addressing husband] They sort of said, and we agreed first time, so... [Laughs]
Well, did you feel bad about it not going like the birth plan?
No! [Laughs] We'd been quite you know open, if this happens then we'll do that or the other, do you know what I mean, we'd thought about the options.
That's good, yeah.
I didn't really want a ventouse, but that rather than forceps was better.
No, no.
Because I think it's the speed, how quickly you are ready, your labour's quite slow and then it speeds up "You're having a ventouse" - right that's the decision, legs in stirrups and go for it!
That's it yeah. OK, so the birth was different from what you thought it would be,

Rachel

basically, wasn't it? In lots of ways.
Yeah, I think it was probably.
How did you feel when you first held him? You said that he was kind of slapped onto your tummy and then whisked off, that's not really holding him, so...
No, I think it was almost like "This is your child" sort of thing. And then errm... He had some oxygen and then he was wrapped up and then, they bathed him first and then they got him dressed and then I held him. And he was squealing, you know crying, for about an hour, but it didn't seem to matter! And then errm... I breast fed him, and he just went to the breast and...
And was that all right?
Yeah, that was fine. It was quite painful at first but after a bit it was, yeah it was fine. Yeah it was quite nice really, because I'd had him at like half four in the afternoon so I was in time for the auxiliary nurse coming with the tea round! [Laughs]
[Laughs] How convenient!
Yeah it was very convenient! But it was really nice that I could actually show him off straight away, I was tired but... [Laughs]
So, when you were showing him off, how did you feel at that time?
Proud. [Shows in her face too]
Chuffed with yourself? Chuffed with him?
Yeah, really, because he is a big baby. He was ten pounds and a bit when he was born, and he was like... [Uses hands to show just how big he was]
Oh God yeah, I remember!
Yeah so he wasn't a fragile baby, he wasn't... He was always hungry, I'd just be putting my boob back and he'd want them to come back out! [Laughs] Quite an amazing feeling really! I'd just put him in the cot next to me and he was a very, he was always so long, he filled the cot!
Yeah? And in what ways was James involved in the pregnancy? Again, we'll deal with the pregnancy first and then we'll move onto the birth.
Errm... He went to all my classes with me.
Was he curious about what was, all the changes that were happening to you?
Yeah I mean, errm... He went to the scans with me, when I had a my bleed, when I went in to hospital seven weeks before I was due, he came in then straightway. And I would talk to him about things, and he was involved in the NCT classes, he came when the other couples were there and took part in the cross-couples exercises and that was, that was quite good too. And also it allowed us to have an opportunity to say how we felt in a supportive context, without it being confrontational. I remember James at one point wanted to bring the placenta home, he wanted to bury it in the garden! [Laughs and rolls her eyes] I was like "Don't be stupid!" [Laughs] I was like really shocked because it wasn't something that we had talked about at home! So... [Laughs] But yeah he was really supportive, he was involved quite a lot.
Yeah and the thing is when you are feeling physically and emotionally over sensitive or

Nine Women, Nine Months, Nine Lives

hyper sensitive, you talked about that?
Yeah, but at the beginning I think it was difficult, especially you know because of the circumstances. Yeah James was far more into babies than I was really, and that was quite difficult. I was like battling with my own emotions really, I felt guilty about not wanting the baby, but I couldn't help how I felt. After we'd decided to have him, I felt guilty.
How long did you feel guilty for? For feeling unsure?
Until the nineteenth of March. [Laughs]
[Laughs] So right up until 'B' day then!
Yeah, I mean even when I used to go to the NCT classes. You know they'd all be there cooing over pictures looking forward to 'being a mummy' and I'd just go home and cry. I had all of these mixed up expectations of what life was going to be like.
Did you talk to anybody who felt like that? Someone else who felt ambivalent too? Or perhaps your mum?
Errm... No, no I think I'm, I think I felt guilty and so couldn't talk to family about it. I actually spoke to my friend at work who wasn't a mum, so I could kind of talk to her about it. You know, everybody else, my other close friends are mums and I think they'd feel or think... I think they have an expectation of you as a mum, of how a mother feels, and they didn't change, but...That's why, if we can afford it and have another child, then I would like that to be a positive experience rather than a negative experience.
What would happen, do you think, if you got pregnant again, would you feel that it would be a positive experience?
Errm... I'd hope so.
Do you think it was the unplanned sort of side of it?
Yeah, because we hadn't been together all that long, and it was quite a big, there was a lot of pressure then, you know to be with somebody, and have a baby together. And also work, the thought of giving up work, I mean that's completely changed, my perspective now, when I was pregnant I wanted to be back at work quickly afterwards and now, it's changed, I don't want to work! No! [Laughs]
[Laughs] Sounds like James was quite involved in the pregnancy, what about the birth, was James there?
Yeah, James was there for the whole birth, he was, teachers are allowed five days off paternity leave. So he had that day off came with me, and was there throughout, and he stayed till about nine o'clock. And then I came, I had him on the Tuesday, two nights in hospital, James was there all day on the Wednesday, we went home on the Thursday, so he was very much involved, through the whole process really.
Yeah, sounds like you'd made quite a lot of decisions together, with regards to the birth plan...
Yeah, I mean we'd read up on things. Like I didn't want pethidine, I was quite 'anti' that, I think I was more certain what I didn't want more than what I... I was fairly open-minded about what was best for me at the time and for the baby but I was quite sure of things I didn't like. Like I didn't want my waters broken, but I did, and pethidine well...

Rachel

Also if I needed to have a caesarean then I knew I wanted a local rather than a general, things like that.
Yeah, you'd thought it through.
And I didn't want that scalp clip thing, you know to have the baby monitored. I think that was it, they were talking about my progress, and I'd already had a mobile epidural, which I'd asked for because I'd found out about that. Midwives don't always tell you that it's available so I knew that I would have to ask for it. I didn't particularly want to lay down in that one position, I wanted to fidget about. I mean James, he kind of stayed out of it when it came to those decisions. When I had the ventouse you had to push down with the contractions and he got a bit of shock then when I was gripping him! [Laughs]
And do you think James's support in the birth and the pregnancy was more or less than you had hoped for?
Errm...
It may have been more during the birth and less in the pregnancy or...?
No, I think it was kind of what I'd, what I'd hoped for, I think I'd expected him to be as supportive as he was.
The next chunk is your experiences of early motherhood. Those first few days and weeks, up until the end of the first three months. OK? So probably just before I saw you last time, round about then.
Errm...
Did the pregnancy effect early motherhood? So in terms of sort of like whether you had water retention or...?
Oh I couldn't believe how tired I felt, I had errm... A couple of migraines that week and then I had cystitis which really knocked me out. And I felt really, not really, and I used to have a nap in the afternoon and I would joke with James that I just didn't have normal time like everybody else, I had to go to bed in the middle of the day! [Laughs] But then I was up most of the nights with him. And also you'd give him a feed and that would be a two-hour shift and then he'd be awake for an hour after and would want you to talk with him, and errm... When James went back to work I was doing it all by myself.
All the time, yeah.
And errm...He's never been a great sleeper, I think it was the shift of my sleeping pattern, try to go to bed about ten.
Yep, grab it when you can!
I'd have a shower and, I always used to think I could hear him cry, even though James had him I thought I could hear him cry, I used to think "Is that him or not?" And I spoke to another one of my friends, and she felt the same, she thought she could hear her baby crying in the other room, so it was really strange, a strange instinct really. And I couldn't believe how much I bled afterwards. I expected to bleed but not for as long or as heavy. And one thing I really didn't like about breastfeeding was that once you'd have a shower and you were clean, then you'd start leaking and you'd feel really dirty again. I had a feeling of being dirty for quite a long time, and of feeling quite sore and bleeding

281

and then he would want to comfort feed from about eight till one which was hopeless because I was feeling so sore as well. I think, I think you feel really proud and excited but it's like all the people who come to visit you, you either feel like you're being the hostess and you're not seeing to the baby or you just like... No time for it really. I mean you're trying to keep everybody you like because James's parents live away from here, so trying to give them an opportunity to come and see him. Whereas with your own family it's different. They had spent longer travelling and wanted to stay for longer, do you know what I mean? You would try to be fair but you 'd think "Oh God!" And I think, my mum and James's mum, they'd both bottle fed us, so they didn't accept, my mum especially because she'd seen me sore with feeding. They'd kind of ask me "When is he going to have a bottle?" and "Are you sure he's hungry again?" and not realising, you know, that breastfed babies do it like that. Do you know what I mean they were always trying to put pressure on to not breast feed. You always have to justify why you are breastfeeding. And it wasn't always said in a negative way but, you know, you get the... That was, not a pressure but something that was a bit tiring at times.
Yeah, especially when you have to explain again and again.
Yeah! [Laughs]
Yes, that's understandable.
But it's lovely when they first start smiling and responding to you. I really enjoyed being at home with him. I really wasn't into going back to work, and I wasn't lonely. I mean my mum's really local, and my dad was which I could, I could actually have a life without needing to do... I didn't really go to any sort of organised mother groups, you know sitting there comparing their babies.
Is that what you imagined early motherhood would be like? Being stuck at home and desperate to get back to work?
Yeah.
Feeling a bit isolated?
I think sometimes, I didn't resent James because we were a team with him. I think when he was slightly older, when he was four or five months old, I was looking for something else to keep my mind ticking over, or a change of routine, but errm... because I wasn't into the mother groups, I quite liked to...
Did you go along to any...?
Not really! [Laughs] And also there, I find it really difficult to errm... People who have brought up their children differently, have different ideas, I find it really difficult to not, I think "Well that's not the way that I want to bring up Charlie" and I tend to find that I don't particularly bond with those kinds of people. The friends I have made, they have similar ideas to how I want to bring up Charlie, and we get on well.
Yeah, well that's not that surprising really. I mean I don't like all women just because I'm a woman! [Laughs]
[Laughs] Yeah, I think that people have that thing you know, that you're in a group where everyone is having their baby at about the same time. I think that there is this

Rachel

expectation that you will have all of these really twee coffee mornings together and you're all going to get on really well. And I'm not like that, at all.
OK, so would you say that motherhood matched up to what you'd expected? It may have been different in certain areas, better in other areas, worse in some...
I think it's more tiring than you ever imagine. And you wonder how you'll get things done. But I think it's more rewarding than you think, so I was really kind of not keen on the idea of the actual baby stage when you'd be doing things for him, but the actual bond and love that you have for them is far more than I could have ever imagined really. And especially now that one of my best friends has got a baby it's so nice to be able to talk to her and show her my baby "Look what I've done!" [Laughs]
Here's one I made earlier! [Laughs]
[Laughs] Yeah! Just taking him out and doing things with him, I find I really enjoy that.
Good. So, what would you say was the most difficult thing in those early days? Perhaps the first three or four weeks?
Errm...
Do you look back and think "Oh thank God it's not like that now!"
I think it's the errm... The waking up every two and a half hours, that's probably the hardest part. I think it's the re-organisation of your life and your time-scale that are probably the hardest...And still feeling tender when you're breastfeeding, and when you see people they don't seem to, it doesn't seem to hurt them at all, and you've got to get the position right, and oh! [Laughs] It's almost like a trial you know, but after a while you grow accustomed to it, and they are bigger and they know what they are doing more, it's so much easier. And I think it was the leaking as well with the milk that was like, that was strange, especially at night time because sometimes you'd go longer or he wouldn't go as long, and sometimes you'd leak and you'd wake up sodden. It was like your body wasn't how it used to be, do you know what I mean? All the functions were different?
Did you feel like you had no control?
Yeah! And your hair started to fall out! There were all sorts of things. You just didn't feel particularly attractive at all, and your stomach was a great big blobby thing. I think you need to adjust over the first few months really.
Mmmm. So that was, that was one of the hardest things? A bit of a shock?
Yeah, I think so.
Yeah and what would you say was the best part?
I loved holding him close to me and hearing him breath, and watching him responding to me. And things like you would walk into the room and he would know that it was you, and when you comforted him he sort of knew that it was you who was comforting him, do you know what I mean? You are the special person in their life.
You're the one that he wanted?
Yeah, that was great!
How much was James involved in the early days?

Nine Women, Nine Months, Nine Lives

He had five days paternity leave, and errm... He did like change nappies and, but because he was at work most of the time until the evenings, I did most of those kinds of things, the night duties, really. I think that one of the things that I used to find frustrating was that at the weekends, he'd never know what to dress him in. I think it's still because I've done his food and sorted out all his clothes and things, I think he thinks that children just wear whatever - He'd be like "Oh I dunno!" [Laughs]
So in the beginning James was involved as much as you were, in that first week?
Yeah.
And then after that, when he'd gone back to work?
Me!
Was it just because of the change in the situation?
Yeah, it seemed for the best really. Yeah, because of the circumstances really. I think so. I think that, because I was at home, I was doing the shopping, the cleaning, the ironing, and you know just doing those kind of jobs. And then when I went back to work, things like that didn't get done and caused a bit of conflict, especially because my mum is in another village 8 miles away and she does the child care. So that's quite a big detour as well, to go over there and then have to go back into the city, and trying to get into work early, what with being a teacher. Before I had him I used to get in at eight and now I don't get in until half past eight.
It's all a bit of a rush?
Yeah, and it's all been a big change really, and Charlie still wasn't sleeping when I went back.
So you were a bit zombied?
Yeah, well at that time he was waking between five and six times a night as well!
Oh my God!
Yeah.
Right, OK, had you talked about who would do what? Had you thought about who would do nappy changing for example, in those early few weeks? Things will have changes and evolved once you had him, but before you did?
No, I think we'd just thought we'd try and see how it went. We both like to bath him. I mean nowadays when James comes home from work he'll usually start and do the tea, and give Charlie his tea, and then errm... James'll perhaps bath him and I'll get his things ready for the next day. During that time, it's my only time away from children really so...
Of course, from three year olds to a one year old! [Laughs]
Yeah [Laughs] It's a bit like a busman's holiday isn't it?!
So would you say that that has worked out?
Yeah, there are some roles that we have naturally taken on, like James will do the shopping, I'll do the washing of clothes. It was really an unsaid thing you know we never said "Oh I'm going to do this and you are going to do that".
So you do what you feel you are best at?

Rachel

Yeah, and what your time schedule allows really, what fits. I feel like I'm either cleaning every day because it takes a long time, especially if you have Charlie, to do a job. So you end up doing a job every day and the house never seems clean all at once. So we just decided to get a cleaner. It's made our lives easier by having her. And that used to cause problems too, like the cleaning, you know "When is that going to be done?" So it seemed easier to get a cleaner and that's what we've done.
It brought you a bit of peace of mind as well, the pressure's off, you don't have to worry about the mundane things and now you can get on and play with Charlie.
Yeah, because I think I was really resentful about going back to work really in the end.
How many months old was Charlie when you went back to work?
Errm... I went back the last week in the summer term so that I could get my summer pay.
Oh that's right, yeah.
So, he'd be, about four months old. And by the time I'd gone back fully, he was six months old. And that week I went back I was still breast feeding, and I think that I was, I knew that I was going back for a week to get two months pay, you know for a weeks work, I was kind of almost aware that I wouldn't be able to give him all the feeds he was used to. And feeling the pressure that I was going to have to start bottle feeding him and I didn't particularly want to, and that's why you know... I can't remember what question it was you were asking me!
It's all right, don't worry. I was just asking you about whether you'd talked about things beforehand, and you said that you hadn't really discussed it much. Do you think on the whole that worked out for the better or the worse? That you remained fairly flexible...?
Errm... At Christmas because it was a long term as well, I had quite a lot of work to do, it was a lot of work for me. I never had sort of an opportunity to sort of, I used to get up at half past six and not finish until... Because Charlie used to not go to bed until nine. So from half past six I had no break from children until nine, and I used to go to bed not long after because I was so tired. So errm... We've rearranged it now so that he goes to my mum's on Wednesdays and Thursdays and he picks him up, so that's better. You see I always have a staff meeting after work so I don't leave work until twenty to six so by the time I've been to mum's house it'll be half past six when we get home. You see I can't just go and pick him up I always have to find out what's he been doing in the day, what he's eaten, you know, find out, notice the transitions... So you know that has helped, having had a bit of a heart to heart about what was working and what wasn't, that it needs to be more of an equal split really. And this terms been a lot better, it's worked better.
OK so it's working OK now then?
Yeah! [Laughs] And that's when I'd decided that I wanted to do four days as well. I mean I'd kind of weighed up doing a job share, but this way I work full days, I don't have to liase with someone else I just say this is what you're doing for the day. I think otherwise I'd just end up doing the same amount of work but not be paid for it!
Yeah, quite!

Nine Women, Nine Months, Nine Lives

Yeah so I decided that I'd rather get the money for it really! [Laughs] Better than the extra hassle! I may reduce it again, I'll see how it goes...
Yeah, that's it, things are still flexible so you could always change again. OK so the next chunk is you experience of motherhood up to the present day. How do you think your life has changed since you had Charlie?
Completely!
Yeah?
I think our main difference is that I wouldn't leave Charlie over night, both his grandparents would have him, and he'd be fine. But I can't do that and I think that is because I work five days a week so everything else is just precious time for Charlie and I really don't like, even at the week ends. Because I used to live in London before I moved here and a lot of my friends are still down there. But I really don't like going at the weekends, because I just pine away, I want to be with Charlie, I feel like I should be with Charlie. I feel that I only really see him at the end of the day and I really don't like that. So my time is for Charlie really. I think it's that you put Charlie first in everything you do.
So that's a change?
That's the biggest change. And all the money I earn I spend on him! I'd rather buy Charlie anything than for myself! A new book, some toys, you know. And it's important to have family time, to go out as a family, and playing with him at the end of the day. It's like when you come home and you don't put your feet up, you play with Charlie. So he has a sort of quality, play time. Don't we, we play with you! And errm... I think it's being organised. I think it's, I feel as though at work I do my preparation time whenever, now everything seems to be to a schedule and everything is precious.
So you would say that is how you've changed then?
Yeah I think I was always fairly organised but it's like, if there is a spare minute you might fit something in, whereas before you might sit down, this is when you do it. It's like being more timetabled I suppose. To fit everything in.
So how would you say you've changed in the past year? Good and bad aspects, permanent changes and temporary ones as well...
Permanently tired! [Laughs]
[Laughs] Yeah! Do you think you're perhaps more mature now? More patient, less patient?
Yeah I think in some ways I am more patient although when he has that whinging tone that just grates on me, do you know what I mean? I think since I have had a baby I am far more pre-menstrual than I ever used to be.
Yeah?
I can definitely feel myself getting really... And I only, I mean I've always had bad periods and I've still got them, heavier than I think they were, but I'm more pre-menstrual now too.

Rachel

Yeah, so the emotions and the sort of feeling like you could snap somebody's head off if they say the wrong thing?
Yeah I feel really irritable now, especially at school I can sometimes feel myself being… Not sharp with the children but thinking "You know that could really rattle me", and <u>feeling</u> it rattle you.
Right.
I think that's a physical change. I think errm… I'm a bit depressed about the fact I've not lost all my weight. That gets me down. I would like to lose it but it seems that no matter what I do… But I think I'm more patient yeah, and I'm more aware of needing quality time with him, and doing things together. I don't miss going out at night at all!
No?
I'm quite happy to sit here, staying in. I think I'm too knackered to go out! I think one of the problems as well is that I feel guilty that my mum has him most days, I'd feel too guilty to ask her to babysit.
Yeah, yeah, I suppose that's extra…
Yeah, and I mean my Dad struggles at night with his mobility… And James's parents live so far away and when they tend to come to you during the week you don't need to see them on the weekends. I think also within my job, it's helped a lot too. You have more empathy for parents. I think whereas before you were very much on a professional level, whereas now there is a parental level. And you appreciate that they have concerns, not that you discussed it before, but you realised it was upsetting the child. Say a child is crying and you'll ask them "What's wrong?" and they'll say they want custard on their dinner, you know what I mean, you might think "Oh for goodness sake, what's the big deal?" But to them it's a big deal and upsetting their child. That kind of thing I think has altered in me, you know to understand a little more - parents with their children. When they drop their child off and they are crying, you know that if they go the child will be all right shortly after, but the parents can't do it. And you know sometimes when I've dropped Charlie off and he's cried and I've had to leave him, it upsets you for the whole day, do you know what I mean? You're left thinking "Is he all right?" Whereas before I'd be like "Oh will you make a decision, you either go or you stay!" I think you are not quite as impatient with parents, you know you realise that your child is the most important thing really and their happiness is paramount.
Now you've gone back to work, and you've cut down to four days…
In September I'll cut down to four days.
And do you get any time to yourself? Without Charlie, without James…?
Errm… When I go swimming!
And how often do you manage to go swimming?
It's supposed to be every week but… [Laughs]
I know that feeling, yes!
Other things crop up don't they Charlie? So errm… I kind of feel guilty about that too. That you know, I'm doing it for me, (a) to lose weight and (b) to get some exercise.

Nine Women, Nine Months, Nine Lives

I find I'm watching the clock, using up my time for Charlie.
Mmmm, so is that the only time that you get for yourself? Do you, I don't know, go round and spending the evening with your friends or whatever?
No, no. I did go out the other week for an evening, but it's not very often. It's because I'm too tired the next day at work, and I'm too tired with Charlie really the next day too. And we usually have a bit of a game in the night. Like when I went out a couple of weeks ago with one of my friends, Charlie in the middle of the night, when I went in to settle him down, decided "Hey mums back home!" and he was getting more and more awake...
Oh no!
I was like "No Charlie it's half past two in the morning go to sleep!" So in the end I just had to let him be because he was getting more and more excited that I'd come back. Although saying that, tomorrow I'm supposed to be going out with the staff! So I am trying to make more time sort of, because I still can't leave him through the night.
That's because you feel guilty not because you think he won't be all right?
No, it's for my own selfish reasons really, that I want to see him and sort of...
To know he's OK?
Yeah, and just to be with him really. Although we take it in turns at the weekends to have lie-ins, but I do find myself wanting to just catch up on sleep really! [Laughs]
And how would you say that James has changed? Do you think he has changed?
Errm...
It might be something small, or something that you just...
He's more tired! [Laughs]
Yeah, well there you go!
I think we have a different perspective. I think James seems more keen on the house, he's often in the garden. I think that the practicalities are more his. I like things to be tidy and you know...
Mmm. Different priorities?
Yeah.
So was James always keen on things like that or is it a recent...?
He's always been keen on the garden. Growing flowers, you know, in London few people have a garden so...
Now you have one!
Yeah, so he can! But anyway I think he's got more mature, he's happy to play together with Charlie at night times. I think, you know, we're both grown ups now, do you know what I mean?! [Laughs]
[Laughs] Yeah!
I don't think either of us are, there aren't many of our friends, friends of our age group who actually have children. Some friends of James's are actually pregnant now so their lives are going to change. But we're kind of the first in our age group to have children. Also, because we're both, I mean when I look back, I moved in with James in the July

Rachel

and I was already pregnant, we didn't really have time to be, to build up a close network of friends here, so you know I suppose we're quite isolated from other people. I mean, you know we have family, and that's our social context, so I don't think we have got the pressure of like going out with friends, do you know what I mean?
So everything changed all in one go really?
Yeah, and because we didn't particularly have time to establish friendships beyond school or our workplaces, it's not an issue... Wanting to go out with them all the time.
And would you say your relationship has changed? You just said you feel like you are proper grown ups now...
Yeah we've changed. I think this is the most important time whilst we have Charlie, together. I think we have less time to be our own individuals, make our own choices, like we now have time for the family and I don't think we discuss work like we used to. I don't think we ever used to particularly discuss it a lot but we don't at all.
You don't at all now?
No, it tends to be Charlie goes to bed, we have half an hour and then I am asleep usually! [Laughs] Whereas James tends to stay up a bit later, but I'm... It's just a change in your routine but it, there is less time for us individually, our time is now for Charlie really.
And do you try and make time for the two of you to be together? Like going out for a meal in the evening?
No.
Perhaps putting a video on when Charlie is in bed, or sitting down together?
No, no. I think that now Charlie is going to bed that little bit earlier, we do actually have a bit longer to sit and talk. It's easier now that he goes to bed that bit earlier, and that's just, and he's slept through on eight times out of fourteen – haven't you? Yes! So that means we're not quite so shattered!
Yeah.
And I suppose in some ways we're at home by six o'clock we can share Charlie's bedtime routine and we also all sit at the table for breakfast. For an evening meal Charlie sits with us, so things aren't totally devoted to Charlie but you know... And we go out at the weekend, but it's always to something where he can go. So we are trying to...
Yeah, well it is a gradual thing...
And we're all going away for the week soon, so...
That'll be exciting! [Laughs]
[Laughs] Yeah! It will won't it Charlie?
So would you say that is something you are trying to move towards now with Charlie going to bed earlier?
Not really! [Laughs] I think you know errm... You suggest it more that we should do more just the two of us don't you? [Addressing husband]
Husband: Mmm. But we survive!
Survival's about the best way to put it yeah!

289

Nine Women, Nine Months, Nine Lives

Also I think it will be easier when I'm working just the four days, when I've got a whole day of Charlie to myself really.
Yeah, and perhaps then you won't feel quite so reluctant to leave him, not necessarily over night, but for an evening to start with.
Yeah, I think it might be better when I've had the seven or eight weeks in the summer, you know had him solidly, then I'll perhaps be able to do that more.
OK. The next chunk is your immediate future. So the next twelve months. What do you hope to achieve this next year?
Errm...
Anything... At all?
Errm... What as a family or just as an individual?
As an individual.
I think it is to try and find more time, I don't really see this in the next twelve months but long term I'd actually like to do an art class, but I don't really see that happening until he is six or seven, do you know what I mean? When he's more...
More manageable? Yeah!
Yeah! [Laughs] Another idea, in the long term again, I wouldn't mind doing a masters. But it's all fairly long term really, when I've got time in the evenings, when my life isn't quite so full. You know when I can do that. They're a bit long term but...
No that's fine. And do you think you can achieve it, to start and try and make time for yourself in the coming year?
Yes I think so. Especially with having that extra day as well, I think, it will be easier to try and do it. And not be crashed out. To have him all day, and maybe Friday nights to go out - James and I.
Yeah, yeah. What would you say you have learnt about yourself this past year that you would like to develop next year? Something that you are quite pleased with about yourself and that you would like to keep going...
I don't know, errm... I'm in charge of the, of a unit at the nursery and I'm actually doing a bit of a massive change there at the moment and I suppose it's sort of, restructuring the school as a result of the changes.
Oh wow!
Yeah... So I suppose it would be to do with the changes at work, altering the intake of the school, and overseeing the changes, so that's a good thing!
Yeah, to have more responsibility?
Yeah, because I think you know because I've initiated the changes, it's, I'm supposed to be coming off the timetable sort of to oversee the changes. I don't know about home, social life, taking time for myself...
Is there anything that you have found out about yourself that you would like to change next year? Something that makes you think "Oh my God, aren't I awful?!" You know, "I can't carry on like this!"
I'd like to change my weight! [Laughs] Although I can't really see how that is going to

Rachel

happen. I would actually like to find more time to do keep fit but I hate the gym, and I hate swimming, I just do it because it's quite an easy way to exercise all at once. Errm... What was the question?
Is there something you don't like about yourself that you want to change?
I think it's sometimes, if I'm really tired and I've had a bad day, sometimes... Not taking it out on Charlie but I sometimes feel I've had enough of this noise now and he's trying to play with that thing [noisy toy] and I think that's when I would like a little more tolerance, because it is you know... I mean I go from a one year old to three year olds and back again and the noise level is the same. Because there is 60 children in the unit as well, so when they are all inside the noise level is 'quite' loud. And you know sometimes I think "Oh God!" So I suppose I would like to be more tolerant at times...!
Yeah?
Or when Charlie doesn't want to eat, that's when I can feel myself thinking that he's just messing around, I know that he likes it - he just spits it out, and you can feel yourself getting tense...
"You know you want it really!"
Yeah, I suppose it's that that I really don't like about myself. Everybody else's child seems to be getting a better deal than Charlie is, do you know what I mean? I sometimes feel that way.
OK, right well that's it.
Oh! [Laughs]
That was great. I hope that wasn't too much. We went on for quite a while.
No, no!

Nine Women, Nine Months, Nine Lives

Sadie

Sadie and her boyfriend were 17 years old when she became pregnant accidentally. He said he would support her so they went ahead with the pregnancy and moved in together. Two days before this interview took place, and eleven days before her first son Alex's first birthday, she had her second son. She was working part-time before conceiving for the first time but has not worked since that pregnancy. Her relationship with her partner was strained and on the verge of breaking down at the time of this interview.

The first section is about when you found out you were pregnant with Alex, so it's a long while ago, although I'm sure it sticks in your memory!
Yeah! [Laughs]
OK, so the first question is were you trying to get pregnant at the time?
No.
No. So it was unplanned?
Yeah.
OK. Can you remember what went through your mind when you saw the blue line on the test?
I was scared, worried.
Was anybody with you?
Yeah, my boyfriend, and my friend, I was just upset really.
Yeah, so did you, had you thought before hand that you were pregnant or did you...?
Errm... Yeah I did have an idea.
So you did have a feeling. How many weeks were you when you did the test?
About 2 months.

Nine Women, Nine Months, Nine Lives

Yeah about 8 or 9 weeks, 2 months. So you were sort of expecting it to be positive?
Yeah.
And your immediate reaction was to be scared and upset. And what did you think afterwards, when you'd got over the shock as it were?
I didn't know whether to keep it or have an abortion. But I decided to keep it in the end.
So you were thinking about whether it was actually possible?
Yeah, it seems so long ago now!
Yeah, so it's not really fresh in your mind? [Has just had – in the last 48 hours- her second baby]
Not really!
So your partner and your friend were with you when you did the test. And can you remember your partner's reaction when you found out?
He was shocked but he said he'd stick by me, he was, he didn't really say much.
Is that unusual for him or…?
Probably for a lad, yeah! [Laughs]
So you told him that you were possibly…?
I didn't actually tell him. Well I did tell him a week before I done the test, so he knew what to expect.
Right.
So he knew I might be pregnant.
So he'd had a while to think about it?
Yeah, but he was agreeing with whatever I wanted to do.
OK. The next section is your experience of pregnancy and the birth. So I'd like you to think back to the first time round with Alex. OK did you imagine what pregnancy would feel like before you got pregnant?
Yeah.
You did. And what did you think it would feel like before you got pregnant?
Being big and fat! [Laughs]
Did you think it would feel nice? Did you think it would feel uncomfortable?
Yeah, I thought it would be good.
Yeah? And was that different to your actual experiences?
What when I was actually pregnant?
Yeah.
Sometimes you felt uncomfortable and sometimes it were nice because you felt all the movements, you know, him moving inside you.
So you didn't feel let down or, you hadn't sort of imagined it would be wonderful and it was actually dreadful?
No, no.
So the actual physical experience was OK. What about emotionally?
I did feel down a lot. Yeah I would get down about the slightest thing. Apart from that I was fine.

Sadie

And do you think that was because you were pregnant?
Yeah it was.
And what do you put that down to?
Oh what do you call it postnatal antenatal…depression?
Depression. So you think that was whilst you were actually pregnant? So you actually felt depressed then?
When I was actually pregnant I felt depressed, but then I'd be great some days, so…
So what, you'd get really happy and then you'd get really down?
Yeah, over the silliest, over the slightest thing!
So you were a bit sensitive?
Yeah.
Were you a bit snappy and irritable?
Yeah, definitely.
What did you expect would happen at the birth with Alex? I remember when I spoke to you before that you hadn't been to the hospital very often and it was all a bit much, a bit different and the pain was a bit much…
I don't really know what I expected, I was just scared.
Had you tried to find out about it?
Yeah, I did ask questions of the nurses and my mum. They said <u>painful</u>! I didn't really know what to expect what with it being my first, so it was just the pain.
So, apart from that it was all right?
Yeah, yeah. I slept through most of my labour anyway.
Oh right, so…were you in labour for a long while?
Fifteen hours![Rolls her eyes at the memory]
Oh God! And so the birth, was it as you had thought it would be?
Yes.
It was?
I knew that it was going to be painful.
You knew what to expect and it wasn't that different?
No.
And how did you feel when you first held your baby?
Errm…
Can you remember it?
I was a bit shocked really to actually have him. The real thing! I was scared, but I loved it! I can't really remember much more about it…
So you were a bit, a bit shocked, that this was really a baby?
Yeah, yeah, scared and shocked!
OK. In what ways was your partner involved in the pregnancy, in your first pregnancy, was he supportive?
Yeah.
Was he curious about the changes that were happening to you?

Nine Women, Nine Months, Nine Lives

No, not really... He didn't know how to handle my mood swings. But he were there for me, he were good at the labour, but not much...Errm...
So he, was he perhaps not really interested in the pregnancy?
No, no, it didn't really hit him, what with him being so young.
Right. So how old was he when...?
We were both seventeen.
You were both seventeen. OK. So in what way was he good?
Holding my hand, being supportive...errm
Was that more or less than you hoped for with the pregnancy? And then, again, for the birth?
What, the support?
Yeah, was his behaviour during the pregnancy more or less than you hoped for? Were you perhaps a bit disappointed that he...?
Less [Very definite about this]
So it was less than you hoped for in the pregnancy?
He weren't really supportive until the baby, until he actually came.
And then during the labour, was he...?
He was more supportive then. He'd wised up by then. [Head nodded very firmly]
OK. And what about this time round with Nathan? You had Nathan two days ago, has he been different this time?
Yeah! [Snorts derisively] He wouldn't come in with me, he was scared to come in with me. But he came in at the end.
So why was he scared?
I don't think he liked it, but he was good again.
So how was his behaviour different to what you'd expected? You said that he wasn't very interested the first time with Alex.
Ermm...
So you'd hoped he'd be more supportive of you emotionally, practically, or both?
Both. [Disappointment in her voice]
Both. So you perhaps felt a little bit let down by that?
Yes, yeah.
And which was the most disappointing, would you say, being let down emotionally or being let down practically?
Practical, yeah.
The practical side of things. And did you try and talk to him about it?
[Snorts derisively again] Talking to him is like talking to a brick wall.
Oh right! [Hollow laughter] So you did try?
Yeah, I did try but he doesn't understand.
So what, he didn't understand what you were trying to tell him?
He doesn't listen...[Shrugs shoulders]
He doesn't listen... Right. OK. The next bit is about your experience of early

Sadie

motherhood. So if you could think back up until the time when Alex was about three months old. Do you think that your pregnancy effected the first three months of motherhood? For example, if you had to have stitches. You didn't have to have a caesarean or anything like that?
No, no.
So things like water retention or just being so tired what with having been heavily pregnant?
I was just feeling tired.
Right... And there was nothing else from your pregnancy that lasted into early motherhood?
I just felt down for the first few weeks. Apart from that I felt fine.
You feeling down, was that like a continuation of when you'd been down towards the end of your pregnancy?
Yeah.
So did you notice that it got worse or it got better once you'd had Alex?
I felt better... (eventually)
And do you feel that the birth effected early motherhood, was there anything?
No, no.
OK. How did you imagine early motherhood would be before you had Alex? Had you sort of thought about, I don't know, what he would be like?
Yeah.
Whether he'd be sleeping, whether you'd sleep?
Yeah.
So, what had you imagined about it?
What he would look like, would he be good ...errm
Can't remember?
No, no, not really.
Are you OK to carry on?
Yeah, yeah, really.
And how do you think it matched up, do you think motherhood was as you'd expected?
Yeah, because I'm like, I've always had babies close to me so I was like used to (them) and I've always helped out. My friends have got babies, so I'd seen what they had to do, so I knew what I had to do. When I first had Alex I knew roughly how to do certain things, so I had an idea.
Right so you did have an idea. So rather than sort of imagining what it would be like, you had a pretty good idea of what it would actually be like?
Yeah, yeah.
And so you felt that the reality matched up with your expectations?
Yes, yeah.
So it did match up quite well?
Yeah.

297

Nine Women, Nine Months, Nine Lives

Was there anything that perhaps didn't? Was there anything that was better than you thought? Was there anything that was worse than you thought?
I don't know. Errm... Oh, night feeding.
Yeah?
Yeah, I didn't really expect that. Apart from that I think I knew about everything.
Yeah, so you had a fair idea. OK, and can you remember what was difficult in those early days? Say in those first three weeks, what can you remember being a bit of a shock or something that you thought "Oh my God!"?
Getting up in the night. Definitely.
Yeah, the night feeds?
Yeah, having to get up, making the bottles up, making sure they were all set out ready. That was about all really.
So getting up in the night, getting the bottles ready and the feeds?
Yeah.
OK. And what was the best thing in those early days, say those first three weeks?
I actually had a baby! I enjoyed feeding him, bathing him...
Did you breast feed him?
No, I didn't breast feed him. Errm... I liked taking him out and my mates coming round.
What, showing him off to people?
Yeah! [laughter]
OK. And how much was your partner involved in the early days?
Quite a lot...
So he took his turn doing...?
Errm... Not really. He didn't want to change his nappies. Errm...
And had you talked about who would do what?
No, we hadn't.
So you hadn't talked about it at all?
No, no.
Because you said you had quite a lot of experience and had always been around babies, had hands on experience. Had Paul actually had any...?
No, no... He got bored of that side of things.
So he hasn't got any younger brothers or sisters that he could have learnt...?
He has but he didn't take any interest.
He didn't? Oh right. So you hadn't really talked about what it would be like, having a baby, from the sounds of it?
No, no!
Did you talk about it this time round with Nathan?
No.
And do you think that was perhaps because you already had Alex?
Yeah, because I knew what I was expecting, what I had to do.

Sadie

And did he...?
No.
Did he ask you anything?
No.
Did he ask if things would be different this time round or...?
No, nothing like that.
So would you say that it worked out all right? Do you perhaps wish that you had talked about it or...?
No, it just worked out all right, we knew what we were doing this time.
And the first time, with Alex? Do you think it worked out all right?
Yeah.
It wasn't any more or any less than you expected?
No, it was about the same.
OK. So are you saying that that worked out for the better or for the worse, overall?
For the better, yeah.
Right, the next section is about your experience of motherhood up to the present day. Now your experience will be completely different from any other girl I've spoken to because you were expecting Nathan for much of the time that you had Alex in the last year. So how would you say your life has changed since you've had Alex, your first baby?
An awful lot, in lots of ways...
Were you working before?
Errm... I'd just finished college, I had been working and then I had to quit that because I was feeling a lot tired.
So how do you think you've changed since you had your first baby? You said that you had grown up a lot?
Yeah, definitely, I feel like I can't act silly anymore.
So what you mean you can't act that way or you don't want to?
I find it hard to join in the fun. I'd be worrying about the kid, worrying about Alex.
So in what ways do you think you've grown up? You've obviously noticed changes in yourself. So what about the way you were before and the way you are now? Would you say you are more or less happy, content, patient?
More patient than I have been, now I've got kids of my own.
OK. And would you say that you have had to become those things or would you say there has been a gradual change? Have you had to think about it, make a conscious effort?
Gradually.
Gradually. So you've...?
Over time.
So you haven't had to think about it? About not losing your temper?
Not really.
OK. And would you say that is a permanent change?

299

Nine Women, Nine Months, Nine Lives

Yes.
OK so, sorry did you say that it was a permanent change or...?
Yeah, a permanent change.
OK and do you think that you've changed for the worse in some ways?
No.
OK so you're saying that things like you finding it difficult being silly with your mates, do you, would you say that you wish that you could still be silly?
Yeah, I do wish I could be silly, liked doing daft things.
Yeah, so would you say that you're not as relaxed...?
Yeah I'm not as relaxed around my mates, I can't act daft because I'm used to being round kids and getting on with the job, it's difficult not to be...
Right. And do you hope to go back to work?
Yeah.
You do. And did you want to go back to work before, when Alex was older, and then you fell for Nathan?
Yeah.
So you were hoping to go back when Alex was...?
One, one or two.
So that worked out OK?
Yeah, yeah.
OK, and do you get any time to yourself?
No, not really, unless mum can baby-sit.
OK, and does your mum offer to have Alex, or do you ask her?
No, mum offers.
OK, that's good. So you try and make time for yourself?
Yeah.
And what do you do in your time for your self? Do you just sit there and vegetate in wonderful luxury?
Yeah, oh yeah!
Put your feet up?
Yeah. I go round to my mates, sometimes.
So you go and see your friends?
Yeah, and sit and have a cup of tea and a chat.
OK. And do you think that your partner has changed? Has Paul changed?
No! [Shakes head vigorously]
No? You don't think he's changed at all?
No.
You don't think so, not at all? You don't think he's perhaps got a bit more patient?
Yeah maybe a bit more. He's got quite good with Alex, yeah he's good with Alex, he's got time for Alex.
Do you think that's got better as Alex has got older or...?

Sadie

Yeah, he's more...Errm...
OK. So does you partner ever have him so you've got time for yourself?
No. Not at all really, no.
So he must have changed a little bit because if he's spending more time...if you think in terms of the whole year?
He's changed a bit. [said with reluctance]
But not as much as you?
No, not as much as me.
And have you ever spoken to him about the fact that you have changed, that you feel like you're that bit sort of more mature, like you said?
No, no.
No... Does he ever pass comment, said anything, even jokingly, you know like "You're old for your age" or something?
He says I'm a bit boring now... But if you think about it I've been pregnant for nearly two years!
Yeah! [Laughter]
Apart from that he hasn't said owt.
And would you say that your relationship has changed? From what it was before you had Alex?
Yeah.
And in what way would you say it has changed, both good and bad?
Well I can't really go out gallivanting like I used to, he goes out with his mates, I used to go out with him, but not now.
So... Is there anything that you would say has changed for the better, do you feel closer to him?
Yeah, yeah I do feel closer to him.
Is that because now you've got two children whereas...?
Yeah, yeah definitely.
Do you try and make time together, just you two?
Yeah, yeah.
Without Alex, and now without Nathan?
Yeah...
Does Alex ever go and stay over night at his Nan's?
Yeah, he's going this weekend to his nana's [her mums] and Nathan is going to go to Paul's mum's so we'll both be able to go out. So we've both planned that this week. So we'll be able to go out and do our own things.
Oh right! So you're going out doing your own things separately? You're not going out together?
Yeah, yeah, but we are going to start to do that more.
Oh right, so is that something you haven't done for a long while?
Yeah.

Nine Women, Nine Months, Nine Lives

Yeah, so is that something that you miss?
Yeah, it is.
And do you think he misses it too?
Yeah, because he likes that, he wants to take me out more.
So you do manage it. Would you say that you managed it quite often?
Yeah I do think we manage it quite often because when we do want to go out we've got quite a few babysitters.
OK, well that's good because it is important. Right OK, the next bit is your immediate future, the next 12 months, OK? It must seem like miles away I'm sure, it probably did last year![Laughs] What do you hope to achieve in the coming year?
Not to get pregnant! [said with real feeling]
Right [laughter] I would say that's pretty high on your list!
I do want to start back at work, and I'm going to make sure I have more time for meself, so...
So, do you think that you didn't before?
No, no.
And do you think you suffered a bit for it?
Yeah. I missed out on a lot of things, I'm going to go out more, and get time for myself.
Yeah, well they sound like great things to try and achieve. And do you think you can achieve them?
Yeah...
And what have you learnt about yourself in the past year that you would like to keep going next year? Is there something about yourself that you've felt proud of, and that you want to be as good next year?
I don't know... To feel good in myself, because I always feel down.
Right. So really it's trying to find time for yourself?
Yeah.
So you've started to do it recently, and you want to keep that going?
Yeah.
And what have you learnt about yourself that you want to change next year?
Errm...
Perhaps that you haven't put enough time by for yourself?
Yeah, I didn't have enough time for myself, I had to make sure that he was, that I was there for them first, and then Paul, never myself.
And you think you can change that next year?
Yes, yeah.
Yeah, well that is good, yes that is good. OK, that's lovely, great, I hope it wasn't too much for you, you must be knackered?!
No, no, I'm all right.
OK.